Medical Ethics

Medical Ethics

Accounts of Ground-Breaking Cases

SIXTH EDITION

Gregory E. Pence
Professor of Philosophy
School of Medicine and Department of Philosophy
University of Alabama at Birmingham

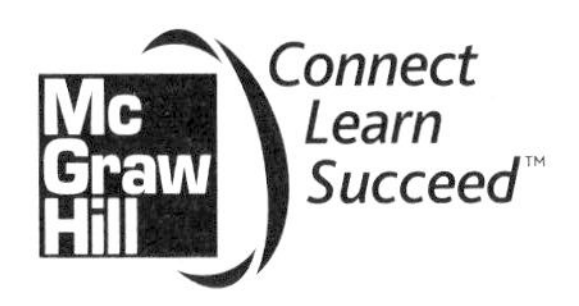

The McGraw-Hill Companies

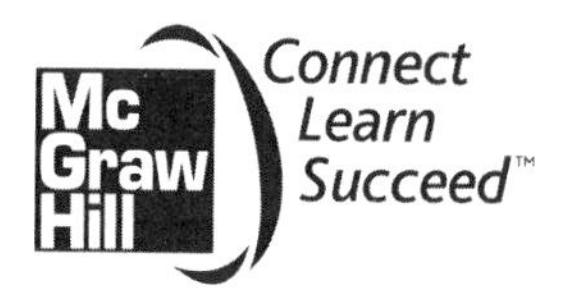

MEDICAL ETHICS: ACCOUNTS OF GROUND-BREAKING CASES, SIXTH EDITION

Published by McGraw-Hill, a business unit of The McGraw-Hill Companies, Inc., 1221 Avenue of the Americas, New York, NY 10020.

This book is printed on acid-free paper.

3 4 5 6 7 8 9 0 DOC/DOC 1 0 9 8 7 6 5 4 3 2

ISBN 978-0-07-340749-4
MHID 0-07-340749-6

Vice President & Editor-in-Chief: *Michael Ryan*
VP EDP/Central Publishing Services: *Kimberly Meriwether David*
Editorial Director: *Beth Mejia*
Managing Editor: *Meghan Campbell*
Executive Marketing Manager: *Pamela S. Cooper*
Project Manager: *Robin A. Reed*
Design Coordinator: *Margarite Reynolds*
Cover Image Credit: © *Creatas/PunchStock*
Production Supervisor: *Sue Culbertson*
Media Project Manager: *Bethuel Jabez*
Composition: *Glyph International*
Typeface: *10/12 Palatino*
Printer: *R. R. Donnelley*

Library of Congress Cataloging-in-Publication Data

Pence, Gregory E.
Medical ethics : accounts of ground-breaking cases / Gregory E. Pence.—6th ed.
p. cm.
Previously published: Classic cases in medical ethics. 2008
Includes index.
ISBN 978-0-07-340749-4 (alk. paper)
1. Medical ethics—Case studies. I. Pence, Gregory E. Classic cases in medical ethics II. Title.
R724.P36 2010
174.2—dc22

2010002490

www.mhhe.com

Preface

Twenty years ago, McGraw-Hill and I published the first edition of *Medical Ethics* and now, 20 years later, I'm happy to be publishing the 6th edition. New to this edition are:

Each chapter has an essential question for discussion by students and professors.

- *John/Joan,* a new chapter, describes the case of David Reimer, born a male, surgically altered and raised female, counseled by psychologist John Money who fraudulently published data, and discusses problems of nature/nurture and the surgical imperative to normalize gender at birth.
- *Animal research* focuses on new evidence that most testing on animals is worthless.
- *Desire to be first* focuses on how the recent race to be the first to transplant a face paralleled the previous race to be the first to transplant a human heart.
- *Assisted reproduction* focuses on whether women using multiple births or giving birth at advanced ages have the best interests of children at heart.
- *Research on humans* now includes the Olivieri and *Constant Gardener*-type cases.
- *Physician-assisted dying* now focuses on the tragic case of New Orleans physician Anna Pou during Hurricane Katrina.
- *Medical finance* focuses on President Obama's attempts to pass universal health coverage for Americans.
- *Genetics* updates include a predictive gene for Alzheimer's, as well as genes for Huntington's, breast cancer, and diabetes, and the question of personal responsibility for gene-linked illness.
- *Abortion* updates the changing emphasis of the Supreme Court on legalized abortion and updates emergency contraception.
- *Comas* discusses new controversies about discovering misdiagnosed PVS patients with fMRI scans and thalamic stimulation.
- *Using one infant for another* has an update connecting the controversy over PVS patients in minimally conscious states to the controversy over using anencephalic babies as organ sources for other babies.

I'm also pleased to announce that this 6th edition has a password-protected Web site for professors with 180 Learning Objectives on all 18 chapters, a test bank of 100 multiple-choice questions, and a special appendix for debating in bioethics, "Argumentative Strategies in Bioethics." This site can be found at www.mhhe.com/pence6e. Please contact your McGraw-Hill representative for access information.

Over the years, several reviewers have been enormously helpful—Stuart Rachels, Charles Cardwell, Kenneth Kipnis, Bonnie Steinbock, and Denise Simonsen—and reviewers for McGraw-Hill:

Craig Jordan, University of Texas at San Antonio
Rebecca Potts, Minnesota West Community and Technical College
Miller Brown, Trinity College, Hartford
Walter Edinger, University of Toledo
Stephen Hanson, University of Louisville
Peter Cvek, Saint Peter's College
Timothy J. Madigan, St. John Fisher College
Janet Binder, Metropolitan State University
Howard Ducharme, University of Akron
Bambi Robinson, Southeast Missouri State University
Mark Christensen, Lourdes College

As always, I'm interested in your feedback, so email me at: pence@uab.edu.

Gregory E. Pence

About the Author

Gregory Pence has taught Bioethics in the philosophy department and medical school at the University of Alabama for 34 years. Since 1994, he has won three teaching awards at UAB.

He has published in *The Wall Street Journal, Newsweek, The New York Times, Atlanta Constitution, Newsweek, Philadelphia Inquirer,* and *the Chronicle of Higher Education.* He has appeared on CNN's *Wolf Blitzer's Washington Review, The Point with Gredda von Susteren, The Early Show with Bryant Gumbel,* and on National Public Radio.

His research focuses on emerging ethical issues in bioethics, including cloning, stem cells, and improved food. He has written six trade books, including *Who's Afraid of Human Cloning* (1998) and *Designer Food* (2002).

In 2001, he testified before a Congressional subcommittee about embryonic and reproductive cloning. In 2006, he won a Pellegrino Medal for lifetime contributions to medical ethics.

Brief Contents

Brief Contents

Brief Contents

Contents

Part Two
GROUND-BREAKING CASES ABOUT THE BEGINNINGS OF HUMAN LIFE

CHAPTER 1

Requests to Die

Elizabeth Bouvia and Larry McAfee

This chapter discusses Elizabeth Bouvia and Larry McAfee, two people with nonterminal physical disabilities who tried to die, who won important cases in court, and who had surprising outcomes. It discusses the lives of people with disabilities, relief of depression, autonomy, disability culture, and philosophers in history on rational suicide. Its essential question for discussion concerns whether physicians should resist the requests of competent, nonterminal, disabled young adults to die.

THE CASE OF ELIZABETH BOUVIA

In 1983, Elizabeth Bouvia's father drove her from Oregon to Riverside General Hospital in California, where psychiatrists admitted her as a voluntary suicidal patient. Wanting "just to be left alone and not bothered by friends or family or anyone else and to ultimately starve to death," she had already attempted suicide once.[1] "Death is letting go of all burdens," she claimed. "It is being able to be free of my physical disability and mental struggle to live."

Almost totally paralyzed from cerebral palsy, Elizabeth was then 25 years old. She had never had the use of her legs, although she could use her right hand to operate a battery-powered wheelchair and to smoke cigarettes. She could control her facial muscles to chew, swallow, and speak.

Her life had never been easy. When she was five years old, her parents divorced. Her mother raised her for the next five years, after which her mother abandoned Elizabeth in a children's home. The following account comes from two physicians:

> For their 18th birthday, some children receive cars and gifts. When [Elizabeth] turned 18, her father, a postal inspector, told her that he would no longer be able to care for her because of her disabilities. The chief of psychiatry at Riverside says that what she did next showed great drive and promise. She gathered her requisite amount of state aid and lived on her own in an apartment with a live-in nurse. Although she earlier had dropped out of high school, she completed her general equivalency degree and went on to graduate from San Diego State University with a bachelor's degree in 1981. She even entered a master's program at the university's School of Social Work, but left in 1982 over a disagreement about her field work placement. . . .

> For eight months, she worked as a volunteer in the San Diego placement program, but she has never been employed for salary or wages. . . .
>
> During the last year, Ms. Bouvia faced a series of devastating events. In August 1982, she married an ex-convict, Richard Bouvia, with whom she had been corresponding by mail. Together they conceived a child, but a few months later she suffered a miscarriage. . . .
>
> Her husband's part-time job did not provide enough income for the two to live decently, so they called her father to ask for help. He declined to aid them, Richard Bouvia said. They next went to Richard Bouvia's sister in Iowa to ask for help. That did not work out for long, and soon they ended up back in Oregon, where Richard still could not find work. At that point, he abandoned her, stating—according to pleadings in the case—that he "could not accept her disabilities, a miscarriage, and rejection by her parents." . . .
>
> A few days later, Elizabeth Bouvia got a ride to Riverside General and wheeled herself into the emergency room, claiming that she wanted to commit suicide.[2]

In addition to her problems with her husband and father, she had painful severe degenerative arthritis. As an indigent resident of California (she had lived in Riverside as well as in Oregon), Medi-Cal, a state-federal program, paid for her medical care.

Donald Fisher, chief of psychiatry at Riverside Hospital, cared for Elizabeth during her first four months there. Since he refused to let her starve herself to death, Elizabeth contacted the American Civil Liberties Union (ACLU) and telephoned a reporter. Richard Scott of Beverly Hills, both a physician and a lawyer, represented her free of charge.

The Legal Battle: Refusing Sustenance

In a hearing before California probate judge John Hews, Dr. Fisher testified that because Elizabeth might change her mind, he would not let her starve and would force-feed her: "The court cannot order me to be a murderer nor to conspire with my staff and employees to murder Elizabeth."[3] Elizabeth Bouvia asked Judge Hews to enjoin Dr. Fisher from forcibly feeding her.

Habeeb Bacchus, associate chief of medicine at Riverside Hospital and Bouvia's second physician, argued that "being allowed to die when there's no need for her to die—this is a dangerous precedent. Patients might wonder, 'Am I next slated to be allowed to die?'"[4]

Advocates for the disabled feared that if Elizabeth were allowed to die, other disabled people would try to do the same thing. A lawyer at the Law Institute for the Disabled asserted that Bouvia symbolized a "social problem" of disabled people who are told they cannot be productive and said, "She needs to learn to live with dignity."[5]

At this point, the case escalated into a public debate:

> Disabled individuals held vigils at the hospital to convince her to change her mind. Bouvia's estranged husband hitchhiked to Riverside from Iowa, retained lawyers, and asked to be named her legal guardian. He charged the ACLU with using his wife as a "guinea pig." She filed for divorce. Columnist Jack Anderson's offer to raise funds for Bouvia's treatment was rebuffed. Richard Nixon sent a letter to Bouvia to "keep fighting." A meeting with President Reagan was

discussed. Two neurosurgeons offered free surgery to help her gain the use of her arms. A convicted felon volunteered to shoot her.[6]

Judge Hews allowed the forced-feeding. Admitting Elizabeth's rationality, sincerity, and competence, he decided based on the "profound effect on the medical staff, nurses, and administration of the hospital," as well as the "devastating effect on other . . . physically handicapped persons."[7] Bouvia's lawyer said Hews accepted "the Chicken Little defense that the sky would fall if Ms. Bouvia wasn't force-fed."[8] Judge Hews held that since the patient was not terminally ill and could live for decades, "there is no other reasonable option."

The columnist Arthur Hoppe argued otherwise:

> I had the feeling that the judge, the doctor, and the hospital had found Elizabeth Bouvia guilty—guilty of not playing the game. It was as though the Easter Seal Child had looked into the camera and said being crippled was a lousy deal and certainly nothing to smile about.[9]

Boston University law professor George Annas blasted Hews:

> The county . . . threatened to eject Ms. Bouvia from the hospital by force, and leave her out on the sidewalk, hoping someone would take her away. Almost from the beginning, the county and hospital made it clear that they did not care whether she lived or died but, because of their own fear of potential legal liability, would not let her die at Riverside Hospital.[10]

Elizabeth appealed, and throughout it, she continued to be force-fed. When aides inserted plastic tubing in her mouth, she bit through the tubing, so thereafter three attendants held her down while another inserted tubing through her nose into her stomach and pumped in a liquid diet. Annas commented on this gruesome scene:

> I do not believe competent adults should ever be force-fed; . . . If a court determines, however, that invasive forced-feeding is required, . . . then to [prevent] hospitals from becoming the most hideous torture chambers, some reasonable limit must be placed on this "treatment."[11]

Elizabeth Bouvia lost her first appeal and left Riverside Hospital in 1984. Different commentators interpreted differently what happened next. Two physicians wrote in a medical journal:

> The standoff continued until April 7, when Ms. Bouvia unexpectedly checked herself out of the hospital. The hospital bill for the 217 days, excluding physicians' fees, was more than $56,000, paid by Riverside County and by the State of California. Ms. Bouvia went to the Hospital del Mar at Playease de Tijuana, Mexico, known for amygdalin (Laetrile) treatments for cancer. She believed the staff would help her die. Her new physicians, however, became convinced that she wanted to live. Two weeks later, Ms. Bouvia left the hospital, hired nurses, and moved to a motel. Three days later, with friends, a reporter, and an intern from Hospital del Mar at her side, she gave up her plan to starve herself to death and took solid food. Ms. Bouvia said that she wanted treatment, including surgery to reduce muscle spasms. As of August 1985, Ms. Bouvia's location and plans were not known. Her case was complicated further by the revelation that the newspaper

> reporter who covered the case most closely had a contract with Ms. Bouvia for a book, television, and movie rights to her story.[12]

This account emphasizes Elizabeth Bouvia's unexpected departure from the hospital, her costly hospital bills at public expense, the agreement of Mexican and American physicians in refusing to allow her to die, her seemingly arbitrary decision to give up starving herself, and a contract for book and film rights to her story.

In contrast, lawyer George Annas writes:

> Two years ago this column dealt with Elizabeth Bouvia's unequal and doomed struggle. . . . After losing both in the hospital and in the courtroom, Ms. Bouvia fled to Mexico on April 7, 1984, to seek her death. She was soon persuaded that Mexican physicians and nurses would be no more sympathetic to her plan than those at Riverside, and so returned to California. Because of the brutal force-feeding she had endured at Riverside, she was afraid to return there. Since no other facility would admit her unless she agreed to eat, she resigned herself to eating and entered a "private care" location. There she remained, without incident, for more than a year.[13]

An advocate for dignified dying, the Hemlock Society's Derek Humphrey wrote even more sympathetically:

> Her troubles multiplied. The graduate school where she had been studying refused to readmit her, and her brother was drowned in a boating accident. Not long after, Elizabeth had a miscarriage, and she learned her mother was dying of cancer.
>
> . . . Determined once again to be in charge of her fate, she asked her father to take her to the county hospital in Riverside, near Los Angeles (an area where she had friends), for an examination. She checked herself into the psychiatric ward and told physicians she wanted to die by starvation. Elizabeth specifically asked that, until she died, she be looked after normally and given painkillers when her arthritis was troublesome.[14]

Disability advocate Paul Longmore offered a very different perspective on Bouvia's case, arguing that it reflected rank prejudice against the disabled. He wrote:

> The very agencies supposedly designed to enable severely physically handicapped adults like her to achieve independence . . . become yet another massive hurdle they must surmount, an enemy they must repeatedly battle but can never finally defeat. . . .
>
> [When she tried to go on internship,] the SDSU [San Diego State University] School of Social Work refused to back her up. They wanted to place her at a center where she would work only with disabled people. She refused. Reportedly, one of her employers told her she was unemployable, and that, if they had known just how disabled she was, they would never have admitted her to the program. . . .
>
> The attorneys brought in three psychiatric professionals to provide an independent evaluation. None of them had experience or expertise in dealing with persons with disabilities. In fact, Elizabeth Bouvia had never been examined by a psychiatric or medical professional qualified to understand her life experience. . . .
>
> Her examiners prejudicially concluded that because of her physical condition she would never be able to achieve her life goals, that her [physical] disability was

> the reason she wanted to die, and that her decision for death was reasonable. . . . [Judge Hews] too declared that Ms. Bouvia's physical disability was the sole reason she wished to die.[15]

Each account appeared in scholarly journals, implying objectivity, yet the physicians portray her as irresponsible; Annas and Humphrey portray her as a heroine fighting a cold bureaucracy; and Longmore portrays her as a victim of a prejudiced system and of misguided, do-gooder lawyers. Physicians refer to her as "Bouvia," Humphrey calls her "Elizabeth," and Longmore uses "Elizabeth Bouvia" or "Ms. Bouvia." The physicians say that, "she got a ride" to Riverside, as if she had hitchhiked to somewhere arbitrary; Humphrey says that her father took her to a place "where she had friends." Longmore emphasizes her desire to be independent; Humphrey emphasizes her physical pain and social trauma. Longmore suggests that society is prejudiced against disabled people and thus that Elizabeth Bouvia's disability is not so much her problem as society's problem. Humphrey writes from a point of view inside Elizabeth Bouvia; the physicians write from the viewpoint of hospital staff members who deal with problematic patients. Longmore critiques an inadequate system that forces terrible, desperate decisions.

In 1985, Elizabeth entered Los Angeles County-USC Medical Center, where physicians installed a morphine pump to control pain caused by her worsening arthritis. Because she declared she would eat, they did not force-feed her.

After two months, physicians transferred her to nearby High Desert Hospital, another public facility. Although she ate, her physicians there decided that she wasn't eating *enough* and again force-fed her. They reasoned that, "since she is occupying our space, she must accede to the same care which we afford every other patient admitted here, care designed to improve and not detract from chances of recovery and rehabilitation."[16] Critics objected: must all patients who occupy High Desert hospital's space do as they are told?

Elizabeth petitioned courts to stop her forced-feeding. At this time, she weighed only 70 pounds. A consultant on nutrition noted that a weight of 75 or 85 pounds "might be desirable." Her physicians wanted her to weigh about 110 pounds.

At a hearing, Judge Warren Deering interpreted her low weight as "not motivated by a bona fide right to privacy but by a desire to terminate her life."[17] He said the right to privacy did not cover suicide by starvation and ordered forced-feeding because, "Saving her life is paramount."

Elizabeth appealed and the California Court of Appeal ruled in her favor: "A desire to terminate one's life is probably the ultimate exercise of one's right to privacy."[18] This court found "no substantive evidence to support the [lower] court's decision."

Judge Deering had been concerned that Elizabeth could live for decades more, but his concern was dismissed: "This trial court mistakenly attached undue importance to the amount of time possibly available to her, and failed to give equal weight and consideration for the quality of that life; an equal, if not more significant, consideration."

The appeals court concluded:

> This matter constitutes a perfect paradigm of the axiom: "Justice delayed is justice denied." Her mental and emotional feelings are equally entitled to respect. She

> has been subjected to the forced intrusion of an artificial mechanism into her body against her will. She has a right to refuse the increased dehumanizing aspect of her condition. . . . The right to refuse medical treatment is basic and fundamental. It is recognized as part of the right of privacy protected by both the state and federal constitutions. Its exercise requires no one's approval. It is not merely one vote subject to being overridden by medical opinion. . . .
>
> [A precedent has been established that when] a doctor performs treatment in the absence of informed consent, there is an actionable battery. The obvious corollary to this principle is that a competent adult patient has the legal right to refuse medical treatment. [Moreover,] if the right of the patient to self-determination as to his own medical treatment is to have any meaning at all, it must be paramount to the interests of the patient's hospital and doctors. . . . The right of a competent adult patient to refuse medical treatment is a constitutionally guaranteed right which must not be abridged. . . .
>
> In Elizabeth Bouvia's view, the quality of her life has been diminished to the point of hopelessness, uselessness, unenjoyability, and frustration. She, as the patient, lying helplessly in bed, unable to care for herself, may consider her existence meaningless. She is not to be faulted for so concluding. . . . As in all matters, lines must be drawn at some point, somewhere, but that decision must ultimately belong to the one whose life is in issue.

Building on some prior decisions in other states,[19] this state court said that a competent adult patient had a constitutionally guaranteed right to refuse medical treatment and that it must not be abridged. This court also had strong words about forced-feeding: "We do not believe it is the policy of this State that all and every life must be preserved against the will of the sufferer. It is incongruous, if not monstrous, for medical practitioners to assert their right to preserve a life that someone else must live, or more accurately, endure, for '15 or 20 years.' We cannot conceive it to be the policy of this State to inflict such an ordeal upon anyone."

The court concluded that, "no criminal or civil liability attaches to honoring a competent, informed patient's refusal for medical service."

If nothing else, Elizabeth Bouvia, frail, small, alone, and barely able to move, won a remarkable victory for other patients. Preceding the U.S. Supreme Court's *Cruzan* decision by five years and with the national press focused on her case, she wrested from the courts a clear statement that competent, adult patients have a constitutional right to refuse medical treatment.

Yet after her victory, Elizabeth did not kill herself. When some caring people offered to help her die, she changed her mind. Most important, by giving her control over her life, they gave her a reason to live.

A decade after her victory in court, she described her body as "gnarled and useless."[20] She lived in California on Medi-Cal, in a private hospital room with 24-hour-day care at a cost in 1994 of $300 a day. A morphine pump controlled her pain, and she weighed 100 pounds. She said her life was "a lot of needles and bags," and she spent her time watching television. "I wouldn't say I'm happy, but I'm physically comfortable, more comfortable than before. There is nothing really to do. I just kind of lay here."

Robert Scott, the physician and lawyer who represented Elizabeth Bouvia, battled depression most of his life and committed suicide in 1992. When he did Elizabeth Bouvia said, "Jesus, I wish he could have come in and taken me with him."

In 1996 Elizabeth appeared on "60 Minutes" on the tenth anniversary of a previous "60 Minutes" story on her. For a decade, she had lived in Riverside County hospital, but in 1997, her new pro bono attorney, Griffith Thomas, M.D., got her disability payments put into a trust fund that allowed her to live in her own apartment with 24-hour-a-day in-home assistants. Even though it was cheaper for the public to do this than to house her in a hospital, it took a decade for someone to make this arrangement for her.

Elizabeth still had pain each day in 1996 and still needed a morphine drip. She wished to be left alone and did not intend to be alive for another story by "60 Minutes" in 2006. Not thankful for being forced to live, she felt ambivalent about being alive. An obituary for a disability rights advocate in 2008 in the *Los Angeles Times* mentioned that Elizabeth Bouvia was still alive.[21]

THE CASE OF LARRY MCAFEE

At 29-years-old, in 1985 Larry McAfee became almost completely paralyzed (a C-2 quadriplegic) in a motorcycle accident. He had studied mechanical engineering at Georgia State University in Atlanta. On a dirt road, he fell over his motorcycle, snapped his head, and crushed his two top vertebrae. Left with use of only his eyes, mouth, and head, he could not clear his throat and sometimes choked. He could not breathe on his own and needed a ventilator. He lacked control over bladder and bowels and could feel no pleasure from sexual activity. He had not married.

McAfee had a $1 million health insurance policy and remained for over a year at Shepherd Spinal Center in Atlanta, where the average stay for C-1 to C-4 patients is 19 weeks. After that year, he moved to an apartment in Atlanta, where he insisted on certified nurses who were three times more expensive than home health aides. After living like this for 16 months, he exhausted his insurance. His family offered to take care of him, but he did not want to burden them.

With no resources, he became eligible for Medicaid, the fund in each state that funds medical care for the indigent. McAfee wanted Georgia Medicaid to pay for his care in his apartment and refused to enter a state nursing home. Because Georgia had no nursing home beds for ventilator-dependent patients, it paid for a bed in a facility in Ohio that could care for such patients. That facility accepted McAfee on a temporary basis until Georgia could find a permanent bed for him.

Only a small number of nursing homes in America admit ventilator-dependent patients. Even fewer take such patients on Medicaid because Medicaid's reimbursement is not enough to cover the number of staff needed to care for such labor-intensive patients.

In Ohio, Larry wouldn't make appointments for vocational rehabilitation. The administrator there said, "Larry was very demanding, wanted things precisely the way he wanted them. . . . I had nurses toward the end who just couldn't work with him anymore because they were just extremely, extremely frustrated."[22] He noted that McAfee's family and friends remained in Georgia.

McAfee was housed in Ohio with demented, senile, and brain-damaged patients who were being cheaply warehoused with only one or two staff for as many as 40 patients. The easiest way to warehouse such patients is to keep them heavily sedated. McAfee said that he experienced intense loneliness and received inadequate personal care.

After two years, when it became clear that McAfee had been dumped on them, Ohio officials angrily hustled him onto a plane and left him in the emergency room at Grady Memorial Hospital in Atlanta. "You're just a sack of potatoes," McAfee said.[23]

After he returned to Atlanta, and because no other facility in Georgia would take him, Larry spent several miserable months in the intensive care unit of Grady Memorial Hospital. In 1989, Briarcliff Nursing Home in a suburb of Birmingham, Alabama, finally accepted him as a medical patient.

Russ Fine, a disability advocate and director of the Injury Control Research Center at the University of Alabama at Birmingham, listened when Larry called his weekly radio talk show, hosted by Russ and his wife, Dee. According to Russ, McAfee's treatment on Medicaid represented "everything that's wrong about the system that serves disabled people."[24]

On first meeting Larry, Fine found him lying in bed staring at the ceiling, with no voice-activated telephone and no television. All he could do was stare "at whatever happened to be in front of his face. From a quality of life standpoint, it was a devastating commentary on a society with a very advanced health-care system."[25]

A reporter once arrived to find McAfee's urinary catheter not connected to a container and spilling urine on the floor. Fine says, "These facilities were not equipped to take care of a patient such as Larry, with labor-intensive health-care requirements."[26]

In 1989, four years after the federal court ruled for Elizabeth Bouvia, Larry filed suit in federal court in Atlanta to exercise his right to die. Because his ventilator had once been dislodged accidentally and he had experienced terrifying suffocation, Larry did not want it disconnected. Instead, he had designed a puff-sip switch for his IV line, by blowing and sucking in a specific pattern, which would enable him to turn on an electric switch activating the flow of lethal drugs into him.

In 1989, after a heart-wrenching 45-minute hearing in Fulton County Superior Court, Judge Edward Johnson found in Larry McAfee's favor. Johnson ruled that physicians could prescribe lethal drugs that McAfee would take, using his switch to die.

Everyone assumed that with his legal victory, McAfee would kill himself within days. Like Elizabeth Bouvia, he did not.

Russ Fine had convinced McAfee to stay alive. But then his financial problems began.

Larry first qualified for SSI assistance. Social Security, besides providing income to retired Americans, provides financial assistance to disabled people as Supplemental Security Income (SSI). In 2009, SSI payments averaged $674 a month and were paid to about 7 million elderly, disabled, or blind Americans.

In 1989, Russ Fine persuaded Birmingham's United Cerebral Palsy to let Larry live temporarily in its nine-person group home for the severely disabled that had a supported-employment program. Larry stayed there on-and-off until late 1990, but because he required expensive nurses, he soon had to look elsewhere to live.

Federal regulations surrounding Medicaid block using its payment for people such as Larry to live in group homes. Disability advocates claimed that this structural discrimination forces people like Larry or Elizabeth Bouvia to live in public hospitals or to be warehoused in huge public nursing homes.

When President George Bush, Sr., refused a waiver of these Medicaid regulations to help Larry, the Georgia legislature created an independent-living facility for him and the five other patients as an exception to Georgia's disability law and Medicaid plan. Larry then lived in Augusta, near its medical school.

In 1993, his accident and fight were portrayed in *The Switch*, a CBS movie. To keep his disability payments, McAfee could not accept any money from the movie.

A few months later, Georgia omitted funding for McAfee's group home in its state budget. Once again, Russ Fine held Georgia's feet to the fire for Larry, pointing out that the cost per person in the group home was only $52 a day. Georgia found funds to continue the home for another year.

In 1993, a kink in his catheter caused urine to back up. Being paralyzed, Larry could not feel what was happening; the backup caused toxicity and high blood pressure. This caused two devastating strokes.[27] Larry survived, but the strokes injured his brain and he was left with just a little short-term memory.

He had planned to leave the group home for his own apartment but instead officials transferred him to a long-term nursing home. Larry McAfee died in 1995 at age 39, ten years after his accident. He died not by his own hand, but after being comatose for many months. Tragically, this was just the kind of place and just the kind of end that Larry had wanted to avoid.

THE CASE OF DAX COWART

Another famous case in bioethics, 29-year-old bachelor Dax (Donald) Cowart suffered burns over two-thirds of his body in 1973 in Texas. He was treated against his will for 14 months in a burn unit in Parkland Hospital in Dallas. Dax's physicians ignored his refusal to be treated; instead, they honored the wishes of his mother, who overruled him. He was left blind, disfigured, and with only partial use of his fingers.[28]

After winning a million dollars from an out-of-court settlement with a gas company, Dax hired a plane, flew to Mexico, and spent several hours on a landing strip with a gun in his hand, debating whether to kill himself. Like Elizabeth Bouvia and Larry McAfee, once he obtained the power to take control of his life, he decided not to kill himself.

Instead, he graduated from law school in 1986 and has been married twice. He became interested in ham radio and raising golden retrievers. He has been active as a trial lawyer and has won cases for plaintiffs in lawsuits.

In retrospect, he rejects the decision of his physicians to keep him alive. He frequently tells his story in public, emphasizing the cruelty of his physicians, who made him endure 14 months of terrible pain. He argues that even though he is glad to be alive today, his physicians were wrong to treat him against his wishes.

As he once said to this author, "If I should be so unlucky as to be burned that way again, and if I knew what was waiting at the end, I wouldn't go through that pain to get there."[29]

BACKGROUND: PERSPECTIVES ON SUICIDE

Greece and Rome

Ancient Greek aristocrats strove not simply to live, but to lead lives of nobility, honor, excellence, and beauty. Believing that "the unexamined life is not worth living," they thought the "important thing is not to live but to live well." They thought that study of philosophy would provide wisdom to approach death (*philosophy* means "love of wisdom"). Plato records Socrates as saying, "True philosophers make dying their profession, and . . . to them of all men, death is least alarming. . . . So if you see one distressed at the prospect of dying, it will be proof that he is a lover not of wisdom but of the body."[30]

Socrates died famously. Sentenced to die for impiety and corrupting the young, he could have fled Athens, but chose instead to drink hemlock, a poison. At his death scene, he discussed death with a friend.

The friend says that if one is convinced of life after death, it is easy not to fear death, but what if the soul is "dispersed and destroyed on the very day that the man himself dies [and] may be dissipated like breath or smoke, and vanish away, so that nothing is left of it anywhere. . . . No one but a fool is entitled to face death with confidence, unless he can prove that the soul is absolutely immortal and indestructible."

Socrates replies that the soul may be immortal, but if it is not, then death is like a sleep from which one never awakes. If so, we should not fear it, because no one will exist to feel pain or to miss life.

After this discussion about death, Socrates takes hemlock, which acts as a poison by decreasing circulation at the extremities, creating distal numbness, and eventually stopping the heart.

As his friends begin to cry, Socrates says, "Calm yourselves and try to be brave!" He dies moments later. His admiring follower, Plato, and the author of this account, writes, "Such . . . was the end of our comrade, who was, we may fairly say, of all those whom we knew in our time, the bravest and also the wisest and most upright man."

Centuries later in Rome, emperor Marcus Aurelius (portrayed in the 2000 movie *Gladiator*) wrote that suicide surpassed undignified dying. These Roman Stoics defended the argument for the open door: "If the room is smoky, if only moderately, I will stay; if there is too much smoke, I will go. Remember this, keep a firm hand on it, the door is always open."[31]

Seneca, another stoic, wrote about old age: "If it begins to shake my mind, if it destroys my faculties one by one, if it leaves me not life but breath, I will depart the putrid or the tottering edifice."[32]

In the twentieth century, existentialist philosopher Jean-Paul Sartre revived the argument for the open door.[33] He emphasized that choice—even the choice of staying alive each day—is inescapable. He famously wrote, "Not to choose is always still a choice."

Christianity and Voluntary Death

The Bible does not explicitly prohibit suicide and seems to condone the suicides of Saul and Judas. During the fourth century, Augustine condemned suicide, basing his condemnation on the sixth commandment, "Thou shalt not kill" (Exodus 20:13).

Augustine distinguished between private killing and killing endorsed by God or divine authority. Killing undertaken on one's own authority is never right, but when God commands killing, humans must obey. So Abraham had to obey when God commanded him to kill his son, Isaac. Individuals who so kill are instruments in God's hand.

This reasoning underlies the permissibility of killing in capital punishment and in just wars. The worldly Ambrose had already said that Christians could kill in war, and Augustine went further by condoning war against heretics. Frederick Russell in *The Just War in the Middle Ages* says that through Augustine's interpretation of killing for Christians, "the New Testament doctrines of love and purity were accommodated to the savagery of the Old Testament and pacifism was defeated."[34]

Augustine does not explain how he knows when God orders humans to kill and when God orders humans to abstain. In particular, how do we know that God forbids suicide for people with terminal illness?

The thirteenth-century philosopher and theologian Thomas Aquinas held that suicide is sinful. It is so because it leaves no time for repentance; because life is a gift from God and only God can take it back; because it deprives the community of talented people; because it deprives children of their parents; and because it is unnatural, going against the instinct of self-preservation.

Three thinkers who allowed suicide were the French essayist Michel de Montaigne in the sixteenth century, the Dutch philosopher Baruch Spinoza, and the English poet John Donne in the seventeenth. Montaigne concluded his essay "To Philosophize Is to Learn How to Die" by saying, "If we have learned how to live properly and calmly, we will know how to die in the same manner."[35] Spinoza wrote, "A free man, that is to say, a man who lives according to the dictates of reason alone, is not led by the fear of death."[36] Donne wrote, "When the [terminal] disease would not reduce us, [God] sent a second and worse affliction, ignorant and torturing physicians."[37]

David Hume In the eighteenth century, Scottish philosopher David Hume argued that suicide "is no transgression of our duty to God." Hume hated vanity and observed, "The life of a man is of no greater importance to the universe than that of an oyster."[38]

In his "Essay on Suicide," Hume disagreed with Augustine and Aquinas. For dying patients, Hume argued, voluntary death is not a sin: "A house which falls by its own weight is not brought to ruin by [God's] providence."[39] Hume argued that if God made the world through the laws of causality—the laws of biology, medicine, and physics—then disease belonged to the natural working of such laws.

Hume attacked the idea that suicide is blasphemous. Immanuel Kant argued that we have a station in life assigned to us by God which we must not give up, but Hume replied, "It is a kind of blasphemy to imagine that any created being can [by taking his own life] disturb the order of the world. Any suicide is insignificant to the workings of the universe and it is blasphemy to think otherwise." To Hume, only narcissists believe that the world's smooth functioning requires their continued existence.

Hume disputed Aquinas's argument that suicide harms the community,

> A man who retires from life does no harm to society; he only ceases to do good; which, if it is an injury, is of the lowest kind. All our obligations to do good to society seem to imply something reciprocal. I receive benefits of society, and therefore ought to promote its interests; but when I withdraw myself altogether from society, can I be bound any longer? But [even] allowing that our obligations to do good were perpetual, they have certainly some bounds; I am not obliged to do a small good to society at the expense of a great harm to myself: when then should I prolong a miserable existence, because of some frivolous advantage which the public may perhaps receive from me?

Immanuel Kant Hume's contemporary, the German philosopher Immanuel Kant, opposed suicide for several reasons. First, an act is right for Kant if it represents or is based on a rule that can be universalized, that is, a rule we would want everyone to act on. Kant argued that suicide cannot be universalized because we cannot accept the rule for all humans of self-termination.

Moreover, if the motive of suicide is self-interest (for instance, escaping pain), then that is not a moral justification. For Kant, moral decisions are not justified by what furthers one's self-interests.

More generally for Kant, suicide is immoral because people should always be treated as ends in themselves, never as mere means. For Kant, that means they should treat their own lives and bodies as ends in themselves, even to the extent that Kant seems to frown on giving another person one of one's kidneys.[40]

Kant reasoned that treating oneself as an end in itself entails recognizing one's free will as an absolute (rather than as a relative) value, but destroying oneself entails destroying that freedom of will. "Man's freedom cannot subsist except on a condition which is immutable. This condition is that man not use his freedom against himself to his own destruction."[41]

Third, a person "who does not respect his life even in principle cannot be restrained from the most dreadful vices." If I do not respect my own life, I will not respect anything else. To respect the sacred value of the lives of others, I must respect the sacred value of my own.

Finally, Kant wrote, "Human beings are sentinels on earth and may not leave their posts until relieved by another beneficent hand. God is our owner; we are His property."[42]

John Stuart Mill In one of the most famous passages in political philosophy, John Stuart Mill expressed "one very simple principle" in his 1859 essay, *On Liberty.* It grounds the political and ethical autonomy that enables competent patients to end their own lives. Mill writes that,

> One very simple principle [is] entitled to govern absolutely the dealings of society with the individual in the way of compulsion and control, whether the means

> used is physical force in the form of legal penalties, or the moral coercion of public opinion. That principle is, that the sole end for which mankind are warranted, individually or collectively, in interfering with the liberty of action of any of their number, is self-protection. That the only purpose for which power can be rightfully exercised over any member of a civilized community, against his will, is to prevent harm to others. His own good, either physical or moral, is not a sufficient warrant. . . . The only part of the conduct of any one, for which he is amenable to society, is that which concerns others. In the part which merely concerns himself, his independence is, of right, absolute. Over himself, over his own body and mind, the individual is sovereign.[43]

According to this principle, so long as others are not harmed, we can do whatever we want with our own lives and bodies.

Mill distinguished between *self-regarding* and *other-regarding* acts, and argued that we may censure others only for their other-regarding acts. Paradoxically, Mill's analysis can be used both for and against suicide. On one hand, taking one's own life is clearly self-regarding; suicide is often described as the ultimate personal issue. On the other hand, suicide is other-regarding because it deeply affects others, especially when they believe they have been abandoned or they believe they should have acted differently to prevent it. If a suicidal person desired to make others feel guilty, sorry, or incompetent, then Mill's principle condemns him, because the person killed himself to harm others.

The Modern Era When American feminist Charlotte Perkins Gillman killed herself in 1935, she left a note saying that she preferred "chloroform to cancer." In an essay published posthumously, she wrote: "The record of a previously noble life is precisely what makes it sheer insult to allow death in pitiful degradation. We may not wish to 'die with our boots on,' but we may well prefer to 'die with our brains on.'"[44]

A century ago, only the poor and people without families went to a hospital to die. Before the Harrison Act of 1914, Americans could purchase heroin and opiates to lessen the pain of terminal cancer and die at home on their own terms. Today, physicians control such drugs, death has been medicalized, and most people die in hospitals or nursing homes.

The nature of deadly diseases has also changed. Before World War II, most people died of sudden-onset, acute diseases such as pneumonia and cholera. Today, people live longer and die slowly from chronic diseases such as emphysema, diabetes, dementia, cancer, and coronary artery disease. Because such diseases slowly erode the quality of life, death at a time of one's own choosing remains a moral issue.

The Concept of Assisted Suicide

One question raised by the cases of Elizabeth Bouvia and Larry McAfee is what to call their intended action: suicide, rational suicide, assisted suicide, euthanasia, voluntary death, or self-deliverance? Let us clarify some terms here.

First, *euthanasia* usually means the killing of one person by another for merciful reasons. The preceding cases do not involve euthanasia, then, since in each case the death would be initiated by the person herself or himself.

Second, it is inaccurate to say that a terminally ill patient who forgoes medical treatment "commits suicide." It is true that the definition of suicide is now often broadened to include indirect ways of bringing about one's own death.[45] Nevertheless, we should distinguish between: (1) cases where an underlying disease is incrementally leading to death, and by choosing not to do everything possible, the patient accepts death at an earlier date; and (2) cases where a competent adult without a terminal illness causes his or her own death. The second kind of case is appropriately called suicide.

One reason to maintain the distinction between forgoing treatment in terminal illness and committing suicide is that if a death is classified as a suicide, life insurance companies refuse to pay benefits. Another reason is that in all states it is illegal for nonphysicians to assist in suicides (Washington and Oregon now allow physicians to assist terminal patients to die: see Chapter 3).[46]

The issue for physicians and nurses in the Bouvia and McAfee cases is therefore best called *assisted suicide*. Neither Elizabeth Bouvia nor Larry McAfee had a terminal disease, hence the term *suicide*. They could not easily kill themselves, and so they needed help from others, especially medical staff members; hence the term *assisted*.

ETHICAL ISSUES: FOR AND AGAINST ASSISTED SUICIDE

Easy to Kill Oneself?

Why don't patients such as Elizabeth Bouvia and Larry McAfee simply go off somewhere and kill themselves? Answer: it's difficult to commit suicide when you want to die painlessly and aesthetically, and when you need to be sure that you accomplish what you intend. When you are disabled, it's almost impossible to kill yourself without someone's help.

During the Iran-Contra hearings in 1987, national security advisor Robert McFarlane tried to kill himself and took 30–45 tablets of 10 mg Valium. When he didn't die, people inferred he hadn't wanted to, but in reality, he didn't know how to. Most people don't.

Even most physicians don't know how to help someone commit suicide. In 1985, physician Robert Rosier didn't know how much morphine to give his terminally ill wife to help her die. If physicians don't know, what about ordinary people?[47]

Whenever people botch suicides, critics infer ambivalence, but this inference is often mistaken. Emergency medicine contains many stories of bizarre survivals.[48] The hand holding the gun wobbles a fraction of an inch and leaves the would-be suicide a drooling zombie. Because the drugs they take for courage also relax muscles, some leapers survive jumps from the Golden Gate Bridge. One jumper hit a parked car and not only did not die, but didn't even lose consciousness.[49]

Although suicide attempts by teenagers increased 300 percent between 1967 and 1982, only one in 50 attempts succeeded.[50] The elderly know more and succeed one in three times; Miami Beach leads America in successful suicides. Women attempt suicide more than men, but are less successful. Men use violent means, such as guns; women use drugs.

Methods available for committing suicide present a grim picture. People taking benzodiazepines usually take them, like McFarlane, in insufficient quantities to cause death, instead rendering themselves anoxic, comatose, or brain-but-not-bodily dead.

People using other methods may only end up in the ER. Carbon monoxide (CO) poisoning may fail because the car can stall, run out of gas, or the CO may not concentrate enough, so the person becomes merely comatose.

Slitting wrists in a warm tub, like the famous scene in *The Godfather*? Not easy: the cuts are painful, must be made deep and in the right place, and between unconsciousness and death, the arm may move out of the water and then the blood coagulates. One ER physician observes, "Most slashers just get a trophy: a claw hand."

Failed suicides wake up in the ER with a nasogastric tube down their throat, into which ER doctors pump syrup of ipecac to induce vomiting. They follow this by injecting saline solution and alternately flooding and suctioning out the stomach (gastric lavage), finally pumping granulated charcoal in the stomach to absorb remaining drugs. For patients who return to consciousness while physicians are doing these procedures, the feelings are painful, undignified, and messy, and afterward, the patients will be viewed as children who need careful monitoring lest they try again.

If they want to spare the feelings of others, or if they want to be found in a reasonably dignified state after death, potential suicides must avoid certain methods. Overdoses of sedatives not only decrease respiration, but relax bowels and bladders. Jumping off a building or shooting oneself in the head leaves a big mess. Hanging is not so great: difficult to do correctly—because the neck may not break and the victim, kicking in agony as he partially asphyxiates—may not die, it relaxes bowel and bladder control. Men who die by hanging are also found with an erection.

Rationality and Competence

The play and movie *Whose Life Is It, Anyway?* featured quadriplegic hero Ken Harrison, who wants to die and offers rational arguments for suicide to his psychiatrist. However, because Harrison is intelligent and sane enough to formulate a convincing case, his psychiatrist decides he's too intelligent and sane to die. Harrison can prove his rationality only by deciding to live.

In Bouvia's case, psychiatrist Nancy Mullen testified that since Elizabeth was suicidal, she was incompetent to make decisions about her life. Mullen said that she could conceive of no situation where a person could make a competent decision to take her own life.[51] Carol Gill, a clinical assistant professor of occupational therapy who used a wheelchair, criticized the ACLU for accepting the decision of "a handful of medical experts" that Bouvia was competent when she decided to starve herself.[52]

These experts may have begged the question of rational suicide. A question is begged when the answer is assumed to be true rather than proved. In these cases, the question or point is whether a decision to die rather than lead an unsatisfactory life is irrational: whether it indicates misinformation or faulty reasoning. Just assuming that a decision to die is always irrational begs that question.

This is not to say that a decision to die is always rational. Elizabeth Bouvia may have been depressed, and psychological tests might have shown this. But Mullen and Gill did not base their arguments on such tests. They were not Elizabeth's therapists and were not treating her. Mullen and Gill reacted to the content of Elisabeth's decision, rather than to psychological tests. Indeed, three psychiatric professionals who tested Elizabeth found her competent.[53]

In America a patient is legally competent until proven otherwise in a hearing. No patient can be held in a hospital against her will without having been proven legally incompetent. In practice, hospitals sometimes break such laws. Although Dax Cowart was never declared incompetent, he was treated against his will for 14 months in a burn unit.

Autonomy

At the start of bioethics, autonomy fueled the patient rights movement. Applied to the right to die, a person who has not been proved incompetent has a right to end his life based on his general autonomy (or personal liberty) to control his life, his body, and his personal affairs.

Opponents of assisted suicide argued that Elizabeth Bouvia and Larry McAfee did not want to die because they did not kill themselves quietly but made dramatic demands on public institutions. They were "acting out" and pleading for attention. In such cases, physicians must not accede to wishes of unstable patients, because doing so may not represent the patient's best interests. It would be foolish to assist in the suicide of every distraught patient who came to an ER wishing to die.

The Roman Catholic Church opposes autonomous suicide. In 1990, Father Kevin O'Rourke argued that humans are not in control of their lives.[54] O'Rourke argued that God has a plan for each person and that such a plan never includes suicide.

One problem with uncritical acceptance of autonomy is the famous SUPPORT study (Study to Understand Prognoses and Preferences for Outcomes and Risks of Treatments). It studied predictions about advance directives and end-of-life care and discovered that competent people do not accurately predict what they will later find unacceptable as quality of life.[55] People who predicted that they would rather die than go on a ventilator most often did *not* choose to die but instead, did ultimately choose the ventilator. It's one thing to say abstractly that one would "rather be dead than live like that," but when actually faced with death, most people decide to live.

In another study, some people predicted that patients who expressed strong attachment to religion would be more likely to forgo aggressive treatment at the end of life. But the opposite was true: Devout patients were three times as likely to want everything done, to avoid signing advance directives, and to request CPR and treatments in intensive care units.[56]

In rehabilitation medicine there is the equally famous *adaptation effect*, in which after six months or so, patients like Larry McAfee or Dax Cowart, who were disabled in accidents, change their views. What they once considered unacceptable then becomes acceptable.

Given the SUPPORT study's results, for people with severe disabilities whose life seems to have some pleasure and who are not in too much pain, helping them die cannot be justified solely by appealing to their present wishes. Chances run high that they incorrectly forecast their future preferences.

On the other side, supporters of assisted suicide argued that providing such assistance finishes a continuum of good medical care. Normally, leaving a patient untreated is abandonment and considered unethical (and for physicians, a crime). But when quality of life diminishes, the fact that a patient does not have a terminal disease is irrelevant. The real issue is whether a quality of life is acceptable to the person who must endure it, and that is an evaluative judgment that can be made only by the patient herself. If physicians refuse to assist in suicide and make this evaluation for patients, that is vile paternalism.

Although autonomy creates bad results in some cases, honoring it leads to the greatest good for the greatest number. The death rate for humans is 100 percent. Each of us will die, and each of us wants control over how we do so. We value autonomy in our life and in our dying.

If physicians ignore autonomy, patients can be "flogged to death" with unnecessary tubes, surgery, and radiation. Such barbaric end-of-life treatment differs little from involuntary commitment of competent people in psychiatric wards.

Autonomy is both an ethical and a political value in bioethics. As we have seen, both Kant and Mill argued for autonomy as the source of values and individual choices.

Unlike Kant, Mill argued that the state should have no power to force an individual to act in his own best interest. In essence, Mill saw individual rights as conditions limiting what government may do to citizens.

The key question was not whether Elizabeth Bouvia was demonstrably competent or incompetent, but where the onus of proof should lie. For rugged individualists and libertarians who abhor the growing powers of government and physicians the onus should be on those who would take away autonomy.

In 1990, the United States Supreme Court decided in *Cruzan* that no state may pass a law limiting the right of competent patients to decline medical treatment, even if declining treatment would hasten death. *Cruzan* built on the *Bouvia* and *McAfee* decisions and was a victory for the right of competent adults to control how they died.

Treating Depression, Pain, and Symptoms Well

Although every decision to die is not irrational, many suicidal people suffer from treatable depression. Humane physicians will not let patients die because of chemical imbalances in their brains.

This is especially true of the three patients in this chapter, who were young, nonterminal, competent adults. Although it is understandable to want to die after being horribly burned or after losing physical abilities, people in the throes of depression do not understand how much better they can come to feel. Antidepressants lift moods and change outlooks on life, and therefore, they should be given to all nonterminal patients who wish to die.

A different clinical issue concerns relief of symptoms. In this regard, psychiatrist and palliative care physician John Shuster says it is always important to ask patients who want to die, "What is the chief symptom that makes you want to die?"[57] He observes that often that chief symptom is not what outsiders would predict. One of his patients suffered obviously from air hunger but that was not his chief complaint. Instead, he missed going to a public park in his trailer, so visits to the park were quickly arranged by hospital volunteers. Moreover, with well-financed coverage, almost any symptom can be controlled, including pain, air hunger, itchiness, fatigue, and even boredom.

Social Prejudice and Physical Disabilities

Disability advocate Paul Longmore, whose commentary was quoted earlier and who is himself a ventilator-dependent quadriplegic, opposes voluntary death for people with disabilities. He believes that the Bouvia case shows how a prejudiced system destroys the independence of disabled people rather than nurturing it.

By creating intolerable conditions for disabled people, society paints them into a corner. Society leaves such patients with only one autonomous decision consistent with their former autonomous selves: they can decide to die. Others make every other decision for them and keep them passive and dependent. In Longmore's words:

> Given the lumping together of people with disabilities with those who are terminally ill, the blurring of voluntary assisted suicide and forced "mercy" killing, and the oppressive conditions of social devaluation and isolation, blocked opportunities, economic deprivation, and enforced social powerlessness, talk of their "rational" or "voluntary" suicide is simply Orwellian newspeak. The advocates of assisted suicide assume a nonexistent autonomy. They offer an illusory self-determination.[58]

To see Elizabeth Bouvia as simply a case of a right to die is to miss a much bigger issue. What made Elizabeth Bouvia want to die was the cumulative effect of centuries of prejudice against people who are physically disabled—prejudice that is virulently expressed in modern American society, which idealizes youth, beauty, sex, athleticism, fitness, and wealth. Yet other values also make life worthwhile, such as caring for others, erudition, creativity, and community, but our culture does not idealize such values.

Longmore attacks films that encourage disabled people to view killing themselves as a rational response to their low quality of life. He cites *Annie Hall*, *Elephant Man*, and (could have cited) the 2004 film *Million Dollar Baby*. He claims that watching *Whose Life Is It, Anyway?* depressed Elizabeth Bouvia.

Some critics of autonomy see Bouvia as society's failure: a case where someone slipped through the cracks of an uncaring, impersonal system. They see Elizabeth Bouvia as a tragic figure not because of her physical situation but rather because of her *social* situation. Even as a hospitalized patient, she remained alone, and it was her terrible aloneness that underlay her fierce assertion of her right to tear herself away from life.

Structural Discrimination against the Disabled

In 1990, the Americans with Disabilities Act (ADA) passed and in the following years, began to go into effect. This legislation represents one of the most sweeping changes in American law. Although not always enforced, its long-term effects are designed to integrate Americans with disabilities into normal life.

Raising the issue of inadequate resources puts physicians in an awkward place. On the one hand, they do not want to be instruments of torture to disable people who want to die. On the other hand, they do not want to acquiesce to unnecessary deaths of the disabled people because a prejudiced, cheap society has the wrong attitude toward people with disabilities. In this regard, it is important to recognize that most institutions are still not anywhere near compliance with the ADA, despite it being passed nearly two decades ago.

The bulwark against structural discrimination is great care, but to get it is not easy. To do so, patients must be rich, have good insurance, have hard-working relatives or spouses, or society must become generous. If the true measure of a society is how it treats its least well-off members, then our society is not magnanimous, at least toward the disabled.[59]

As a result of childhood polio, Paul Longmore's arms were paralyzed, his spine is curved, and he uses a ventilator as much as 18 hours a day.[60] He is an associate professor of history at San Francisco State University. His success would not have been possible if he weren't able to live independently on his own, which required lots of home health care aides. Fortunately, California's generous Medicaid program paid for his domestic aides (costing $15,000 a year) and he managed to avoid being disqualified from Medicare disability, which paid for his ventilator (costing $12,000 a year). Had he lived in Georgia or Michigan, Longmore, too, might have wanted to die, as he would not have been able to find a group home and he "probably would have found my life unendurable."

Longmore maintains that Elizabeth Bouvia's problems resulted in part because she did not receive the maximum payments she was entitled to; he says that her county is notorious for its stinginess in benefits to disabled people. The hospital where she was supposed to do her internship refused to comply with laws designed to ensure her disability rights.

California's In-Home Supportive Services program allowed Elizabeth to manage her own life at home while she was single; when she married, however, she became ineligible: her husband was expected to care for her. If she had found a job, she also would have been ineligible. Longmore concludes:

> This is a woman who aimed at something more significant than mere self-sufficiency. She struggled to attain self-determination, but she was repeatedly thwarted in her efforts by discriminatory actions on the part of the government, her teachers, her employers, her parents, and her society. Contrary to the highly prejudiced view of the appeals court, what makes life with a major physical disability ignominious, embarrassing, humiliating, and dehumanizing is not the need for extensive physical assistance, but the dehumanizing social contempt toward those who require such aid.

Russ Fine believes that McAfee's desire to die resulted from his inadequate care. Public officials were controlling costs by requiring patients like McAfee to live in the most cost-effective facilities, but McAfee said that if he couldn't get his own apartment he would rather die. According to Fine, McAfee "was very vocal about inferior nursing care, which was the rule, not the exception, in these marginal health-care facilities that had accepted these contracts."[61]

One Thanksgiving, Fine had brought McAfee dinner and the two were watching a televised football game while waiting for McAfee's family to arrive. Fine was drowsing in an armchair when he suddenly realized that McAfee had stopped breathing. By the time the family arrived, nurses and aides were swarming over McAfee, trying to get him breathing. When he finally revived, Fine saw tears streaming out of his eyes. "He didn't really want to die," Fine concluded. "He was just terrified."[62]

It should be noted that McAfee, like Bouvia, wanted to work, but getting paid for working would have made him ineligible for most publicly funded assistance in housing or Medicaid.

Cases such as Bouvia's and McAfee's suggest that society often does give severely disabled people only three limited, grim choices: to become a burden on their families or friends, to live miserably in a large public institution, or to kill themselves.

In small-group homes, a few home health aides can help disabled residents lead productive lives. Both Elizabeth Bouvia and Larry McAfee wanted such arrangements, and giving them this would have been cheaper than the care they did receive in hospitals. (Elizabeth Bouvia's care cost at least $300 a day between 1986 and 1996.)

Not many group homes exist. A major reason is a reaction called NIMBY—"not in my backyard." In the case of group homes for the disabled, such resistance seems to be based on prejudice. Neighborhoods argue that group homes create dangerous situations and lower property values. Prejudice should not be allowed to prevent communities from giving their disabled citizens better choices than imprisonment in hospitals or death.

The Rule of Rescue

The campaign to obtain a presidential waiver for Larry McAfee provoked criticism. Two citizens complained when McAfee said that he would not return to a nursing home to "vegetate" and wanted Georgia to pay for his private apartment.[63] They wrote:

> But why should McAfee be the only one singled out and given special attention, not to be in a nursing home, or that Medicaid should "open up" for? . . . McAfee "understands" that life is preferable, but it must be life with some dignity; in this case, his way or no way. McAfee says that if someone else won't pay for him to live where and how he chooses, he'd rather be dead. What about all the other people in the same situation?[64]

Critics like these hold that American society rescues only someone like McAfee, who gets into the national spotlight; it ignores all the others whose needs are just as great. In McAfee's case, there were some 75,000 to 85,000 others.

Larry McAfee and Elizabeth Bouvia both illustrate *the rule of rescue.* When one person's plight is made prominent by the news media, society tends to feel compelled to rescue that person, even if the rescue entails spending enormous amounts of scarce medical resources. In contrast, obscure people quietly go "unrescued" and live in abysmal conditions until they die. The rule of rescue in effect turns some crucial decisions over to the media: the editors of local newspapers and television news departments become gatekeepers, determining who will and will not be rescued. This is hardly the most rational way to distribute scarce medical resources.

Disability Culture

During the last decades, people with disabilities increasingly protested against society's discrimination. They asserted their right to 24-hour-a-day attendants, public transportation, and good housing.[65] People with disabilities think they have a condition, not an illness. For them, "disability culture" is not a bad thing, but a source of pride and identity.

They argue that the disabled community is the only minority that anyone may join at any time. Just as James Meredith had to sue in 1962 to become the first black person admitted to the University of Mississippi, quadriplegic Edward V. Roberts had to sue to be admitted to the University of California. Has society more successfully integrated the races than the disabled?

Many people with disabilities see their life as a call to action to help their less assertive, disabled friends. They despise Mattel's "Share-a-Smile Becky" in a wheelchair (sold in some hospitals' gift shops) and demonstrate outside the classes of Princeton bioethicist Peter Singer, whose views on quality of life, they fear, will allow society to easily kill the disabled or deny them adequate resources.

Disability groups hectored the Hemlock Society (once, Compassion in Dying, now Compassion and Choices), accusing it of being too sympathetic to the assisted death of nonterminal patients. They cite psychologist Faye Girsh, this society's executive director, who testified on behalf of Bouvia, on behalf of Jack Kevorkian when he killed some nonterminal, women who were beset by economic hardship; on behalf of George DeLury, who in 1996 in Manhattan killed his wife in her late stages of multiple sclerosis; and on behalf of Canadian Robert Latimer, who in 1993 killed his 12-year-old daughter with cerebral palsy. Disability groups accused Girsh and her society of being on the side of rich, well-insured, autonomous elites, not in securing better conditions for the disabled.

CONCLUSION

As our cases showed, requests to die from nonterminal, young patients involve more than viewing as cruel physicians who refuse to honor these requests on demand. Much more is often involved here, including issues about justice in the design of medical services in our society for people with disabilities and issues about adequate treatment of depression and symptoms.

FURTHER READING AND RESOURCES

"A Man of Endurance," *20/20* television show on March 22, 1999, on Dex Cowart's case. Call 1-800-CALL-ABC to order tape (around $30).

"Elizabeth Bouvia: 10 Years Later," *60 Minutes,* Special, www.cbs.com

Pat Milmoe McCarrick, "Active Euthanasia and Assisted Suicide," Scope Note 18, *Kennedy Institute of Ethics Journal,* no. 1, March 1992.

James Rachels, *The End of Life,* Oxford, Oxford University Press, 1986.

Lonnie Kliever, ed., *Dax's Case: Essays in Medical Ethics and Human Meaning,* Dallas, TX, Southern Methodist University Press, 1989.

David Anderson, "A Right to Die: The Dax Cowart Case—An Ethical Case Study on CD-ROM," New York, Routledge, 1996.

DISCUSSION QUESTIONS

1. Can decisions be justified by their outcomes? What if Bouvia or Cowart had killed themselves when they had the opportunity? Would that mean the physicians who prevented their earlier deaths were wrong?
2. How do you know when you've really treated depression and "debilitating symptoms" when a patient has sustained a terrible accident or is dying? Isn't that a Catch-22, where you only know you've successfully treated it when the patient decides to live?
3. Is the right to die glamorized in movies? What if the paralyzed fighter, portrayed by actress Hillary Swank in *Million Dollar Baby,* had to suffocate slowly for 20 minutes in dying? What if her reflexes kicked in and her body resisted? She lost bowel and bladder control? It didn't work and she was left comatose or brain-damaged?
4. Right now, society seems to exalt young bodies, sexiness, athleticism, and wealth. Do these images set young people up for failure? As most people can't have these goods, what message do these images send to people who are the opposite? Is this a good set of values to live by?
5. How do diversity and autonomy go together, or not? Will some ethnic groups be more interested in autonomy in medicine than others? Is autonomy more meaningful to some than others? Should autonomy be defined as a check or balance against the power of the medical establishment over the individual?

CHAPTER 2

Comas

Karen Quinlan, Nancy Cruzan, and Terri Schiavo

Built on previous cases of Nancy Cruzan and Karen Quinlan, the famous case of Terri Schiavo exploded in 2005. All cases involved incompetent adults and whether treatment could be removed to let them die. The Quinlan case started in 1975 in New Jersey courts. Fifteen years later in 1990, the U.S. Supreme Court decided the landmark case of Nancy Cruzan. Fifteen years after that in 2005, the Schiavo case showed that problems still remained.

The Quinlan case sparked the public's interest in medical ethics and asked many questions: Does a person die when only machines keep her body alive? Can families alone decide when medicine ceases to be treatment and becomes torture? Does killing patients differ from intentionally letting them die? In making decisions, what role should courts take? What should be the standard of brain death? The definition of personhood? How should we safeguard incompetent patients from overzealous families? When families want treatment continued for relatives, should we force them to accept medical realities?

The essential question for this chapter concerns whether we should give patients in persistent vegetative state (PVS) every chance of recovery and whether misdiagnosis and financial pressure might pressure physicians to let such patients die early.

THE QUINLAN CASE

In April 1975, after just turning 21, a perky, independent young woman named Karen Quinlan became comatose from drinking alcohol after taking either barbiturates or benzodiazepines, or both.[1] Karen had also been dieting, and at admission, weighed only 115 pounds.

Benzodiazepines—antianxiety drugs such as Valium, Librium, Ativan, and Xanax—act on specific nerve receptors in the brain and are considered safer than barbiturates. The latter have been around since 1912, when physicians first used phenobarbital.

Both benzodiazepines and barbiturates intensify with alcohol, an effect called *synergism*. Alcohol *potentiates* (intensifies the effects of) these drugs, and an empty stomach increases the effects. Actor River Phoenix unintentionally killed himself in 1993 by mixing barbiturates, alcohol, and benzodiazepines.

Karen lost her brain from a synergistic reaction of barbiturates, benzodiazepines, and alcohol taken on an empty stomach. These drugs suppressed her breathing, caused loss of oxygen to her brain, and after 30 minutes, destroyed her higher brain.

At St. Clare's Hospital, a Catholic institution in New Jersey, a small ventilator, also called a respirator, kept Karen breathing. It also prevented aspiration of vomit, which could cause pneumonia.

Ventilators began to be used in medicine during the 1960s and by 1975 had become common in cases of emergency and trauma. The ventilator's use in this case showed that the *criteria of death* needed clarification. Because the brain must have a fresh supply of oxygenated blood to live, lack of such oxygenated blood (anoxia) quickly damages the brain and over enough time, destroys it. The traditional definition of death—where the body stops breathing and the person is declared dead—indirectly *assumed* brain death to be inevitable, but now a ventilator prevented this.

Karen's appearance shocked her sister, who said:

> Whenever I thought of a person in a coma, I thought they would just lie there very quietly, almost as though they were sleeping. Karen's head was moving around, as if she was trying to pull away from that tube in her throat, and she made little noises, like moans. I don't know if she was in pain, but it seemed as though she was. And I thought—if Karen could ever see herself like this, it would be the worst thing in the world for her.[2]

Sometimes Karen would choke, sit bolt upright with her arms flung out and her eyes wide open, appearing to be in intense pain. Eventually her breathing stabilized, but even then she didn't breathe deeply enough to sigh. Without breathing to a sigh, the lower sacs of her lungs risked infection. Hence she was put on a larger ventilator for a "sigh volume." This larger ventilator required a tracheotomy (a hole cut surgically in the throat or trachea) to which her mother, Julia Quinlan, reluctantly agreed.

This more powerful ventilator altered her appearance. At a later hearing, her lawyer testified about Karen in September 1975 that:

> Her eyes are open and move in a circular manner as she breathes; her eyes blink approximately three or four times per minute; her forehead evidences every noticeable perspiration; her mouth is open while the ventilator expands to ingest oxygen, and while her mouth is open, her tongue appears to be moving in a rather random manner; her mouth closes as the oxygen is ingested into her body through the tracheotomy and she appears to be slightly convulsing or gasping as the oxygen enters the windpipe; her hands are visible in an emaciated form, facing in a praying position away from her body. Her present weight would seem to be in vicinity of 70–80 pounds.[3]

Karen Quinlan was in a coma, but what exactly does that mean? The word "coma" is vague. Despite popular belief at the time, under New Jersey law in 1975 Karen was not brain-dead, which required *all* of her brain to be nonfunctioning.

Karen Quinlan was in a serious form of coma called persistent vegetative state (PVS), a generic term covering a type of deep unconsciousness that, if persisting for a few months, is almost always irreversible. In this case, her eyes were *disconjugate*, i.e., they moved in different, random directions at the same time. Despite eye movements, she was thought to be *decorticate*: her brain could not receive input from her eyes. Karen had slow-wave—not isoelectric or flat—electroencephalograms (EEGs).

At one time, a patient in such a condition would simply starve to death, but in the late 1960s, crude intravenous and nasogastric feeding tubes began to be used. Initially, an intravenous tube fed Karen, but as her condition persisted, the rigidity of her muscles made it difficult to insert and reinsert such a tube into her veins. Five months after her admission, in September 1975, she required a nasogastric feeding tube.

The Quinlans never allowed a picture to be taken of Karen in PVS. So the public never saw a realistic picture of her with a shaved head on her ventilator and feeding tube.

In the fall of 1975, the Quinlans decided that Karen would never regain consciousness, so they decided to remove the ventilator and let Karen's body die. They had no idea that their struggle to reach this decision would be the easy part.

The Quinlans averred that Karen had twice said that if anything terrible happened to her, she did not want to be kept alive as a vegetable on machines. But was she really a "vegetable"? We now know that a rare patient may recover from PVS.

Recall that the use of ventilators in the Quinlan case revealed new ethical problems about brain death. In combination with a feeding tube, the question arose of how active could ethical physicians be in *withdrawing* such devices? To some physicians and family members, such withdrawals *felt* like they were killing a vulnerable patient. The Catholic Church asserted such. Were such feelings justified? Isn't it a physician's job to look out for vulnerable patients? What if the patient's family feels differently from the physician? How should such a conflict be resolved?

Robert Morse, a resident in internal medicine, and Arshad Javed, a fellow in pulmonary medicine, were the physicians of record. The Quinlans asked them to disconnect Karen's ventilator. The doctors feared charges of criminal misconduct if they complied. Why?

First, in 1975 the American Medical Association (AMA) seemed to equate withdrawing a ventilator with euthanasia, and then equated that with murder. Back then, no federal or state court had clarified the rights of dying patients or their families.

Second, the physicians feared that the Quinlans might later change their minds and sue them for malpractice. One common definition of malpractice is "departure from normal standards of medical practice in a community," and in 1975—when most physicians continued treatment until the last moments of life—assisting in the deaths of comatose patients would have been such a departure.

Paul Armstrong, a young lawyer interested in Constitutional law and also a Legal Aid attorney, represented Karen Quinlan and her parents.

Dr. Morse testified that no medical precedent allowed him to disconnect Karen's ventilator. Neurologist Julius Korein described Karen as having no mental age at all and as being like "an anencephalic monster."[4] Famous neurologist Fred

Plum described Karen as "lying in bed, emaciated, curled up in what is known as flexion contracture." Every joint was bent in a flexion position and making one tight sort of fetal position. It's too grotesque, really, to describe in human terms like fetal.[5]

Because Karen had never written down her wishes in an advance directive, the judge did not know what she would have wanted, so he decided that her ventilator must continue. He further ruled that her parents' testimony about her wishes could not be taken as final, because it entailed her death. He also ruled that a right to die could not be found in the U.S. Constitution.

Several weeks later, the New Jersey State Supreme Court heard the case on direct review. Physicians testifying there surprised these justices when they distinguished between disconnecting a ventilator and not starting it. They argued that once they accepted patients, they had an absolute duty to pursue patients' welfare, such that they could never cause death. But neurologist Julius Korein countertestified that physicians privately used "judicious neglect" in letting terminal patients die.

The justices pressed the hospital's lawyers about the physician-patient relationship. Why couldn't Morse and Javed allow Karen to be transferred to another hospital, where other physicians could disconnect her? St. Clare's lawyers hemmed and hawed, but finally said that they thought it would be immoral to do so. The justices found all these lines of reasoning "rather flimsy."

The U.S. Supreme Court in 1965 cited a right to privacy in *Griswold v. Connecticut,* when it found unconstitutional those state laws that banned physicians from giving contraceptives to married couples. In 1942 *Oklahoma v. Skinner* had noted a fundamental right to reproduction and control of one's body to block a law allowing involuntary sterilization of habitual criminals. The *Griswold* court said that for a state government to say couples couldn't use contraception to avoid having children violated the *fundamental liberty to lead one's personal life as one saw fit,* which was assumed throughout the Constitution and which made the lives of Americans the envy of many people around the world.

The U.S. Supreme Court further strengthened the right to privacy or personal liberty in its 1973 *Roe v. Wade* decision on abortion (see Chapter 4). In *Roe v. Wade,* the Court decided that the same liberty included the right of a woman to decide whether she wanted to stay pregnant or to abort her fetus, or put differently, whether a state could pass a law prohibiting such abortions, which most had previously done.

In January 1976, after two months of deliberation, the New Jersey Supreme Court ruled unanimously in favor of the Quinlans. The right to privacy allowed the family of a dying incompetent patient to decide what she would have wanted and in this case, to let Karen die by disconnecting her ventilator. The Supreme Court of the United States had not yet made a comparable decision about the end of life, so the New Jersey Supreme Court's decision was a major ruling about the right to privacy in a case of letting die.

The New Jersey court allowed Joseph Quinlan to become Karen's guardian, gave legal immunity to Morse and Javed for disconnecting Karen's life support, and suggested (though it did not require) an advisory role for ethics committees in hospitals composed mostly of lay people to help in future cases.

Pulling the Plug or Weaning from a Ventilator?

In April 1976, four months after the higher-court decision, a ventilator helped Karen Quinlan's body breathe. By then, decubitus ulcers had eaten through her flesh, exposing her hip bones. But why was Karen still alive four months later? This is the least understood and most controversial aspect of this case.

According to the Quinlans, Morse resisted implementing the decision of the New Jersey Supreme Court, because "this is something I will have to live with for the rest of my life."[6] The head nun lectured Mrs. Quinlan more bluntly: "You have to understand our position, Mrs. Quinlan. In this hospital we don't kill people."[7] To this, Julia Quinlan replied, "Why didn't you tell me ten months ago? I would have taken Karen out of this hospital immediately."

The administrators at St. Clare's, and those at other Catholic hospitals, saw the *Quinlan* decision as another step down a slippery slope that had started three years earlier with the legalization of abortion by *Roe v. Wade* in 1973. During the trial, the Vatican theologian Gino Concetti had criticized the Quinlans: "A right to death does not exist. Love for life, even a life reduced to ruin, drives one to protect life with every possible care."[8] A pulmonary specialist at Catholic University in Rome said, removal of the ventilator "would be an extremely dangerous move by her doctors, and represents an indirect form of euthanasia."[9]

Instead of simply disconnecting Karen's ventilator, Morse and Javed weaned her from it. By building up different muscles, they gradually trained her body to breathe off the ventilator. The tired, confused Quinlans probably did not understand what this meant, but the real implications would become painfully clear over the next ten years. Eventually, Javed had Karen off the ventilator for four hours; then, after intensive work over many weeks, for twelve hours. By late May of 1976, Karen was off the ventilator altogether.

This weaning confused the public: Some people took it to mean that Karen had gotten better. Others thought that Karen's physicians had "pulled the plug," but a miracle had prevented her death. Both impressions were false.

St. Clare's hospital now wanted Karen transferred and in June 1976, New Jersey's Medicaid office forced a nursing home to accept her. At this point, Karen had been in PVS for 14 months.

After more than ten years in this nursing home, Karen Quinlan's body expired in June 1986. For several months before that, Karen had had pneumonia; and the Quinlans had declined antibiotics to reverse it.

Substituted Judgment and Kinds of Cases

The *Quinlan* decision ran two different kinds of cases together.[10] As noted, the Court based its decision partly on the right to privacy, a right that in medical contexts would presumably apply only to competent patients. But the standard of *substituted judgment* also grounded *Quinlan*, according to which relatives or friends could say what they believed to be the wishes of the incompetent patient.

Consequently, this decision had at least two major problems. First, how did family's right to exercise substituted judgment derive from *Griswold* and *Roe v. Wade?* Critics felt that the New Jersey court had jumped too quickly from married people's right to control their own reproduction to the parents' right to decide that an adult, comatose, incompetent child wanted to die—especially because few intervening decisions had been made about whether competent adults had a right to hasten their own death by refusing medical treatment. Given that quick, huge jump, critics wondered what was next? Giving parents the right to make life-or-death decisions for permanently incompetent patients? For retarded babies?

Second, substituted judgment is a notoriously subjective criterion.[11] It presumes that decisions made by a patient's family will reflect what the patient herself would have wanted done. In the Quinlan case, like the later Cruzan and Schiavo cases, it was unclear whether these women had really expressed a wish not to have their lives prolonged or whether the families just wished it so.

Finally, the right to privacy most obviously applies to competent patients and their rights to determine their own medical destinies. Ideally, the U.S. Supreme Court would have first laid out that right and then tackled incompetent patients. But life is messy and things didn't happen that way, so the *Quinlan* decision tackled incompetent patients first. It took 15 more years before things were straightened out, when the U.S. Supreme Court finally decided the Cruzan case.

THE CRUZAN CASE

The Cruzan case led to a landmark decision by the United States Supreme Court in June 1990.[12] Before this decision, twenty states had recognized the right of competent patients to refuse medical life support, and all these states (with the exception of New York and Missouri) had recognized the right of surrogates to make decisions for incompetent patients.[13] The *Cruzan* decision first explicitly recognized the rights of competent dying patients.

On January 11, 1983, 24-year-old Nancy Cruzan lost control of her car at night on a lonely, icy country road in Missouri.[14] Thrown 35 feet from the car, she landed face down in a water-filled ditch. Paramedics arriving on the scene found that her heart had stopped beating. Injecting a stimulant into her heart, they restarted it, but because her brain had been anoxic for 15 minutes, Nancy did not regain consciousness.[15]

Over seven years, Nancy's body became rigid—her hands curled tightly, and her fingernails were claw-like. Like Karen Quinlan, Nancy could take nothing by mouth and somebody had to turn her every two hours to prevent ulcers. She drooled much of the time, causing her hair, pillow, and sheets to be wet. Her care cost the state of Missouri $130,000 a year.

Where the Quinlan case focused on withdrawal of a ventilator, the Cruzan case, like the Schiavo case 15 years later, focused on withdrawal of a feeding tube. Because she could not swallow, Nancy could not be fed by mouth. Loss of ability to swallow signals a key decision in the care of incapacitated patients, especially those with dementia or neurological diseases. Before feeding tubes began to be used in the 1960s, such patients died naturally by starvation. Feeding tubes prevent this natural deterioration of the body and can put degeneration on hold for years or even decades.

Legally or morally, the question then arose: Is a PVS patient *owed* food and water forever? Karen Quinlan's parents thought so; they never withdrew the nutrition that kept her body alive. Nancy's parents, Joe and Joyce Cruzan, thought otherwise: they sought permission in court to disconnect her feeding tube.

In discussing the Cruzan case, it is necessary to understand standards of legal evidence. The minimum standard is *preponderance of evidence;* a more rigorous standard is *clear and convincing evidence;* the most rigorous standard—the one used for serious felonies—is *beyond a reasonable doubt.*

Preponderance of evidence simply means that there is more evidence one way than the other; in some cases, this means there is some evidence rather than none. *Clear and convincing* denotes more rigorous evidence; in death, it requires an advance directive (living will) or durable power of attorney. Finally, *beyond a reasonable doubt* requires the most evidence and, of course, is used in trials of homicide to establish guilt and where the accused is presumed innocent.

The Cruzans won their case in lower (probate) court, but upon direct review, the Missouri Supreme Court reversed that decision, and its reversal had to do with the standard of clear and convincing evidence. Because Nancy had no advance directive and because only her parents and a sister testified about her alleged wishes, the Cruzans did not produce enough evidence to be "clear and convincing" about Nancy's true wishes.

Missouri felt it had a duty to protect an incompetent adult child against parents who might be merely seeking financial and emotional closure. The Missouri Supreme Court agreed and concluded that the state had an interest in preserving life, regardless of quality of life, and no matter how strongly the family felt otherwise, that before medical support could be withdrawn from an incompetent patient, the family had to meet the standard of clear and convincing evidence.

In this case, the United States Supreme Court declared three things. First, it recognized a right of *competent* patients to decline medical treatment, even if such refusal led directly to their death. *Cruzan* emphasized that competent Americans had the freedom at the end of life to refuse unwanted medical support.

Second, the Supreme Court found that withdrawing a feeding tube did not differ from withdrawing any other kind of life-sustaining medical support. Some state laws, which permitted forgoing or withdrawing ventilators but not artificial nutrition, were hence unconstitutional.

Third, with regard to *incompetent* patients, the Supreme Court held in *Cruzan* that a state *could, but need not,* pass a statute requiring the clear and convincing standard of evidence about what a formerly competent patient would have wanted. Because Missouri had such a standard, its law was constitutional. Because the Cruzan family had not met that standard, Nancy's feeding tube could not be removed.

Cruzan said nothing about never-competent patients, such as people with profound mental retardation. Because of past abuses, it is reasonable to expect that in these cases only state laws with the most rigorous standards of proof would pass the Supreme Court's review. For such cases, the Supreme Court could require the standard of beyond a reasonable doubt.

Reactions to the Supreme Court *Cruzan* decision ran along two lines: legal commentators welcomed it; medical commentators hated it.

Most legal scholars supported the new conservative position of the Rehnquist Court on its role with regard to the Constitution. The proper function of the Supreme Court, according to the law professor Charles Baron, was not as a super legislature over the states or even "to promulgate uniform rules of state law." Instead, the U.S. Supreme Court should strike down only state laws that conflict with either federal law or the U.S. Constitution.[16] So not every bad or undesirable state law is unconstitutional.

Texas law professor John Robertson went so far as to say that Nancy Cruzan could not be harmed and hence had no interests in the case. He argued that the real claim in *Cruzan* had nothing to do with Nancy Cruzan's right to die or her right to privacy (her liberty interests); instead, the case was about the Cruzan family's right to be free of the emotional burden of maintaining her body in a state institution.[17]

Both Baron and Robertson agreed that the previous legal standard of *substituted judgment* was a mockery "[leading] us to pretend that we are merely complying (however reluctantly) with the wishes of the patient. The result in most states is mere lip service to substituted judgment. Almost any evidence is deemed sufficient to establish a preference for death over PVS and/or families are empowered to express patient preferences for death—with few questions asked."

The case of Nancy Cruzan illustrates this problem. Joe, Nancy's father, said that because Nancy was strong willed and a fighter, she wouldn't want to exist in PVS. But others might infer a different conclusion: that she might have wanted to fight for any chance to return to normalcy.

In contrast, another standard used in such cases was that of *best interests of* the patient. So in the Cruzan case, would the best interests of Nancy be to live on in such a state? Some people would say no, although this judgment is not open and shut, especially as Missouri argued that Nancy's best interests entailed continued feeding, as activists argued in the later Schiavo case.

A different kind of reaction came from physicians who worked with families of vegetative patients. Neurologist and bioethicist Ronald Cranford of Minnesota, who would later testify in the Schiavo case, predicted that, "many families will experience the utter helplessness of the Cruzans." Allowing the standard of clear-and-convincing evidence would "place an enormous burden on society," which will spend hundreds of millions of dollars each year for a condition that no one in their right mind would ever want to be in.[18]

Hospice physician Joanne Lynn emphasized that in Missouri and New York, "the suffering of the patient and family, the costs, the kind of life that can be gained, are all to count for nothing. If life can be prolonged, then it will have to be."[19]

Nancy had been divorced just before her accident, and some of her old friends knew her only by her married name, Davis. When her case first became widely known, her friends had not realized who she was. After the major decision, the case was reheard in a lower court and Nancy's old friends testified. In that hearing, the lower court decided that Nancy Cruzan's parents had met the clear-and-convincing standard.[20] So five months after the Supreme Court decided *Cruzan*, on December 14, 1990, physicians legally removed Nancy Cruzan's feeding tube, and her body died.

THE HUGH FINN CASE

Controversy erupted in 1998 when the Republican governor of Virginia disputed a wife's right to remove the feeding tube of her husband, Hugh Finn, who had been in PVS for three years.[21] A former television anchorman in Louisville, Kentucky,

Finn had prepared a document stating that he would not want to live in a persistent vegetative state sustained by a feeding tube. Unfortunately, before he could sign it, an automobile accident severed his aorta and left his brain anoxic for many minutes. His resulting coma left him unable to eat, care for himself, or communicate.

Or so it seemed, until a nurse claimed that, when she smoothed his hair, he had said "Hi" to her, so Hugh's brother, John, challenged a request by Hugh's wife, Michelle, to remove Hugh's feeding tube. Hugh's parents joined John in the suit. They lost in court, but Governor James Gilmore asked the Virginia Supreme Court to continue Finn's feeding tube. Gilmore stated that its removal would be "mercy killing or euthanasia." The high Court disagreed, deciding that removal would merely "permit the natural process of dying" and would not be euthanasia.

Hugh Finn's body died shortly thereafter, but Governor Gilmore had set a precedent for escalating a private family dispute about a dying patient into a sensationalized, national debate. Seven years later, Governor Jeb Bush in Florida intervened in another such dispute.

THE TERRI SCHIAVO CASE

During the months of 1990 when the U.S. Supreme Court was deciding its *Cruzan* decision, another coma case was beginning. On February 25, 1990, Terri Schiavo, a 27-year-old, anorexic Caucasian woman went into a coma because of anoxia, a lack of oxygen to her brain, perhaps from a heart arrhythmia caused by extreme hypoalkemia (an imbalance of potassium in her body), causing severe hypoxic ischemic encephalopathy (brain damage).[22]

Before her heart attack, Terri Schiavo seemed to suffer from anorexia. People with such eating disorders may suffer from an imbalance of potassium. According to documents filed in a malpractice suit by her family, a three-stage imbalance of potassium led to Terri's heart attack, which led to anoxia and subsequent brain damage.

Many diets today contain too little potassium; the average American woman consumes less than half of the 4,700 milligrams a day considered to be adequate.[23] Among other medical conditions, chronic lack of potassium can cause heart attacks and strokes. Moreover, blood tests for potassium can be normal even when real symptoms occur from chronic potassium insufficiency. As a result, physicians often fail to diagnose a chronic lack of potassium.

To keep her alive, physicians inserted a percutaneous endoscopic gastronomy (PEG) feeding tube. When a patient lacks the reflex to swallow, a PEG tube is placed through the abdominal wall into the stomach, allowing a nutritious, slushy mixture to feed the patient. PEG tubes are sometimes inserted to buy time after an emergency, with the implicit understanding that they may be temporary and may be removed later.

Once attached, feeding tubes can be emotionally difficult for people to remove. Years later, removal of the feeding tube became the central issue of this case.

Two months later in April 1990, her husband Michael transferred Terri from the hospital to a rehabilitation center. In May, and with no objection from her parents,

Robert and Mary Schindler, he became her legal guardian. Later, her parents took her to their home for care but they were overwhelmed by the task and subsequently returned her to the center. Michael also flew Terri once to California for a two-month experiment with a "thalamic stimulator implant" in her brain. After that experiment, Terri returned to the Mediplex Rehabilitation Center in Brandon, Florida, and for months 13–18 into her coma, three shifts of workers worked 24 hours a day trying to rehabilitate Terri.

In July 1991, Terri went to Sable Palms, a skilled care facility, where neurologists continued to test her and where speech, occupational, and physical therapists worked on her for another three years, from 1991 to 1994. At this point, Terri had received nearly five years of intensive efforts to return her to consciousness.

Michael Schiavo and Terri's parents had stopped living together in May 1992. That August, Michael received a settlement from the malpractice case against Terri's obstetrician for failing to diagnose her potassium imbalance. He got $750,000 from the hospital for a trust fund specifically for Terri's care and $300,000 for loss of her companionship.

The three adults then fought over money. Michael owed the Schindlers $10,000 and the Schindlers believed they were entitled to part of the $300,000 for loss of spousal companionship. After the dispute, their relationship seemed to sour.

Based on what several physicians told Michael, at this point Terri had no chance of meaningful recovery. Michael agreed to a "Do Not Resuscitate" order for Terri, but her parents violently disagreed and he later rescinded the order.

The Schindlers then tried to remove Michael as Terri's guardian, but a court-appointed special guardian investigated and determined that Michael had acted appropriately toward Terri, which the court accepted.

Three years passed, during which Terri's condition did not improve. During this time and in order to help care for Terri, Michael became certified as a licensed respiratory therapist.[24]

In May 1998, eight years after Terri's heart attack, Michael asked a court to allow removal of the PEG tube so that Terri could die. Michael testified that, while watching television many years before, Terri had once remarked that she wouldn't want to live in a vegetative state. The Schindlers retorted that their daughter wanted to live.

Nearly two years after Michael Schiavo's request to have Terri's feeding tube removed, Judge George Greer in 2000 approved the request. He ruled that clear and convincing evidence existed that Terri would not have chosen to live under such circumstances. Legally, this ruling seemed to lack support, because Terri's parents disputed this claim and because she had no living will.

The Schindlers appealed, which took a year, but they lost. They appealed again, this time to the Florida Supreme Court, which in April 2001 denied their appeal.

Over the next few years, the Schindlers began to allege that Michael caused Terri's condition, perhaps because of domestic abuse. An autopsy after her death proved that no such abuse occurred. Moreover, if Terri had arrived at an emergency room with this kind of trauma, Michael would have been reported—as required by law—to authorities for domestic violence, battery, or possible manslaughter. Moreover, if such evidence had existed, the hospital and its physicians would have been unlikely to settle a malpractice case or to allow Michael to become Terri's guardian.

The Schindlers testified that, even if Terri had asked them to do so, they would not remove Terri's feeding tube under any circumstances. They said that even if she developed gangrene and all her limbs had to be amputated, they would still keep her alive.[25]

A year later in the fall of 2003, having exhausted all appeals in Florida, the Schindlers appealed in federal court to prevent removal of Terri's feeding tube. The Schindlers also appealed to the public through the media, and several physicians publicly joined their side, including a pathologist and a physician who hoped to try exotic "coma stimulation" therapies.

Lawyers for Florida

Governor Jeb Bush, a Catholic, filed a brief on the side of the Schindlers; he praised the parents in the media for defending their daughter's right to life. President George W. Bush praised his brother's stand. The Advocacy Center for Persons with Disabilities filed a lawsuit claiming that removal of Terri's feeding tube would abuse a person with disabilities. The antiabortion group, Life Legal Defense Fund, helped the Schindlers hire lawyers, eventually paying bills of $300,000.

Three neurologists, including distinguished neurologist Ronald Cranford, testified that Terri was in PVS (Cranford substituted "permanent" for "persistent" to emphasize the irreversibility of her condition). The Schindlers cited Terri's ability to swallow saliva as evidence that she was not in PVS; Cranford rebutted and testified that such swallowing was controlled by primitive functions in her brain stem.

Physicians William Mayfield and William Hammesfahr, champions of hyperbaric oxygenation therapy (HBOT), claimed HBOT would benefit Terri.[26] Neurologist Ronald Cranford retorted, "Increase the blood flood to dead tissue, and what do you get? Dead tissue."[27] Others found Hammesfahr unprofessional and noted that he required cash in advance for his hyperbaric treatments and had published no articles documenting success.

Another disagreement among these physicians concerned what Terri's movements meant. Ability to respond to a squeeze or pinch is consistent with PVS. In the Cruzan case, when neurologist Cranford examined Nancy, her lawyer William Colby described what happened:

> Cranford next grabbed hold of Nancy's stiff right leg and tried to bend it straight. Nancy grimaced. Then he reached for the soft skin on the inside of the upper part of her right arm, and held the pinch. Slowly, as if she were a robot, Nancy's head lifted off the bed and turned. Her face locked on her father's for about ten seconds, before she lowered just as slowly to the pillow.[28]

Despite being there and witnessing this phenomenon in this case, Dr. Cranford insisted that Nancy Cruzan's biography was over, that no one was conscious within the reflexes of her body, and that further treatment was futile.

In the fall of 2003, the Florida legislature passed a special bill, *Terri's Law*, which allowed the governor to issue a one-time stay of a judge's order to remove a feeding tube in certain cases where a patient is in PVS. After its passage, Governor Bush immediately issued such a stay.

Michael and the American Civil Liberties Union appealed in state court and won, but Governor Bush appealed to a midlevel appellate court, lost, and appealed again to the Florida Supreme Court.

On September 23, 2004, Florida's Supreme Court ruled 7-0 that Terri's Law was unconstitutional. It based its decision upon two constitutional canons: the separation of powers and the unlawful delegation of authority. "It is without question an invasion of the authority of the judicial branch for the Legislature to pass a law that allows the executive branch to interfere with the final judicial determination in a case," wrote Chief Justice Barbara Pariente.[29]

About two months later, the top U.S. Court let stand without comment the decision by the Florida Supreme Court against Terri's Law.[30] Activists predicted Terri's imminent "brutal murder" and claimed that she was a "purposefully interactive, alert, curious, lovely young woman who lives with a very serious disability."[31]

Much of these claims came from an edited video, clips of which cable television often showed (because such stories need *some* visual background). These pro-Schindler clips can be easily seen on YouTube or by searching for videos on Terri Schiavo.

At the end of February 2005, 15 years after the case began, the Schindlers filed a variety of motions in Judge Greer's court. Judge Greer ordered the feeding tube removed. The Schindlers appealed, but a Florida appellate court again rebuffed them.

Extraordinary events, of a kind never before seen in the history of modern bioethics, then ensued. As the Schindlers lost in court, they became desperate; they turned to the media for their cause, enlisting their other son and daughter to go on television. Catholic priests dressed in robes of monastic orders appeared with them. Antiabortion activist Randall Terry showed up. People flooded Florida legislators with email and phone calls.

Activists and the Schindlers then turned to the U.S. Congress. First House leaders tried to compel Terri to appear before a House committee as a witness and fall under protection of the federal program that protects such witnesses. Judge Greer ignored this subpoena.

Activists next turned to Congressional leaders and President Bush. House Speaker Tom DeLay faced an ethics scandal and indictments in his home state of Texas for getting money in illegal ways, exactly the kind of scandal that had forced previous speaker Jim Wright out of Congress in 1989. (DeLay also failed to reveal that his family had agreed to remove a ventilator from his father, who had been injured in an accident in 1988 in Texas.)[32]

In the Senate, Senator Bill Frist, the physician, may have planned to run for president in 2008 and may have wanted to align himself with the same culture-of-life constituency that had helped George W. Bush narrowly win. So the two of them worked to have Congress pass a federal version of Terri's Law, which they did, having President Bush fly back during a Congressional recess and sign a bill passed at midnight by a vote of 203 to 58.[33]

Some critics said that Senator Frist crossed a dangerous ethical line and committed virtual malpractice by declaring—merely by watching the edited video clip and never actually visiting or examining Terri—that Terri "did not seem to be" in a persistent vegetative state. As one critic fumed, "It's quackery. It'd be hilarious if it weren't so grotesque, how his presidential ambition and pandering to the right wing is clashing with his life's work."[34] Congressman Dave Weldon, a physician and also a pro-life Republican, agreed with Frist. So these high-ranking politician-physicians publicly contradicted the neurologists who had actually examined Terri.

Congressmen Frist and Weldon had one problem here: the federal government cannot order a physician to insert a feeding tube. The only thing it could do is order a federal judge to review the case again, which was done. The federal judge, James Whittemore, reviewed the whole case over two days and concluded, like two dozen appellate judges before him, that nothing was amiss, that Terri had no chance of recovery, that Michael was properly motivated, and that previous courts had made no errors. An appeal to the U.S. Court of Appeals for the 11th Circuit in Atlanta, a conservative group, produced the same conclusions.

During March 2005, media exposure escalated, producing what *Newsweek* later called "a public spectacle airing nonstop on cable and playing on front pages around the world."[35] Terri's supporters traveled to Pinellas Park, Florida, to hold prayer vigils, while others threatened to kill Michael and his lawyer, George Felos. Various members and friends of both sides went on cable television shows and endlessly discussed the family's problems.

A juggernaut for Terri ensued: soon, four Schindlers, plus recovered coma patients, shady physicians, activist monks, Patrick Mahoney, director of the Christian Defense Coalition, and antiabortion activist Randall Terry campaigned on television, radio, and the Internet against Michael Schiavo, who was media shy and had only his brother, Scott, and lawyer George Felos to help him.

Barbara Weller, an attorney working with the Schindlers, said that she herself had seen Terri trying to talk, and thus went from a lawyer to a witness. Protestors called Judge Greer a "judicial murderer" and Republicans blasted the "imperial judiciary." The Reverend James Kennedy urged Governor Jeb Bush to ignore the federal judges the way Alabama's Governor George Wallace did in defying federal orders to integrate.[36] Soon after, the FBI arrested a man offering $250,000 to kill Michael Schiavo and $50,000 to do the same to Judge Greer. Another two people were arrested trying to break into the hospice.

Terri was said to be "suffering terribly" by starving, even though physicians in palliative care repeatedly denied that when feeding tubes are removed, terminal patients suffer, and that in this case, any person was still present who could be said to suffer.[37]

The case again showed the limitations of the media, of television, of Internet and radio, because what made great visuals (people praying and screaming outside Terri's hospice), what made great drama (the Schindlers crying on television), and what made great tension (various people claiming that Michael was evil), distorted facts of the case. What had been a private family dispute suddenly became total war, playing out on national television.

On March 18, the last appeal to the U.S. Supreme Court failed (which had already twice refused to review the case) and Terri's feeding tube was removed for the last time. Palliative care physicians predicted it would take about two weeks for Terri to die and emphasized that, in terminal patients such as Terri, it would not be painful. Opponents outside decried "murder by starvation." After 13 days, while protestors prayed and rallied outside, Terri's body expired, on March 31, 2005.

What Schiavo's Autopsy Showed

Chief Medical Examiner for Pinellas County, Florida, Jon Thogmartin, M.D, released Terri's autopsy on June 13, 2005. It answered some questions and left others as mysteries.

First, he cleared up the mysterious bone scan of 1991 introduced by the Schindlers in 1992 with the claim that Terri's coma had been caused by trauma, possibly by Michael. Here is what happened: when Mediplex admitted Terri in early 1991, her physicians there ordered a bone scan to rule out degenerative changes in her bones. The bone scan was done at nearby Manatee Memorial Hospital. The form there about the bone scan *erroneously* listed Terri Schiavo as a case of "closed head injury" and said, "the patient has a history of trauma." Thogmartin writes, "It appears that with little or no knowledge of the admitting diagnosis or clinical situation of Mrs. Schiavo, Manatee Memorial staff and radiologists completed the report."[38]

The coroner writes that it is true that the bone scan showed a compression fracture of the spine, but it was *due to osteoporosis*, a common condition in paralyzed patients. Moreover,

> In summary, any rib fractures, leg fractures, skull fractures or spine fractures that occurred concurrent with Mrs. Schiavo's original collapse would almost certainly have been diagnosed in February, 1990, especially with the number of physical exams, radiographs, and other evaluations she received in the early evolution of her care at Humana Hospital-Northside. During her initial hospitalization, she received twenty-three chest radiographs, three brain CT scans, two abdominal radiographs, two echocardiograms, one abdominal ultrasound, one cervical spine radiograph, and one radiograph of her right knee. No fractures or trauma were reported or recorded. . . . By far the most likely explanation for the bone scan findings in Mrs. Schiavo are prolonged immobility induced osteoporosis and complicating H.O. [hypertopic ossification[39]] in an environment of intense physical therapy.[40]

In sum, there was no evidence of trauma or abuse by anyone. Michael was wrongly accused of hurting Terri. Everyone misunderstood what the 1991 bone scan revealed and how it had been mistakenly labeled.

The big surprise of the autopsy was that "Mrs. Schiavo's heart was anatomically normal without any areas of recent or remote myocardial infarction. Her heart (including the cardiac valves, conduction system and myocardium) was essentially unremarkable. . . ." That was a surprise because, although people debated the cause of her heart attack, few doubted that she had had one.

Probably we will never know exactly what happened to Terri's heart. Two crucial pieces of evidence are that she may have consumed as much as one gram of caffeine a day and that she had hypoalkemia. Perhaps this combination, after the extreme weight loss, stressed her heart too much that night.

The night of her original collapse, no other drugs were found in her system.

Another surprise was that the autopsy showed no clinical evidence of bulimia, especially the kind of wear on the enamel of the back teeth that is often caused by this condition. Despite the fact that the malpractice suit was settled on the assertion that Terri had an undiagnosed eating disorder, the coroner's report showed no physical evidence of it.

However, it still could be true that 15 years before, she had been anorexic. Certainly her low potassium level, the fact that her weight dropped over 100 pounds in a few months, combined with her drinking gallons of iced tea, give evidence to this hypothesis.

The autopsy by the coroner also implied that Terri Schiavo was not in a minimally conscious state. It said that she had massive brain damage. Mrs. Schiavo's brain showed global anoxic-ischemic encephalopathy resulting in massive cerebral atrophy. Her brain weight was approximately half of the expected weight. Of particular importance was the hypoxic damage and neuronal loss in her occipital lobes, which indicates cortical blindness. Her remaining brain regions show severe hypoxic injury and neuronal atrophy/loss. No areas of recent or remote traumatic injury were found.[41]

Finally, without the PEG feeding tube, she would have died. "Oral feedings in quantities sufficient to sustain life would have certainly resulted in aspiration." Aspiration of food in such patients is a serious, even lethal, complication, causing infection, choking, and possible suffocation.

ETHICAL ISSUES

Standards of Brain Death

People have always feared that they might be declared dead prematurely and buried alive. In the eighteenth century, gruesome stories circulated about exhumations that found frantic scratches on the inside lids of coffins. In the nineteenth century, some legislatures required a delay before burial, and in 1882 an undertaker named Kirchbaum attached periscopes to coffins so that a person who woke up after being buried might signal for help.[42] Many people were buried with cowbells that they could ring if they awakened underground.

This whole-body standard became inappropriate when ventilators allowed respiration of brain-damaged patients. Before them, heart-lung machines could maintain immobilized patients. As early as 1967, surgeon Christiaan Barnard transplanted Denise Darvall's heart into a dying patient named Louis Washkansky (discussed in Chapter 10), and the question then arose whether Denise Darvall had really been dead before her heart was removed. Because a healthy heart was exactly what was wanted for transplantation, Denise obviously hadn't been declared dead by the whole-body standard. Medicine needed a new standard of death, specifically of *brain death*, to determine when organs could be removed from a still-living body.

Although first described in the medical literature in 1959, brain death did not really become operational until Barnard transplanted a heart in late 1967.[43]

Shortly after that event, an ad hoc committee at Harvard Medical School developed the Harvard criteria of brain death.[44] The Harvard criteria operationally defined brain death as behavior that indicated unawareness of external stimuli, lack of bodily movements, no spontaneous breathing, lack of reflexes, and two isoelectric (nearly flat) EEG readings 24 hours apart. These criteria required loss of virtually all brain activity (including the brain stem, and hence breathing).

The Harvard criteria personify that no one declared dead by these criteria has ever regained consciousness. (One could truly say, "If you're Harvard dead, you're really dead.") The extreme conservatism of the Harvard standard disappoints people waiting for organ transplants from donors: during the last 25 years, the standard has covered relatively few patients.

Another standard of brain death is the *cognitive criterion.* This criterion identifies a philosophical core of properties of persons and assumes that without such a core, a human body is no longer a person; the core properties commonly include reason, memory, agency, and self-awareness. For example, neurological disorders such as Alzheimer's or Lewy body dementia destroy brain cells at a high rate, so that over a decade, none of the higher person remains.

The cognitive criterion has the greatest potential to generate organs for transplantation. So far, however, this criterion has been too controversial and too vague to be adopted by any state, although countless families in fact act on it when they use it to agree to reduce treatment to speed a patient's death.[45]

A third standard of brain death is *irreversibility,* and it falls between the Harvard and cognitive criteria. According to this standard, death occurs simply when unconsciousness is irreversible. Operationally, this judgment would be made by a neurologist and by another physician. The irreversibility standard would allow PVS patients to be declared dead after several years (perhaps, in some cases of anoxia, after several months). At the time of the first heart transplant in 1968, this standard was thought to be too broad.

In popular culture, some people believe that a uniform, metaphysical event with physical manifestations, and perhaps as the counterpart of a similar event at the beginning of life, marks death. Some people would have described these metaphysical events as the entrance and departure of a soul. The occurrence of such metaphysical events of course cannot be proven, and even if they do occur, they seem to have no physical manifestations.

So in medical reality, the definition of death is often not so much a *discovery* as a *decision* that families and their physicians can make. It is not an event, but a process.[46] Unfortunately, many families lack preparation to make such decisions and find it easier to believe in the view that physicians "discover" that a patient has died.

As it turns out, the phrase "brain death" misleads us in many ways. Newspapers commonly refer to someone as being "brain dead" for months until "life-support" is removed, after which the patient is said to "expire." Reformers such as North Carolina medical ethicist Lance Stell believe that such terms incorrectly imply that a patient could be dead in two different ways and that there are degrees of being dead. Such equivocation creates confusion about the epistemological criteria for declaring death, and implies that someone might die more than once. Stell thinks a more accurate phrase would be "death by neurological criteria." A being that meets these criteria, he says, "is not a patient but a cadaver."[47]

Proposals to redefine brain death create controversy. On the one hand, reformers want to end public uncertainty over brain death, expand the number of organs available for transplantation, save the medical system money by not maintaining comatose patients, and help families move on after the death of a relative by having a universally accepted, practical definition of brain death. On the other hand, advocates for vulnerable patients want to give them every chance of recovery.

Chances of Regaining Consciousness from Coma and PVS

The question—whether the movements of PVS patients are intentional behavior or merely reflexes—raises philosophical as well as medical issues. *Intentional* behavior indicates an organism seeking a goal, such as freedom from pain, and might indicate awareness. As the seventeenth-century philosopher Rene Descartes noted, consciousness in others is always an inference from outward behavior; it cannot be directly observed.

Permanent lack of consciousness is also an inference. If we claim—as some people do—that shrimp aren't conscious, this is an inference from the behavior of shrimp and from the comparative anatomy of shrimp and humans.

Consider four surprising cases of long-term unconsciousness. First, after an automobile wreck in Arkansas, Terry Wallis emerged from such a state after 19 years, and 3 years later, continued to improve.[48] In 1996, ex-police officer Gary Dockery of Tennessee emerged out of his coma of *eight years* to talk for a few hours to his family, after which he lapsed back into a coma and died a year later in April.[49] Third, Patricia White Bull became comatose while giving birth to her fourth child and could not speak, swallow, or move much, but suddenly awoke 16 years later to full consciousness on Christmas Eve, 1999. Fourth, after a car accident, Sarah Scantlin of Kansas went into a coma from which she emerged 19 years later.[50] These cases where patients recovered were caused by trauma, not anoxia.

Ethically, the fact that anyone at all comes out of a long-term coma is crucial because it changes the prognosis from a certainty to a probability. Families who want emotional closure on a case prefer to hear physicians say that the patient has **no** chance of recovery. The emotional weight changes when a patient has a **tiny** chance of recovery rather than no chance.

A review of these cases reveals an interesting conceptual disagreement among neurologists. Some claim that any patient who emerges from PVS was not really in PVS. But this is a nonfalsifiable, circular argument: if you awaken, you weren't in PVS. If you never awaken, you were in PVS.

In a then-definitive study in the *New England Journal of Medicine* in 1994 by the Multi-Task Force on PVS, 7 of 434 adults with traumatic head injuries who were in PVS for more than a year made good recoveries and regained consciousness, some with normal quality of life.[51] Should traumatic PVS befall some people, they might want this 7/434th chance of recovery. Several other studies have shown that, although few patients ever emerge from PVS, some people do within the first year, and once in a thousand times, after three years.[52] All these patients suffered *traumatic* injuries, not coma from anoxia.

In a 1995 study of 19 patients with severe head injuries and persisting post-traumatic unawareness, 58 percent (11 patients) recovered within the first year and 5 percent (1 patient) within the second.[53] In a 1996 study of 34 patients with *anoxic* coma, 2 patients with "malignant EEGs" (the worst classification, where patients were expected to die based on lack of brain wave activity), eventually made a "good recovery."[54]

So whether anoxia or trauma caused the coma makes a big difference in prognosis. Some patients emerge, especially in the first few months, after coma caused by trauma, but rarely in coma caused by anoxia. "It's the difference between taking a blow to the brain, which affects a local area—and taking this global, whole-brain hit," asserted New York bioethicist Joseph Fins in explaining the difference.[55]

Some neurologists proposed in 2005 a new category of *minimally conscious state* (MCS) for patients in long-term coma-like states, a category between the previous ways of classifying them as either *comatose* or *vegetative*.[56] After working with brain-damaged patients at several facilities around New York City, neurologists Nicholas Schiff, Joy Hirsch, and Joseph Giacino, along with seven other coauthors, proposed this new category.[57]

These claims generate a great deal of passion in neurology. Alan Shewmon, a famous pediatric neurologist, calls the new category "an inaccurate name for an invalid concept." Shewmon argues that there is no scientific or philosophical way to distinguish between minimal consciousness and full consciousness, implying that consciousness is something one either has or does not have; he compares to being a "little bit pregnant."

But maybe that's the wrong analogy. Why can't a light bulb be, not on or off, but bright or dim? Why can't consciousness be a *gradient*? Terri's defenders retort that people are minimally conscious all the time—in sleep, or after injury—and what is important is the potential for recovery of consciousness. If it's impossible to prove any difference between minimal consciousness and consciousness, it also must be impossible to *disprove* a difference. So if Terri was in MCS, she might at times feel something. After all, the brain does not get injured in neat taxonomic lines.

By 2007, the claims centered not so much on ability to recover from anoxia-caused PVS as on patients classified as in PVS but who were *misdiagnosed*. In one 1996 study in England, Andrews estimated that 17 of 40 patients in PVS had been so misdiagnosed. Could Terri Schiavo have been misdiagnosed?

An important study in 2007 by Owen et al. noted that,

> The assessment of patients with disorders of consciousness, including the vegetative state, is difficult and frequently depends on subjective interpretations of the observed spontaneous and volitional behavior. . . . However, it is becoming increasingly apparent that in some patients damage to the peripheral motor system may prevent overt responses to command although the cognitive ability to perceive and understand such commands may remain intact. Recent advances in functional neuroimaging suggest a novel solution to this problem: in several cases, so-called activation studies have been used to identify residual cognitive function and conscious awareness in patients who are assumed to be in a vegetative state yet retain cognitive abilities that have evaded detection using standard clinical methods.[58]

In this study, a PVS patient was asked to imagine playing tennis and walking through a house, and every time she was asked about playing tennis, an important part of her brain lit up, whereas it did not when she was asked about walking through rooms.

The latest claims focus on MCS, fMRI scans, and deep-brain stimulation of supposed PVS patients. Through an intense program with probes that stimulated the thalamus, a deep part of the brain, they enabled one or two patients to return to MCS. Using fMRI scans of blood flow to the brain, physicians have identified dozens of patients with this potential, and improved one or two remarkably.[59]

In 2009, Belgian researcher Steven Laureys awoke Rom Houben, who for 23 years had been conscious and falsely diagnosed as in a vegetative state, but unable to move. "Once someone is labeled as being without consciousness, it is very hard to get rid of that," Laureys said.[60]

The potential for recovery of such a patient is probably best when maximal efforts are made *in the first six months* after injury. This potential diminishes as the years increase. At the beginning, physicians should always act as if the brain-damaged person is minimally conscious, but after many years (15 years for Terri), chances of recovery approach zero. This seems especially true for patients in comas caused by anoxia.

Terri's Chances of Reawakening

No case exists of anyone emerging from PVS of three years' duration. In Terri Schiavo's case at the end, when activists shouted the contrary at cameras, she had been in PVS for *15 years,* and hence, according to clinical evidence, had no chance of returning to normal consciousness. Physicians who have seen her CT scan said that her brain, instead of being filled with normal brain tissue, then only contained cerebrospinal fluid, an indication of gross neurological damage and vegetative status.[60]

Terri's EEG was flat and her CT scan showed severe atrophy in her cerebral hemispheres. Schindler-friendly physicians suggested vasodilators, but the autopsy showed what professional neurologists had said: nothing would have helped her regain consciousness.

Dartmouth neurologist James Bernat agreed, but understood why laypeople rallied behind Terri. "Just looking at a videotape of someone propped up in bed, with their eyes blinking and so on, it look's like they're aware," he said.[61] They are awake, he said, but not aware. With an intact brain stem, their eyes can still follow things, but only slightly to the left or right.

Mercy and Compassion

In cases like Karen Quinlan's or Nancy Cruzan's, the Golden Rule might imply that, "If I ended up in a condition like Karen's or Nancy's, I would want to die, and I hope that those around me would be merciful enough to let me die. If I could somehow possibly be 'conscious' in such a state, I wouldn't want to go on. I wouldn't want to be imprisoned in such a body for months or years, which would be worse than being buried alive. Mercy requires us to make dying humane, not an endless torture."

Such a thought illustrates how the Golden Rule can be interpreted in different ways—some people might want a chance to recover, even if it is very slight. "Doing whatever someone else wants" must take into account that people differ in their personalities and wants.

The Quinlans and the Cruzans did argue that allowing Karen and Nancy to die would be merciful. The issue of mercy is relevant in these and similar cases because we can't know for certain that such patients do not feel—we cannot be certain that they do not experience sensations such as pain and discomfort; we may not even be certain that they do not experience distress, fear, frustration, loss, or other tormenting emotions.

Eventually, the cases of Karen Quinlan and Nancy Cruzan came to symbolize mercy as an issue for both patients and families. These cases seemed to represent an inversion of values in medicine: instead of doing what families wanted, medicine did what bureaucracies required; instead of a dignified death, breathing machines and feeding tubes maintained existence; instead of a quick death, there was slow withering over a decade of an emaciated body. On top of all that, the chance that a shell of a person might still exist in pain was too much for most people. For many people, the long dying of these two patients lacked mercy.

Would not most people abhor such a life? Abhor the thought of inhabiting 15 years inside a body in which they could not scratch an itch, express a wish, or perform any human act? No one knows what might be going on in such a mental remnant. Whatever destroyed the original mind might have left it in disarray, such that Terri's mental life was an endless nightmare.

If Terri Schiavo could have awakened for 15 minutes and could have understood her condition, what she looked like, and what the case was doing to her family, can anyone think that this shy, weight-conscious woman would have wanted her brain-damaged, disfigured body exhibited to the world this way? If emotional revulsion is going to count in ethics, what about *her* revulsion?

Her parents saw this differently. They felt she would have wanted to live, even in such diminished circumstances. This shows the problem with simplistic interpretations of the Golden Rule or substituted judgment.

Religious Issues

In 1957, Pope Pius XII had told a group of anesthesiologists that they were not obligated to provide extraordinary care to dying patients. As we saw, the Catholic Church opposed withdrawal of a ventilator for Karen Quinlan. Over the next 30 years, the Catholic hospitals in North American softened their opposition to such withdrawals, and indeed, some such hospitals became models of compassionate dying. In this context, feeding tubes had been routinely removed from patients in Catholic hospitals.

As the Schiavo case received greater coverage in the print and visual media, different groups took stands on the case. Within the Christian community, and especially within the Catholic Church, people disagreed about the ethics of removing artificial nutrition and hydration (ANH) from Terri Schiavo.

Perhaps after having seen the videotape of Terri on international television news, and referring to her case, Pope John Paul II said in 2004 that removal of feeding tubes from patients in PVS was "euthanasia by omission."[62] Although not delivered *ex cathedra*, the pope's remark cast doubt on that practice. Several Protestant leaders and some U.S. Catholic bishops also denounced Michael Schiavo's attempt to have Terri's feeding tube removed, saying it was murder.

In contrast, Father Kevin O'Rourke, one of the leading Catholic medical ethicists in North America, argued that providing ANH was extraordinary care and should not be used to prolong the life of PVS patients. He noted that both Catholic ethicists working in hospitals, as well as doctors and nurses there, routinely allowed removal of life support from patients in PVS.

Father John Paris, a leading Jesuit bioethicist and professor of ethics at Boston College, noted that the pope's remarks targeted a specific audience and predicted they would have little impact in America. "I think the best thing to do is ignore it, and it will go away," Paris said. "It's not an authoritative teaching statement."[63]

Catholic hospitals re-doubled their efforts to have every patient sign an advance directive and assign durable power of attorney. Some such hospitals quietly ignored the pope's statements and their physicians quietly removed feeding tubes and ventilators from dying patients.

Bobby Schindler, employed as a science teacher in a Catholic high school, frequently claimed on television that his sister Terri wanted to live. James Dobson's Focus on the Family issued daily news updates on the case. The Family Research Council emailed its subscribers with headlines such as "Terri Communicates" and solicited donations. Gary McCullough, a bearded Floridian who often escorted Mary Schindler to a microphone, owned Christian News Wire and his service issued daily stories.[64]

Before this case, Catholics and Catholic hospitals had great flexibility about withdrawing feeding tubes. The Schiavo case changed that. Now Catholic patients and their families can ethically remove life-sustaining care under very few conditions.[65] The case also had other effects. A director of education for the Catholic Diocese of Birmingham, Alabama, said that the Catholic Church now refuses to recognize the diagnosis of a vegetative state, saying that, "a person is never a vegetable."[66]

Nagging Questions

Not everything in the Schiavo case adds up. First, as the attorney general for Missouri said about the case of Nancy Cruzan, "We generally don't allow a life to be ended on hearsay." He was referring to statements by Nancy's father and sister that they thought they remembered her saying she wouldn't want to live on a feeding tube.

Michael Schiavo's very late recollection of a comment by Terri years before to the same effect seems ad hoc, that is, remembered for the purpose at hand. Regardless of its veracity, it simply does not meet the standard of clear and convincing evidence, especially when directly contradicted by both Schindler parents and her brother, Bobby. Three-to-one *against* doesn't add up to clear-and-convincing evidence *for*.

Second, why not relinquish guardianship to the Schindlers? Michael's position was that, first, he had long ago exhausted all his money on her care, and second, she had died long before. But if that were so, why not let her parents care for her body? After a few years, like Karen Quinlan's mother, they would probably come to agree, but why not let them get closure that way? If Terri was already dead, she couldn't be harmed anymore.

Third, although the coroner's report closed some questions, it opened others: how did she lose so much weight so fast? Just by drinking ice tea? That doesn't add up. Why did she suddenly stop breathing? If not a heart attack, then what? Somebody isn't telling the full truth here somewhere.

Disability Issues

As interest grew in the Schiavo case, advocates for disabled people began to take notice. While the Quinlan and Cruzan cases had never been conceptualized as involving discrimination against disabled persons, the last decades have witnessed the growing influence of disability culture, leading to interest of disability advocates in the Schiavo case.

Advocates for Terri Schiavo claimed that this severely cognitively impaired person was *a victim of discrimination against the disabled*. Since passage of the Americans with Disabilities Act (ADA) in 1990, denial of medical resources to a disabled person because he is disabled violates federal law. However, the ADA has never specified end-of-life cognitive deterioration (which also would include Alzheimer's disease) as a covered disability.

Groups such as Not Dead Yet, the World Association of Persons with Disabilities, the National Spinal Cord Injury Association, and Joni and Friends opposed removal of Terri's feeding tube. Of course, to claim that Terri Schiavo is a victim of discrimination against disabled persons assumes that she is still a person and could emerge from her coma. That is exactly what disability advocates and her parents claimed. Given the increasing acceptance that a patient in PVS for a decade cannot revert back to consciousness, Terri's advocates increasingly *claimed that she is not in PVS at all but in a state of minimal consciousness*.

Charleston disability rights lawyer Harriet McBryde Johnson charged that, "Ms. Schiavo has a statutory right under the Americans with Disabilities Act not to be treated differently because of her disability. Obviously, Florida law would not allow a husband to kill a non-disabled wife by denying her nourishment. Because the state is overtly drawing lines based on disability, it has the burden under the ADA of justifying those lines."[67]

Disability advocates say modern culture presents a prejudiced view of life that works against disabled people. This view extols youth, health, beauty, wealth, lifelong sexuality, maximal functioning, and intelligence. Such advocates abhor the invidious messages given by television shows emphasizing scantily clad young women and men performing challenging physical feats.

They criticized also the indirect *rationing* that occurs when the medical system does not provide enough financial and medical resources for people with disabilities to function on their own. As in the cases of Bouvia and MacAfee (discussed in Chapter 1), such advocates also criticize the idea of encouraging disabled persons to exercise their right to die only when a stingy medical system has made their lives so miserable that the only autonomous decision left for them is to give up and die.

Medical Futility

In December 1991, Helga Wanglie, age 87, had been in PVS for eight months, sustained by a ventilator and a feeding tube, at Hennepin County Hospital in Minneapolis, Minnesota.[68] At the hospital the physicians (who included Ronald Cranford) who decided to withdraw treatment opposed the wishes of the patient's husband, Oliver Wanglie, who refused his permission to discontinue her ventilator and feeding tube.

The Wanglie case was unusual for two reasons. First, since Helga Wanglie's medical insurance covered her hospitalization, the hospital would actually lose money by withdrawing artificial life support. Second, the case involved an ethical and philosophical dispute about whether a medical team could be forced by a family member to continue care it regarded as futile. When Helga Wanglie died, the legal case ended, and the Hennepin County physicians did not continue to seek a precedent in the courts; however, about half a dozen other cases of medical futility were heard by courts and hospital ethics committees.[69]

Physicians in Massachusetts were sued in the 1989 *Gilgunn* case for removing medical support that they unanimously believed to be futile. Even though the jury agreed that Caroline Gilgunn would have wanted to remain on life support, the physicians won because the jury agreed that patients could not force physicians to render futile treatment.

In the 1990s, some physicians believed that medical futility was a descriptive concept that could help physicians and families easily make decisions about treatments of minimal benefit at the end of life. Today, most bioethicists believe that medical futility is not entirely descriptive and may contain controversial assumptions about the value of continued treatment.[70] The Schiavo case is a good example: competent neurologists unanimously agreed that, after three years, further treatment was futile for Terri, yet some staff, her parents, and rogue neurologists disagreed.

Most American patients and their families now decline treatment when their physicians advise them that further treatment is hopeless. A study in 1994 that followed over 4,000 patients whose condition was diagnosed as life threatening or terminal found that only 14 percent of them were resuscitated after being near death. This figure was far less than most physicians predicted and far less than it would have been a decade earlier, when most of those patients would have been resuscitated.[71]

Extraordinary versus Ordinary Treatment

In the years between the Quinlan case and the Cruzan case, physicians and philosophers debated whether certain levels of medical support had moral significance. The first concerned whether patients could be harmed by not receiving extraordinary, as opposed to ordinary, treatment. In 1957, a group of anesthesiologists asked Pope Pius XII what they owed dying patients. The pope said that they need not take heroic steps to keep such patients alive: patients were owed merely ordinary, but not extraordinary, treatments.

Second, "extraordinary" is equivocal and really has meaning across the end points of a continuum that shifts with medical progress. In 1967, when Christiaan Barnard first transplanted a human heart, his heart-lung bypass machine was extraordinary. That machine was the forerunner of the large, bulky ventilator that kept Karen Quinlan breathing. Today, miniaturized ventilators—some small enough to be used with premature babies—are used everywhere in medicine. Yesterday's extraordinary treatment has become today's ordinary treatment, rendering the distinction much more fluid and unhelpful than it might at first seem.

Artificial Nutrition and Hydration

In the 1980s, some people believed that whatever might be said about extraordinary and ordinary care in the future, providing food and water would always be considered ordinary and humane. They felt that such basic care was morally owed to PVS patients. This issue arose in the Schiavo case.

Artificial feeding is done in three basic ways: (1) by a temporary nasogastric tube run up the nostrils and down into the gastrointestinal tract; (2) by a permanent intravenous feeding line, surgically attached to one of the major veins of the chest; (3) by a surgically implanted gastrostomy tube. With many kinds of feeding tubes, patients must be tied down to avoid dislodging the line. All feeding tubes carry the risk of infection; with many, such a large volume of fluid is needed to supply the nutrients that other problems are caused.

The reality of feeding a chronically vegetative patient is not like spooning chicken soup into the mouth of a patient who is simply weak. Most vegetative patients have no swallowing reflexes, so they cannot be fed by mouth. Therefore, an artificial liquid diet must be mechanically introduced into their bodies.

The chicken soup image can distort people's impression of a PVS case. Karen Quinlan's sister, for example, thought that her comatose sister would look like Sleeping Beauty and was shocked by the emaciated figure she saw. By the time of Nancy Cruzan's case in 1990, improvements in artificial feeding would create the opposite effect: because of retention of fluids, PVS patients now had the rotund Porky Pig face seen in Terri Schiavo.

As said, neither dehydration nor starvation distresses semiconscious, dying patients. Patients near death not on nutritional support seem more comfortable than patients on whom such support is forced. One important national commission noted in 1983 that loss of appetite is "almost the norm in the latter stages of terminal illness" and concluded, "Only rarely should a dying patient be fed by tube or intravenously."[72] Indeed, such feeding may actually make the patient suffer and thus harm her.

Furthermore, artificial feeding also requires medical support. Many physicians involved in caring for PVS patients during the late 1970s decided that artificial nutrition was by no means natural feeding, and that the artificial procedures were not simply "care" but highly sophisticated medical treatment.

Arguments abounded in the 1980s for and against withdrawing nutrition and hydration. Some states allowed removal of ventilators but not of feeding tubes, and champions of a sanctity-of-life worldview saw removal of feeding and hydration tubes as the immediate cause of death and hence as mercy killing. One such philosopher argued in 1983 that providing food and water to PVS patients is the ordinary care "that all human beings owe each other"; another argued at about the same time that such feeding involves "the most fundamental of all human relationships," and that "to tamper with, or adulterate, so enduring and central a moral emotion" is "a most dangerous business."[73]

By the 1990s, most physicians had come to feel that artificial IV feeding lines for PVS patients compared to ventilators: both were advanced medical technology. They saw artificial feeding as prolonging the inevitable—dying—or as sustaining the body of a patient who is already dead. They saw little symbolic value in such feeding and thought that equating withdrawal of nutrition with murder was conceptually confused. According to this view, the moral question here is simple: Does artificial feeding and hydration benefit or burden the patient? The *Cruzan* decision in 1990 agreed.

Not everyone agreed with the emerging idea that artificial nutrition and hydration is just another form of medical treatment, which can ethically be withdrawn for PVS patients. Several physicians and members of the clergy in conservative religions opposed such withdrawal.[74] However, most state courts now allow withdrawal of ANH.

Withdrawing and Forgoing Treatment

During the last three decades, a central moral debate has concerned the degree to which a physician may be involved in hastening the death of a dying patient. One cause of this debate was a declaration by the AMA in 1973 (two years before Quinlan):

> The intentional termination of the life of one human being by another—mercy killing—is contrary to that for which the medical profession stands and is contrary to the policy of the American Medical Association.[75]
>
> . . . The cessation of the employment of extraordinary means to prolong the life of the body when there is irrefutable evidence that biological death is imminent is the decision of the patient and/or immediate family.

In this statement, the word "extraordinary" is ambiguous, and AMA policy did not clarify it. Are all patients on ventilators receiving extraordinary care? Is a physician who withdraws a dying patient's ventilator without the family's consent with the intent of termination of life guilty of mercy killing? What if the physician withdraws a feeding tube?

Concern about the possibility of being considered guilty of mercy killing led some physicians to forgo the use of ventilators and artificial feeding. Since withdrawal of such care might be seen as intentional termination of life (mercy killing), it was far easier to forgo medical support than to withdraw it. This reasoning created an odd situation, in which physicians would forgo the same treatment that they would not withdraw.

To others, it seemed that patients could be harmed both by the AMA's policy and by the interpretation that an extraordinary treatment could be forgone but not withdrawn. They believed that because the outcome is never certain, a patient is morally owed extraordinary treatment—both a ventilator and artificial feeding, for example—in order to see if recovery is possible. Also, some people argued that, regardless of whether a ventilator or a catheter was ordinary or extraordinary medical support, nobody really thought that a physician who withdrew such a device killed a terminally ill patient. In such a situation, we would say—if the patient had cancer—that cancer killed the patient, not the physician.

In 1975, Karen Quinlan's physicians—Morse and Javed—were upholding the official position of the AMA: that withdrawing medical support from a patient was the same as "active euthanasia." In 1986, the AMA changed its policy to reflect a new understanding of chronically comatose patients supported by ventilators and artificial nutrition. Now it was ethically possible for a physician, after consulting with the family, to withdraw a ventilator and feeding tubes from an irreversibly comatose patient.

This new AMA policy did not say that being irreversibly comatose was equivalent to being brain dead. Criteria for ethical removal of medical support differ from a state's legal standard of brain death. Physicians, under AMA policy, can remove support from patients who are not legally dead under a state's laws.

Advance Directives

The Quinlan case caused written advance directives to become popular. Such advance directives can take several forms. A *living will* informs physicians about conditions under which a person would or would not want medical support continued. A *values inventory* specifies what a person values in life and may be useful to a patient's family and physicians if they must make decisions for that person. A *durable power of attorney* assigns to someone else the right to make financial and life-and-death medical decisions if the person becomes incompetent. In those states that allow it to be applied to medical decisions, durable power of attorney is the most powerful device for protecting the rights of dying people; however, not all states have statutes creating powers of attorney for proxy medical decisions. By 1990, 43 states had statutes recognizing some version of advance directives.[76] The decision in the Cruzan case emphasized that such a document would be crucial in meeting the "clear and convincing" standard required by New York and Missouri. After the Schiavo case, many Americans rushed to sign advance directives.

In December 1991, the Health Care Financing Administration required all American hospitals to ask incoming patients if they had, or wanted to sign, an advance directive. This requirement increased the use of advance directives and has forced hospitals to specify their policies about honoring such directives.

Advance directives contain two major problems. First, most people do not accurately predict how they will feel later when they are actually near death. According to the famous SUPPORT study (Study to Understand Prognoses and Preferences for Outcomes and Risks of Treatment), most competent people change their minds when actually faced with a decision to decline treatment and die, despite having predicted the opposite about themselves many years before.[77]

If this is true for competent patients, what can we infer about the wishes of incompetent patients? Neither the best interests standard nor the substituted judgment standard are decisive: If a patient has a small chance of coming out of a year-long coma, aren't his best interests in being kept alive? If he had known these odds, would he have wanted to be given the chance? Whose judgment substitutes for his, especially if his choice was made in semi-ignorance?

Worse, evidence has been accumulating that spouses or others designated as legal proxies cannot accurately predict the wishes of previously competent but now incompetent patients.[78] As frequently as they wrongly predict a desire for mere palliative care they just as frequently wrongly predict desires for aggressive treatment.[79]

Advance directives often do not cover nonterminal, though permanently comatose, patients. Only a few advance directives are thorough enough and specify whether food and water are included under unwanted medical treatment or name a specific person to be a proxy for the incompetent patient. Because such directives are only requested of patients upon admission to hospitals, most people under 30 do not have one.

The Schiavo Case, Bioethics and Politics

Outsiders made things worse in the Schiavo case. Not understanding the history of the false report of abuse and trauma on the 1991 bone scan, outside experts guessed that something malevolent had happened to Terri, making Terri's advocates suspect a cover-up by her husband and the courts. Outside physicians, pushing their own exotic, for-profit schemes, exploited gullible parents and friends. Outlier neurologists, pushing a new category of consciousness not in journals of neurology but on the front pages of the *New York Times* and the *Hastings Center Report*, a bioethics journal, also didn't help any.

When the parents went to national media, especially in an age of fierce competition among cable news stations for sensational topics, the floodgates opened. And because politicians on the national scene love media attention, and as Florida Senator Mel Martinez predicted, U.S. senators, songressmen, and even the president got involved.

Since 1997 when scientists announced the cloning of the lamb Dolly, bioethics had become increasingly politicized, with social conservatives extolling the personhood of human embryos and opposing all forms of cloning. The Schiavo case landed on this pedigree and exploded. Whether it's good for bioethics to have its subjects covered all evening on cable news outlets remains to be seen.

FURTHER READING AND RESOURCES

Margaret Battin, *The Least Worst Death: Essays in Bioethics at the End of Life,* New York, Oxford University Press, 1993.

Joanne Lynn, ed., *By No Extraordinary Means: The Choice to Forgo Life-Sustaining Food and Water*, expanded ed., Bloomington, Indiana University Press, 1989.

Joseph Quinlan and Julia Quinlan with Phyllis Battelle, *Karen Ann: The Quinlans Tell Their Story*, New York, Doubleday, 1977.

William Colby, *The Long Goodbye: The Deaths of Nancy Cruzan,* Carlsbad, CA, Hay House, 2002.

Robert Schindler and Mary Schindler, with Suzanne Schindler Vitadamo and Bobby Schindler, *A Life That Matters: The Legacy of Terri Schiavo*, New York, Time Warner Books, 2006.

Michael Schiavo and Michael Hirsh, *Terri: The Truth,* New York, Dutton Adult Books, 2006.

Mark Fuhrman, *Silent Witness: The Untold Story of the Death of Terri Schiavo,* New York, William Morrow, 2005.

Arthur L. Caplan, James J. McCartney, and Dominic Sisti, eds., *The Case of Terri Schiavo: Ethics at the End of Life,* Buffalo, NY, Prometheus, 2006.

"Between Life and Death: The Terri Schiavo Story," A & E films. $25. This excellent 45-minute summary of the case, made by CBS news, has good photos of Terri in various stages of her life and pictures of Patricia White Bull and Terry Wallace (coma patients who awakened after many years). http://store.aetv.com/html/search/index.jhtml?search=Terri+Schiavo+Story&x=12&y=6

Downloadable video of Terri Schiavo: http://www.glennbeck.com/news/09092003-1.shtml

Other websites about Schiavo Case: http://www.apfn.org/apfn/Terri_doctor.htm http://www.pbs.org/newshour/bb/law/july-dec03/lifesupport_10-22.html

Legal Issues about Schiavo Case: http://abstractappeal.com/schiavo/infopage.html http://www.sptimes.com/2003/11/02/State/How_Terri_s_Law_came_.shtml

Timeline in Schiavo Case: http://www.miami.edu/ethics2/schiavo/timeline.htm

Coma Recovery Association, Inc.: www.comarecovery.org/

Karen Ann Quinlan Hospice, Inc.: www.karenannquinlanhospice.org/

DISCUSSION QUESTIONS

1. If you had only a 1 percent chance of coming out of a long-term coma or PVS, would you want physicians to keep treating you or would you rather they let you die?
2. In the above case, what burdens or benefits would continuing treatment place on your family and loved ones?
3. Many elderly people will succumb to coma-like states in their final years as they decline into neurological conditions such as Alzheimer's disease. Can society afford long-term care for millions of such people? Is there a morally relevant difference between such care for a 90-year-old with dementia and a 25-year-old in PVS?
4. If families won't or can't make decisions about death, is it permissible for physicians to act as if they've discovered that death has occurred in a relative, to help out the family? Is this a white lie? Would Kant approve?
5. Are worries about a slippery slope legitimate in the coma cases of this chapter? If society starts triaging such marginal people, will it lead to a "culture of death" rather than a "culture of life?" What will happen if society faces a great financial crisis over paying for medical care for cognitively impaired patients and we don't have a strong culture of life? Will society fail this new test?
6. Rachels (next chapter) argues that it's morally irrelevant whether physicians withdraw or forgo ventilators and feeding tubes, but the two actions certainly feel different to families and physicians. Are these feelings relevant to accessing the morality of letting die?
7. How do expanded definitions of death by neurological criteria depend on great trust in the integrity of the transplant community not to abuse such definitions?
8. What is the proper role of state and federal government in cases like Nancy Cruzan and Terri Schiavo? Should it protect vulnerable patients and assume the worst of families or should it assume the best of families and give them wide latitude to decide?
9. Given the SUPPORT study, (see Chapter 1), would it help to avoid family disputes if most people had an advance directive? What are the limitations of such directives and hospital ethics committees (HECs) to resolve these cases?

10. Is it fair to conceptualize the cases in this chapter as "disabled people" needing protection under the Americans with Disabilities Act (ADA)? If we do so, what problems arise?
11. In the Schiavo case, did Michael Schiavo meet the standard of clear and convincing evidence for removal of Terri's feeding tube? Why didn't he turn the case over to her parents and let them take care of her, as they volunteered to do?

CHAPTER 3

Physician-Assisted Dying: New Frontiers

In a dark, humid space with no electric power that had been damaged after Hurricane Katrina struck New Orleans in 2005, physician Anna Pou stood her post, caring for dozens of critically ill patients who had been abandoned by other physicians and staff of the hospital. With overflowing toilets, no fresh water, a flooded first floor preventing delivery of new supplies, and temperatures inside the hospital above 100°F, Dr. Pou allegedly killed four patients who could not be evacuated by giving them a painless overdose of morphine and midazolam (trade name, Versed). The essential discussion question of this chapter is this: Was Ana Pou a hero or a villain?

SOME HISTORY

Thirty-four years before, in 1971, a Dutch physician killed her terminally ill mother, leading Holland to become an ethics laboratory for physician-assisted dying. In 1998, a physician legally assisted a terminally ill Oregonian to die, culminating a decades-long battle. During the same decade, Dr. Jack Kevorkian assisted over 100 patients to die before being jailed in 1999. In 2009, five terminal residents of Washington State used a new law, which allowed a physician to help them die.

Critics saw these deaths in Oregon, Holland, Washington, and those by the hands of Kevorkian and Pou, as the start of a new culture of death. They had fought each of these measures and vowed to keep fighting.

This chapter reviews these developments and focuses on the morality of physician-assisted dying. Anna Pou's case unifies the various sections and is the focus of the chapter's discussion on whether it is dangerous to let physicians help terminal patients die.

Voluntary Euthanasia in the Netherlands

In 1973, the Dutch began guidelines for physician-assisted death: (1) Only competent patients can request death; (2) Requests must be repeated, unambivalent, unpressured, and documented; (3) Physicians must consult another physician for a second opinion; and (4) Patients must be in unbearable pain or suffering, without likelihood of improvement.[1]

Holland has universal medical coverage, including long-term nursing home care. Dutch patients see physicians who've known them for years.

So did Holland's mercy killings create a slippery slope into barbarism? To answer, the glass may be seen as half empty or half full.

In 1990, its Remmelink Commission reported that between 1973 and 1990, 1,000 *incompetent* patients had been killed by Dutch physicians, a direct violation of the guidelines.[2] All the patients killed were terminally ill. Most had cancer or AIDS and when competent, had asked to have physicians help them die painlessly.

So voluntary euthanasia did spread to the killing of incompetent patients. Although patients like Terri Schiavo or Karen Quinlan cannot legally be killed in Holland, 1,000 Dutch citizens were legally put to death.

Some cases pushed the limits, such as when a physician killed a woman in her 20s who had suffered a decade of severe anorexia. In 1993, a physician killed a severely depressed woman who had been traumatized by the death of her two children and the failure of her marriage.

In 2001, after 30 years of agreements and semilegalization, Queen Beatrix signed a law making physician-assisted dying totally legal in Holland. After three decades of experimentation, 90 percent of Dutch citizens supported the law. The law included the right of patients in the early stages of dementia, amyotrophic lateral sclerosis, or other progressive diseases to sign advanced directives allowing them to be killed at a later date.

In the early years, Dutch physicians rebuffed about 66 percent of patients who request death. By 2005, that figure had dropped to 12 percent, with another 13 percent changing their minds and another 13 percent dying before the physician could help them die.[3]

The Dutch Parliament in 2002 extended its previous euthanasia legislation to competent adolescents aged 16 to 18 and, with consent of parents, teenagers aged 12 to 16. The *Groningen Protocol* began in March 2006 where children under age 12 and especially babies could be killed with parental consent when two physicians agree with parents that the child is terminally ill with no prospect of recovery and suffering great pain.[4] This protocol semilegalized secret euthanasia in babies reportedly being carried out previously in Dutch hospitals, especially for babies with spina bifida.

In 2002, Belgium legalized the same protocol as in Holland, and Switzerland legalized some kinds of physician-assisted dying.

The expansion of mercy killing in Holland was driven by what shall be called in this chapter a conceptual slippery slope (more on this topic later). For now, that means that if terminal AIDS in a competent adult justifies killing, then it also justifies it when the patient wishes for it and later becomes incompetent, or when children or mentally challenged people are also terminal from AIDS.

Jack Kevorkian

In 1990, Jack Kevorkian, a retired pathologist, helped Oregonian Janet Adkins to die, setting off an ethical firestorm in America.

Adkins, 54 years old in 1988, became frustrated by her inability to remember. She had early Alzheimer's disease, the fourth-largest killer of Americans. She tried the experimental drug Tacrine, but it didn't work.

Characterized by progressive loss of memory, Alzheimer's results from irreversible degeneration of neural cells. After the onset of symptoms, its victims on average live 10 years. In its final phase, patients will not recognize their own children.

At the time, assisted suicide was not illegal in Michigan, where Kevorkian lived. Adkins flew there with her husband and her three sons. Her family disapproved of her intention to die and hoped she would change her mind, but in the end, they supported her.

Jack Kevorkian, then 63, grew up in Michigan, the son of Armenian immigrants, and graduated from medical school in 1953. After residency, he worked from 1969 to 1978 in Detroit at Sarasota Hospital as director of laboratories. Later, he worked at hospitals in southern California. (Several shows about Kevorkian may be seen on YouTube.)

In the mid-1980s, he retired and lived on his savings and Social Security, $550 a month. He lived simply in a tiny, two-room apartment near his two sisters.

Compassion did not originally motivate Kevorkian. Instead, he wanted to increase organs for transplantation, but this failed because most terminal patients are unsuitable donors.

Always a loner, he mostly scorned membership in medical societies. "Instinctively, as a student, I thought they were corrupt," he says. "I've been independent all my life."

When Adkins arrived in Michigan, Kevorkian and his two sisters interviewed her and her family for two hours. None of the interviewers thought that Adkins was depressed or ambivalent about her decision to die, nor did they think that she could be helped by medicine. She and her family signed documents and made videotapes to prove that they understood what they were doing.

The next day, June 4, 1990, Adkins met Kevorkian alone and the two drove off in his rusty 1968 Volkswagen van. He had revealed his intentions to several clinics, churches, and funeral homes, but none would let him use their facilities. So he drove to a park in Oakland County, Michigan. Inside his van, he had Janet Adkins, a cot, and his suicide device.

The simple device consisted of three intravenous (IV) bottles hung from an aluminum frame; Kevorkian called it a *Mercitron*. At the park, he connected an IV line to Adkins and started a saline solution for fluid volume. Then she pushed a switch that stopped the saline and released thiopental, a powerful sedative. The switch also started a six-second timer that activated a drip of potassium chloride. Thiopental rendered Janet Adkins unconscious, and about a minute later, the potassium chloride killed her. Kevorkian said that Janet had in effect "a painless heart attack while in deep sleep." The whole process took less than six minutes.

Neither the Adkins family nor Kevorkian had anticipated the resultant publicity. The local district attorney prosecuted Kevorkian for murder. Because no law prohibited assisted suicide in Michigan, a local judge dismissed the case but ordered Kevorkian not to use his Mercitron again (but had no legal basis for his order).

After Adkins's death, Kevorkian assisted hundreds of terminal people. Because he was afraid to fly and hated to drive any distance, his patients had to come to him. He also refused to accept money for his services.

In 1991, Kevorkian assisted in the death of a woman with chronic vaginal-pelvic pain. An autopsy showed no physical cause of her pain. Kevorkian was again indicted for murder, but a judge dismissed the charges because no Michigan law prohibited his actions. However, authorities did suspend his medical license.

Without a license, he couldn't obtain sodium pentothal and potassium chloride, so he began using carbon monoxide (CO). Kevorkian claimed the gas "has no color, taste, or smell; and it's toxic enough to cause rapid unconsciousness in relatively low concentration Furthermore, in light-complexioned people it often produces a rosy color that makes the victim look better as a corpse." He taught patients to attach one end of a plastic tube to a canister of CO and the other to the kind of small plastic mask used in hospitals for oxygen therapy. When he turned on the gas and the patient inhaled, death occurred within five minutes. In 1992, he helped another victim of multiple sclerosis, who donned a mask to breathe CO.

Most bioethicists and physicians denounced him. Kevorkian responded, "Why should I care what brainwashed ethicists and non-thinking physicians say?"[5] Nor did he worry about violating the Hippocratic Oath; he called physicians who followed it "hypocritic oafs." He regarded himself as a Socratic gadfly to the sluggish medical profession, saw his struggle in heroic terms, and compared himself to Mahatma Gandhi and Martin Luther King, Jr.

In 1995, he opened a suicide clinic in Michigan, but the building's owner soon evicted him. By 1998, he had assisted 100 patients in committing suicide and had been acquitted in three trials involving five of those deaths.

In 1998, the Michigan legislature passed a law making physician-assisted dying illegal. Kevorkian then assisted in the vidoetaped death of ALS patient Thomas Youk. Shown at the trial, the videotape offered irrefutable evidence that Kevorkian had deliberately broken the law.

The then-70-year-old Kevorkian received a 10–25 year sentence and entered jail in Jackson, MI. After promising to help no more terminal patients to die, Kevorkian was paroled eight years later in 2007 at age 79.

Dr. Quill: Another Approach to Dying

In 1990, Timothy Quill, an internist in Rochester, New York, helped "Diane" to die. She had terminal, acute myelomonocytic leukemia and had experienced three tumultuous months, during which her son stayed nearby.

When Dr. Quill knew that her end had come, he gave her the drugs she needed to commit suicide. He wrote:

> When we met, it was clear that she [Diane] knew what she was doing, that she was sad and frightened to be leaving, but that she would be even more terrified to stay and suffer. In our tearful goodbye, she promised a reunion in the future at her favorite spot on the edge of Lake Geneva, with dragons swimming in the sunset.[6]

Quill wrote of Diane's death in a medical journal and his district attorney then prosecuted him for murder; however, the grand jury refused to indict him.

Quill's case details contrasted with those of Jack Kevorkian. Quill knew Diane well and had treated her for a long time; he first offered her a course of treatment that might allow her to survive; he helped her die privately and without publicity; he presented his account in an established medical forum; and he did specialize in assisted dying.

Dr. Pou's Case, Continued

The seventh floor of Memorial Medical Center had been leased privately to LifeCare, which turned it into a long-term care facility for senior citizens with multiple medical problems. Anna Pou, then 51 years old and a native of New Orleans, worked there as a cancer surgeon and supervised residents at Louisiana State University School of Medicine.[7]

After Hurricane Katrina made the hospital unlivable, most physicians, students, and nurses fled. Dr. Pou's residents called her a hero for remaining. Fellow physicians described her as hard-working and dedicated, one who exerted a "huge presence."[8]

On Tuesday helicopters began evacuating the sickest patients at Memorial. On Thursday, however, someone informed Dr. Pou that further evacuations might not happen. Meanwhile, thousands of survivors in New Orleans had been herded into the Superdome, from which everyone begged for rescue from the appalling conditions.

According to Dr. Pou, at that point, "When we realized that help was not imminent . . . the standard of rescue changed to that of reverse triage. It was recognized that some patients might not survive, and priority was given to those who had the best chance of survival. On Thursday morning, only category 3 patients [the most gravely ill] remained on the LifeCare unit." That left nine patients there, all of whom were eventually found dead.

Oregon's Legalization

After intense battles, Oregonians in 1994 by referendum approved the Oregon Death with Dignity Act, but its legislature refused to go along. Another referendum in 1997 approved the measure with a 60-to-40 percent vote, forcing the act into law beginning in 1998.

The act had draconian restrictions: Patients had to be: (1) clearly competent, (2) have less than six months to live, and (3) to avoid impulsive decisions, wait 15 days before filling prescriptions. Physicians could not administer the fatal dosage, only prescribe it.

Most Oregonians prefer to die at home. Oregon has the lowest in-hospital mortality rate, suggesting many referrals for home health care and respect for advanced directives.[9] Under its groundbreaking Oregon Health Plan, all its previously uninsured, terminally ill citizens could utilize hospice programs.[10]

What about managed care organizations subtly pushing early death to save money? One misperception is that hospice and palliative care are cheap. A 1998 study showed that physician-assisted death might make a difference in only 1/2 of 1 percent of costs at the end of life.[11] Nevertheless, critics worry that state-run plans might encourage early death. In 2009, some Americans feared that mandatory "death counseling" under one Obama plan for public medicine might be a screen for saving money.

Doctors cannot be forced to participate in such deaths. They also cannot *abandon* patients. Like abortion, those who object to participating in the death "must transfer care so that the needs of the patient can be met" and "must not hinder the transfer."[12]

In the decade that assisted death has been legal in Oregon, about 60 to 90 terminal patients a year requested prescriptions, and about 40 to 60 used them to die.[13]

As these data make clear, Oregonian physicians write prescriptions for about 50 percent more patients than those who use them. About a third of patients die before the waiting period or before taking the pills. Over ten years, only 670 of about 100,000 dying Oregonians requested terminal drugs.[14] The most frequent diseases were ALS, AIDS, and cancer. Physicians most commonly prescribed the barbiturates secobarbital and phenobarbital.

The guidebook for Oregonian physicians encourages them to obtain the drugs for the patient, keep them until the time of death, and be there with the patient in his home as he takes them.[15] Such physicians should insist on an advance directive specifying a "Do Not Resuscitate" order for emergency-response personnel, counsel the family that death may not be immediate but may take hours and have complications, be ready to administer antiemetics and analgesics, counsel and support the family during and after the death, sign the death certificate and other papers required by the act, and arrange transfer to a funeral home.

Finally, many terminal Oregonians learned to die simply by not eating. When patients really are dying, the urge to eat disappears. In such a state, fasting is not painful. Although patients must be determined, such dying can be a peaceful alternative to intravenous lines and barbiturates. One dying patient went 11 days without fluids and 51 days without food before succumbing. One study in 2003 discovered that more Oregonians die by ceasing food and water than by asking physicians to give them drugs.[16]

Background: Ancient Greece and the Hippocratic Oath

The Hippocratic Oath, considered the cornerstone of medical ethics, forbids physicians to kill patients, and its origins were in ancient Greece at the time of Socrates in fifth century BCE. But did Hippocratic physicians represent most ancient Greek physicians?

Hippocrates was a disciple of the mathematician Pythagoras, who developed the famous theorem, who worshipped numbers as divine, and who held that all life was sacred. As his follower, Hippocrates did not represent most ancient Greek physicians.

The Hippocratic corpus, or body of writings, does not represent the work of one man named "Hippocrates," but a number of his followers. The practitioners of the Hippocratic school "possessed no legally recognized professional qualifications" and competed with gymnastic instructors, drug sellers, herbalists, midwives, and exorcists.[17]

Many people today misunderstand the content of the original Hippocratic Oath, which makes physicians swear:

> I swear by Apollo Physician and Asclepius and Hygeia and Panaceia and all the gods and goddesses, making them my witnesses, that I will fulfill according to my ability and judgment this oath and this covenant:
>
> To hold him who has taught me this art as equal to my parents and to live my life in partnership with him, and if he is in need of money, to give him a share of mine, and to regard his offspring as equal to my brothers in male lineage, and to teach his art—if they desire to learn it—without fee and covenant; to give a share of precepts and oral instruction and all the other learning to my sons and to the sons of him who has instructed me and the pupils who have signed the covenant and have taken this oath according to the medical law, but to no one else.
>
> I will apply dietetic measures for the benefit of the sick according to my ability and judgment; I will keep them from harm and injustice.
>
> I will neither give a deadly drug to anybody if asked for it, nor will I make a suggestion to this effect. Similarly I will not give to a woman an abortive remedy. In purity and holiness I will guard my life and my art. I will not use the knife, not even on sufferers of stone, but will withdraw in favor of such men as are engaged in this work.
>
> Whatever houses I visit, I will come for the benefit of the sick, remaining free of all intentional injustice, of all mischief and in particular of sexual relations with both female and male persons, be they free or slaves.
>
> What I may see or hear in the course of the treatment or even outside of the treatment in regard to the life of men, which on no account one must spread abroad, I will keep to myself holding such things shameful to be spoken about.
>
> If I fulfill this oath and do not violate it, may it be granted to me to enjoy life and art, being honored with fame among all men for all time to come; if I transgress it and swear falsely, may the opposite of all this be my lot.[18]

With the original oath, the Hippocratic school solidified its membership against competing healers, for example, against those who performed surgery or those who charged students for teaching them.

Ordinary Greek physicians thought like ordinary Greeks, who thought that life had natural limitations, beyond which only fools tried to extend living. The concept of a *meson* or natural limit infused Greek culture, especially architecture and theater. To attempt to go beyond *meson* was hubris and invited the gods to strike one down. So most ancient Greek physicians helped their patients die.

The prohibition against euthanasia by the Hippocratic school thus set its members apart from the majority of physicians in ancient Greece who helped patients die painlessly and with some dignity.

Dr. Pou's Case, Continued

Shocking conditions prevailed at Memorial Hospital after Hurricane Katrina. Over 2,000 people had sought temporary shelter there—neighbors, family members, family of staff, and previous outpatients—crowding the hallways and draining the hospital of food, water, and clean toilets. As staff rushed by, people who sprawled on the floor cried out for water and help.

On the top floor, conditions for the last nine patients worsened each day. One weighed 380 pounds and although paralyzed, the 61-year-old seemed alert, oriented, and interactive. Another aspirated food and suffered a heart attack, but was resuscitated. Others could breathe only on ventilators; others had chronic, nonhealing wounds that required intensive nursing. All sweltered in rooms as hot as 105 degrees.

It is not hard to imagine what an ancient Greek physician would have done in such circumstances: triage the patients "for their own good," and let them die quickly and humanely. He would not believe that the future quality of life of these nine patients justified great efforts.

The Nazis and "Euthanasia"

Debates about physician-assisted dying frequently refer to German physicians during the Nazi era, who in the name of "euthanasia" killed 90,000 patients because of mental or physical inferiority. This so-called Nazi Argument bears some scrutiny.

First, Nazi physicians administered the *Final Solution* to the "problem" of how to cleanse Germany of racially inferior non-Aryan peoples. Physicians kept this program secret, and under it, killed 6,000,000 Jews, 600,000 Poles, thousands of gypsies, and thousands of gay men and lesbians.

Leo Alexander, a New York psychiatrist who observed the Nuremberg trials, famously argued in 1949 that these killing programs by Nazi physicians began with their belief that some people are better off dead than alive because their quality of life is poor.[19]

In 1986, another New York psychiatrist, Robert Jay Lifton, argued similarly, although his "first step" differed from Alexander's:

> The Nazis justified direct medical killing by use of the . . . concept of "life unworthy of life," *lebensunwertes Leben*. While this concept predated the Nazis, it was carried to its ultimate racial and "therapeutic" extreme by them.
>
> . . . Of the five identifiable steps by which the Nazis carried out the destruction of "life unworthy of life," coercive sterilization was the first. There followed the killing of "impaired" children in hospitals, and then the killing of "impaired" adults—mostly collected from mental hospitals—in centers especially equipped with carbon monoxide. The same killing centers were then used for the murders of "impaired" inmates of concentration camps. The final step was mass killing, mostly of Jews, in the extermination camps themselves.[20]

People opposed to physician-assisted dying often cite Alexander's and Lifton's work. They emphasize that in Nazi Germany medical professors in elite medical schools took the first, dangerous step down a lethal slippery slope.

J. C. Wilkes argues differently that the first steps down the Nazi slippery slope came when physicians mercy-killed a few severely handicapped infants.[21] Starting in 1937, a father who killed his mentally retarded child received only a mild rebuke. Two years later, Dr. Karl Brandt examined an infant named Knauer, born blind and missing an arm and a leg. Hitler cleared him to kill Knauer and all similar infants. Wilkes claims these two test cases led to the first phase of deaths in Germany where physicians killed as many as 6,000 (Wilkes's estimate) disabled children.

These cases differ from the so-called Baby Doe cases discussed in Chapter 7 in that most German parents did not consent to these killings. Officials took the babies and children out of the home and the parents never saw them again.

What about claims by Alexander, Lifton, and Wilkes about the first step that leads down the slippery slope to mass killings? In rebuttal, many history professors say this is just bad history. They emphasize that Germany had been blatantly anti-Semitic since the time of the Crusades. Instead of a subtle first step propelling them downward, Nazi physicians rode a tsunami that had been building for centuries.

The Nazi "euthanasia" program had nothing in common with *competent* patients who are *dying* and who *voluntarily* request assistance in dying from physicians. In brief, Nazi "euthanasia" was not "good deaths" but despicable murders.

A little analysis also helps. The Nazi argument contains many different claims, including:

(1) Involuntary killings of people *for medical reasons* led to the Holocaust.
(2) Involuntary killings of people *by physicians* led to the Holocaust.
(3) Justifying medical killings of people *for reasons of quality of life* led to the Holocaust.
(4) *Involuntary sterilization* of retarded, psychotic, and demented people led to the Holocaust.
(5) The *killing of impaired children* led to the Holocaust.
(6) *Eugenics*, the desire of Nazis to create a master race, led to the Holocaust.
(7) Deep *cultural racism and anti-Semitism* led to the Holocaust.
(8) Acceptance by physicians of a *new role as killers* led to the Holocaust.

Because all its victims died *involuntarily*, and because no terminal patients died voluntarily by Nazi physicians, "playing the Nazi card" does not illustrate good reasoning.

MODERN DEVELOPMENTS

Founded in the United States in 1980 by Derek Humphrey, the Hemlock Society helped people with terminal illness to die with dignity. After merging in 2005 with other organizations, it became Compassion & Choices, which advocates legalizing physician-assisted dying.

In the 1960s, two physicians—one working in America and the other in England—changed medicine to help dying patients. Elisabeth Kübler-Ross, working in Chicago, and Cicely Saunders, in Britain, focused on accepting the inevitability of death and making terminal patients comfortable.

Their programs began the *hospice movement*. Hospice tries to give dying patients dignity and maximal control over the final months of their lives. Originally, hospices were separate facilities, but the concept evolved to visiting nurses treating patients at home.

Because of the work of these two women, physicians today relieve pain better and attend better to the psychological needs of dying patients than they did 40 years ago. In the United States, Medicare now pays for six months of hospice care for dying patients.

Around 1986, *palliative care* was created to seek maximal quality during the remaining time of life. Palliative care does not mean giving up on patients but does forgo experimental, torturous treatments in seeking a one-in-a-million cure. Palliative care physicians focus on maximal relief of bad symptoms such as nausea, boredom, itching, feelings of suffocation, immobility, depression, and especially pain.

Recent Legal Decisions

In 1994, a federal judge struck down a law in Washington State banning assisted suicide, holding that the equal protection of liberty guaranteed in the Fourteenth Amendment covered not only a woman's right to end a pregnancy but also a terminal patient's right to physician-assisted dying.[22] The liberty guaranteed to Americans by the Constitution included the right to die, she said, and assistance by physicians in so doing.

Over the next three years and in two important decisions, the U.S. Supreme Court disagreed. Although a state such as Oregon *could* legalize physician-assisted dying, no fundamental liberty existed in the Constitution to this assistance—such that state laws banning this assistance were unconstitutional.

One case alleged discrimination against dying patients because only some could decide to die by removal of a ventilator or feeding tube. If physicians could legally kill by withdrawing treatment, why not by more direct means? The highest Court answered that "the distinction between assisting suicide and withdrawing life-sustaining treatment, a distinction widely recognized and endorsed in the medical profession and in our legal traditions, is both important and logical; it is certainly rational. . . ."[23]

In the second case, the same Court found that no right to assisted suicide existed in American legal or medical traditions. The Court accepted the AMA's claim that legalization of physician-assisted dying threatened the medical profession's integrity, as well as claims that physician-assisted dying would hurt the disabled and poor. It also found "ample concern" for a slippery slope from increased acceptance of physician killings.

These decisions said only that a fundamental right to die did not already exist in the Constitution, such that state laws banning assisted suicide would violate it. They left the door open for a state to legalize physician-assisted suicide, as Oregon did in 1998 and Washington did in 2008. In this way, these decisions mirrored what *Cruzan* said about laws about incompetent patients, i.e., states *could*, but *need not*, pass this kind of law.

ETHICAL ISSUES

Two different kinds of arguments occur in ethics. One focuses directly on the morality of acts and argues that they are intrinsically wrong, "just wrong," or wrong without regard to consequences. The other grants that in a few cases, such acts may be justified, but opposes them based on their negative roundabout effects. These are *direct* and *indirect* arguments.

The main direct argument against physician-assisted dying is that it is always wrong to kill. Most other arguments against it are indirect and predict slippery slopes.

DIRECT ARGUMENTS—PHYSICIAN-ASSISTED DYING

Killing Is Always Wrong

The best direct argument against physician-assisted dying is that such actions wrongly kill vulnerable humans. Of course, it is always wrong to kill humans under all circumstances, and just because a human is dying, no exceptions can be made. Evil occurs when one human ends the life of another. This argument does not claim that what is wrong about killing is that it can become uncontrollable after a few justified cases, for that would be appealing to a slippery slope. Instead, it claims that all killing is *intrinsically wrong*, no matter what the circumstances.

Whether or not an afterlife or God exists, once a person is dead, he's not coming back. Without an afterlife, this life is all a person has, and to take it away is to take away all values because the valu*er* is gone.

For many decisions, such as transplanting a kidney, if mistakes occur, there is backup, for example, hemodialysis. But mistakes in killing have no backup. Once a person is dead, that's it.

For this reason, killing must not be taken lightly. Life must not be cheapened. The ultimate power on earth is to take away life. All life should be valued, not just human life, but all sentience. Life is precious, no matter how low in quality. Of all values in medicine, this one must reign supreme.

Killing Is Not Always Wrong

The most ancient justification of the direct argument is based on religious metaphysics: that God exists, that Scripture correctly reveals his laws for humans, and that one such law is for humans never to kill another human. Based on this view, some Christians and some orthodox prefer death to self-defense, refuse war and the draft, and will never kill.

One should note that Scripture really bans "unjustified" killings, and hence, allows just wars and the death penalty for murderers. The question here concerns whether helping terminally ill patients die is "unjustified" killing. After all, as God presumably allows the person to have a terminal illness and to be dying, in one sense, dying for each of us is His Will.

More important, the background conditions need to be examined for why the rule against killing has been important throughout the millennia of civilization in the West. Throughout this history, most people have wanted to live as long as possible. That fact is less true today. Why?

Medicine has cured the old, acute diseases that killed swiftly, and left us with chronic diseases, such as cancer and heart disease, that kill slowly. In previous centuries, people tried to live as long as possible because most never experienced the disability and dysfunction that came with chronic diseases.

Now consider the rule against killing and physician-assisted dying. When you help me accomplish what I want to do, you do a good thing, and morality encourages you to help me. When you prevent me from doing what I want to do, you hurt my interests and me, and your actions are probably immoral. Whether or not dying assisted by physicians is good or bad may depend, not on what has been traditionally been judged moral or immoral, but on the wishes of the dying patient.

Of course, critics can object that helping me do what I want to do is not a good thing if I want to do something immoral such as steal my neighbor's car. And, they say, helping people die is immoral.

But why should we allow this objection as a good one? Why should we accept the underlying premise that "helping dying people die is immoral" unless some further reason is given? To simply assert this as an objection is to beg the question. It is not an argument against a position to assume that it is wrong.

Killing versus Letting Die

For several decades, bioethicists have debated whether killing differs from letting die. A 1997 survey by the American Hospital Association found that 70 percent of deaths in hospitals involve some decision by a physician or relative to cease treatment.[24] However, intentional termination of a dying patient's life is still considered unethical by the AMA and is illegal in every state except Oregon and Washington.

A leading physician in medical ethics once admitted, "I have had occasion to give a patient pain medication we both knew would shorten her life."[25] Does this differ from killing her?

Would Ana Pou have been a better doctor if, like other physicians, she had left her post and simply *let* her patients die? Why is it better to allow someone to die slowly and horribly, rather than end their anxiety and pain quickly?

In palliative care, physicians practice *terminal sedation*, which stands on the doctrine of double effect where the physician must not intend death but merely the relief of pain. Does such sedation differ from killing the patient? Is the difference only semantic?

In 1975, in a famous article in the *New England Journal of Medicine*, the philosopher James Rachels attacked the distinction between active and passive euthanasia.[26] Rachels argued that this distinction, though still dominant in modern medicine and law, has no inherent moral value and, when it is erroneously taken for anything more than a shorthand pragmatic rule, leads to decisions about death based on irrelevant factors.

Rachels's logic cuts two ways: first, letting a vegetative patient die is just as bad (or good) as killing him or her; second, killing a vegetative patient is just as good (or bad) as allowing him or her to die. There is nothing moral or immoral in the act of passive or active euthanasia itself; instead, morality or immorality is determined by motives and results in the context of that act. Focusing on whether an act is active or passive, he argued, may confuse our judgments, leading us to think that passively allowing people to die slowly and horribly is morally superior to actively bringing about a quick, painless death.

Rachels caused controversy. Is intending death by removing a respirator equivalent to suffocating a patient with a pillow? If a patient is allowed to die, isn't that patient killed by the disease? But if someone acts directly to bring about dying, isn't that human agent the cause of death? One critic argued:

> What is the difference between merely letting a patient die and killing that patient? Does it depend upon activity or passivity? Does it depend on an agent's intentions? I think that neither of these factors is relevant. What is relevant is the cause of death. When the cause of death is the underlying disease process, the patient is simply allowed to die.[27]

So after Hurricane Katrina, diseases didn't kill Ana Pou's patients, the doctor did.

In support of Rachels, it can be argued that in practice the line between active and passive is hard to draw. In some cases, not acting can be considered active; one example might be not giving antibiotics to Karen Quinlan to treat the pneumonia she developed in her final weeks.

This does not entail that killing and assisted dying do not differ; as Jean Davies argues, just as "rape and making love are different, so are killing and assisted suicide."[28]

Relief of Suffering

One of the most persuasive arguments for physician-assisted dying is the appeal to mercy. Ana Pou probably saw panicked patients suffering in terrible heat, dehydration, and discomfort in the aftermath of Hurricane Katrina. Observing another human being in untreatable pain howling like a wounded animal can move even the most callous of us to tears. The most natural response is to end such suffering. We do this for our pets; why can't we do the same for humans? Moreover, the suffering of terminal patients is not confined to physical pain, as bad as that is: it also involves helplessness, stress, exhaustion, terror, loss, and other experiences that are difficult even to imagine.

A big issue here has to do with relief of pain. Is it possible to relieve all pain and make dying patients completely comfortable? Cicely Saunders, who founded St. Christopher's Hospice in London, says her patients never need suffer pain. She gives them Brompton cocktails, a powerful brew of morphine, heroin, alcohol, and cocaine.

On the other hand, Derek Humphrey of the Hemlock Society argued that, "it is generally agreed that 10 percent of pain cannot be controlled. That is a lot of people."[29] Margaret Battin and Timothy Quill acknowledge that 2 to 5 percent of terminal patients experience pain that is incontrollable, even with excellent palliative care.[30] It is also true that not everyone experiences pain in the same way, and a condition that would be acceptable to some patients might be intolerable to others.

A second question concerns what the cost of relief might be, and what costs are acceptable. In this context, we are not talking about financial costs; the issue is the cost to the patient's well-being. Powerful narcotics such as Brompton cocktails numb consciousness and can reduce patients to a vegetative state during their last months of life.

Dying patients must make a tradeoff between consciousness and relief of pain, and not every patient considers that tradeoff acceptable. For some patients, being conscious and able to talk to relatives and friends is more important than avoiding pain. Here again, autonomy becomes relevant. What counts as a benefit or a harm must be defined within each patient's own value system, and who else but patients can make judgments about this tradeoff?

Ethics and medicine commonly distinguish between pain and suffering. *Pain* is physical; *suffering* is a broader and more personal matter. Pain is only one aspect of suffering and relieving a patient's pain does not necessarily relieve suffering.

Peter Admiraal, a physician and one of the leaders of assisted dying in the Netherlands, agrees that uncontrollable pain is rarely the only reason for death:

> There is severe dehydration, uncontrolled itching and fatigue. These patients are completely exhausted. Some of them can't turn around in their beds. They become incontinent. All these factors make a kind of suffering from which they only want to escape. . . .
>
> And of course you are suffering because you have a mind. You are thinking about what is happening to you. You have fears and anxiety and sorrow. In the end, it gives a complete loss of human dignity. You cannot stop that feeling with medical treatment.[31]

In Dr. Pou's case, one could argue that her nine patients were suffering badly and that they would be unlikely to be evacuated or saved. Gravely ill with many medical problems, lying in hot, humid rooms with no fresh water, it is hard to imagine a more uncomfortable place to be while suffering many chronic, now-untreatable medical problems.

Cries for Help

Joanne Lynn, a physician who has cared for over 1,000 hospice patients, believes that most terminal patients who request physician-assisted death seek attention, control, dignity, relief of symptoms, or relief from depression. Sometimes the request is a plea to see "if anyone really cares whether he or she lives."[32]

Physicians trained in palliative care believe aggressive treatment can ameliorate almost all unpleasant symptoms. With such specialists and good medical coverage, dying need not be undignified or painful.

It is especially important with terminal patients not just to deal with physical symptoms. Terminal patients are often bored and depressed; people avoid them. People who once had important work to do now have nothing to do. People who never watched television now are forced to watch it all day long. Good psychiatrists know how to help.

Dying at home cures some problems. It is empowering to be dying in your own home rather than a hospital, which has its own routine and hierarchy.

Allowing physician-assisted dying would be the easy way out on several fronts. First, physicians don't need to aggressively treat symptoms. Second, the system doesn't need to change to train more people in hospice and palliative care.

In a review of the literature, bioethicists Margaret Pabst Battin and Timothy Quill conclude that physician-assisted dying should be an option of last resort after all resources are exhausted of excellent palliative care.[33] Even though they defend legalizing physician-assisted dying, they stress that it must be no substitute for lack of great palliative care.

On the other hand, a recipe for physician-assisted suicide gone wild would be poorly trained nurses and physicians, managed care plans that don't pay for palliative medicine or hospice or long-term nursing care, and young people impatient for their elders to "get on with it and die."

Patient Autonomy

Let's be frank: people believe different things about the sanctity of life and the wrongness of killing, but what if you're not religious? Or don't see religion as against helping people die? What are we to do? Fight about it? Kill each other over who's right about killing?

One way to say that each person should decide things himself is to say that the *autonomy* of patients should count most. "Autonomy" means the ability to be self-governing and self-directed. Its opposite is to be treated paternalistically, like an incompetent child.

Autonomy mattered to John Stuart Mill, who argued in his *On Liberty* that "over his own body and mind, the individual is sovereign." Mill's view implies that government should not impose its view of when and how people should die.

Autonomy raises some questions about risks: Who is best qualified to assess the danger of dying too soon? What degree of risk is acceptable? Who should determine acceptability? How does the risk of dying too soon compare with the risks entailed by alternatives?

Physicians usually believe that they are best qualified to assess risk, and they're right as far as statistical risk is concerned. But *acceptable* risk is evaluative as well as statistical, and many patients want the right to make their own judgments about what is acceptable risk.

When terminal patients make such evaluations, their concern is more than just fear of pain. Derek Humphrey of the Hemlock Society has written, "It isn't just a question of pain. It is a question of dignity, self-control, and distress. If you can't eat, sleep, or read, and the quality of life is so bad, and there is a certainty that you are dying, it is a matter of dignity to be able to end your life.[34]

In order to evaluate acceptable risk, patients need information. Margaret Battin holds that physicians rarely discuss options with dying patients.[35] She believes that patients' informed consent should be sought not only for medical research but also for ways of dying. Especially when experimental drugs and surgery are involved, terminal patients should be informed about different outcomes and different ways of dying so that they can choose the *least worst death.* Alas, few patients get such information and few are allowed to make such choices.

Ana Pou's patients did not seem to ask to die. At least one of them seems to have been oriented and alert, and could have been so asked. Maybe she thought asking was moot, as no rescue was coming and conditions were worsening. Nevertheless, this lack of consent seems to be the most serious charge against her.

INDIRECT ARGUMENTS ABOUT PHYSICIAN-ASSISTED DYING

The Slippery Slope

One of the most famous ideas in ethics is the *slippery slope*, also called the "thin edge of the wedge"—or simply "wedge"—argument. Claims about it figure prominently in debates about physician-assisted dying.

Slippery slope arguments assert that if a preliminary neutral or good step is accepted, a series of other changes then occur, leading to a final terrible result. They metaphorically see society as teetering like a ball perched atop a steep slope and leaning downward, braced only by chocks or wedges on the ground to prevent it from descending. The chocks are our basic moral principles.

There are two general kinds of claims about slippery slopes: *empirical* and *conceptual*.[36] Claims about *empirical slopes* assert that once you take the first step, something bad in human nature is unleashed, which will be uncontrollable. In the article by Leo Alexander mentioned previously, he refers to an empirical slope: "The destructive principle, once unleashed, is bound to engulf the whole personality and to occupy all its relationships."[37]

A *conceptual* slippery slope asserts that once a small change is made in a moral rule, other changes will soon follow, because of the demands of reason for consistency in treating similar cases similarly. Alexander also refers to this kind of slope:

> The beginnings at first were merely a subtle shift in emphasis in the basic attitude of the physicians. It started with the acceptance of the attitude, basic in the euthanasia movement, that there is such a thing as life not worthy to be lived. This attitude in its early stages concerned itself merely with the severely and chronically sick. Gradually the sphere of those to be included in this category was enlarged to encompass the socially unproductive, the ideologically unwanted, the racially unwanted and finally all non-Germans. But it is important to realize that the infinitely small wedged-in lever from which this entire trend of mind received its impetus was the attitude of the nonrehabilitable sick.[38]

Once physicians are permitted to kill one kind of patient because quality of life is so low as to make "life not worthy to be lived," they not only can, but *will* use the same reasoning in similar cases.

An *empirical* slope prediction says that once society changes a rule about protecting one class of patient, powerful forces will be unleashed that cannot be restrained and kept contained to the original class. Something like this was unleashed in Dr. Michael Swango when he started to kill: Charged and convicted in 2000 with killing three patients in New York State, Dr. Michel Swango killed at least 60 patients, possibly hundreds, starting in Zimbabwe in the early 1980s and moving around the world (when arrested, he was on his way to Saudi Arabia for a new job).[39] His diary revealed that he killed for the thrill of the power to kill and "the sweet, husky, close smell of an indoor homicide."

It is just such malice in human nature that could be unleashed with legal, physician-assisted deaths. Law professor Yale Kamisar observes that "not all people are kind, understanding, and loving." Yet they will be making decisions about the elderly and helpless.[40]

And so Anna Pou was charged with second-degree murder after four patients under her care died suspiciously in Memorial Medical Center in New Orleans, four days after Hurricane Katrina hit.[41] The Louisiana Attorney General alleged that they died of overdoses of morphine and midazolam (i.e., Versed), which she later admitted giving them. Although the grand jury declined to indict Dr. Pou, it may have done so in part because other physicians abandoned the hospital and she heroically stayed, because the four patients well might have died anyway and in worse ways, and because she came across as a compassionate person. But it still may be true that, given the changing ethical climate about physician-assisted killing in America, she felt freer to do this than she would have decades ago. To that degree, and under those circumstances, perhaps some slippage has occurred.

Consider another example of a conceptual slope: first we will allow abortion of a fetus because of Down's Syndrome, then we will let a newborn with Down's Syndrome die. In this kind of slope, as opposed to empirical slopes, *it is always the demand of reason to treat similar cases similarly that expands the initial change*.

This kind of reasoning is seen in the following claims. At the time of the Karen Quinlan case in 1976, disability advocate James Bopp said that if you "accept quality of life as the standard," then "first you withdraw the respirators, then the food and then you actively kill people. It's a straight line from one place to the others."[42] Bioethicist Daniel Callahan then said that the logic of the case for euthanasia will inevitably lead to its extension far beyond terminally ill competent adults. If relief of suffering is critical, Callahan said, "Why should that relief be denied to the demented or the incompetent?"[43] In the claims of these people, what justifies one kind of case will soon justify another.

Contrasts may be made among the two kinds of slope claims. The empirical claim is a prediction about consequences if some moral change occurs, whereas the conceptual claim refers to a linkage in reasoning once particular premises are accepted. Where the empirical slope says one small change will create many others because of something innately bad in humans, the conceptual slope says the same kind of change can occur because of something higher in humans—reason's need to treat similar cases similarly.

Claims about slippery slopes are difficult to evaluate because the predicted, final, bad event is so far away. However, critics predicted that slippery slopes would occur during the Karen Quinlan case, with Holland's changes, and with Oregon's legalization, so we can evaluate such predictions.

In 1975, columnist Nat Hentoff predicted that the *Quinlan* decision would bring on an empirical slippery slope. In 1992, he felt vindicated in describing Jack Kevorkian's actions and the decriminalization of physician-assisted dying in the Netherlands, all of which he called a "reckless cheapening of life."[44]

What can we say about these claims? First, if the danger of an empirical slippery slope was real, we would have expected the precedent of the Quinlan case to first, make it easy for competent patients to die, and second, to generalize to other kinds of incompetent patients, such as senile, demented patients in nursing homes. Yet neither happened. It took 22 years after the *Quinlan* decision before the first terminal patient legally died with the help of a physician in Oregon in 1998, and the Schiavo case showed us how far we are from readily accepting the deaths of incompetent PVS patients.

What about Oregon? Physician-assisted deaths there over the first eight years averaged about 35 to 40 a year.

What about Holland? As said earlier, a real expansion of cases occurred there. Teenagers, psychiatric patients, and newborns who are suffering and terminal have been killed with their consent or the consent of their proxies.

Callahan's prediction has come true, but the Dutch regard it not as a downward descent but as a moral elevation: if it's justified to kill a consenting, terminal 64-year-old with terminal cancer, why isn't it also justified to kill a consenting 16-year-old with terminal cancer?

Depression and Unbearable Symptoms

A very difficult question concerns whether terminal patients who request a physician's help to die suffer from reversible depression and symptoms. The easy answer is that they shouldn't be helped until physicians attempt reversal.

But not every terminal patient has great medical coverage and a great physician in palliative care. Fewer physicians each year enter primary care, and palliative care is neither a popular nor a financially rewarding specialty. Should terminal patients be helped to die who, if they had the best coverage and best physicians, wouldn't choose to do so?

In Chapter 1, we raised a similar question about accepting requests of autonomous, young, nonterminal patients to die, such as Elizabeth Bouvia and Dax Cowart. However, in those cases, we had the luxury of time: time for the adaptation effect to occur, time for resources to be found, and time for society to become enlightened. With dying patients in the Northwest who are certified with less than six months to live, we lack that luxury. So, yes, antidepressants should be tried and everyone should try to get the patient the best palliative care, but if all that isn't possible, compromises must be made.

Inefficient Means

Opponents of legalization claim that physician-assisted deaths are botched 25 percent of the time in Holland and therefore they should be illegal.[45] This is a strange argument as it complains about the "how to" part of legalization. In other words, physicians at present aren't good enough to guarantee death.

Of course, death for some patients will not be easy. Some AIDS patients who were intravenous drug users and who attempted suicide at dosages recommended by the Hemlock Society had high tolerances to central-nervous-system depressants and did not die easily or quickly, sometimes merely ending up in vegetative comas.

To avoid this possibility, the patient needed to ask a friend to be present to possibly help at the end by attaching a large plastic bag over the patient's head and securing it with duct tape, such that the patient could suffocate to death. (This is what critic Nat Hentoff calls the "Exit Bag," sarcastically referring to the efficient, self-administered form of it with velcro straps that once could be ordered from the Hemlock Society.[46]) Use of Exit Bags subjects friends to charges of murder and leaves dying patients faced with the dilemma of dying alone and botching the attempt or asking a friend to be present, to assist, and to risk prosecution for assisting in suicide.

This is why Oregonian physicians often attend the deaths of terminal patients. If something goes wrong, they can adjust medications or deal with unexpected complications. In short, this is not an argument for eliminating physician-assisted dying, but for creating *more* of it.

A Financial Empirical Slope?

Will the greed of families and the avarice of physicians conspire to speed sick patients to an early grave? The honest answer is that we don't know. Hard times have not tested American physicians, who are used to aggressively treating patients and being well paid to do so, especially in oncology, cardiac, and cancer surgery.

One nagging worry is that some historians think that the ultimate reason for the rise of Nazi Germany was economic. After losing World War I, the Germans were made to pay huge war reparations, which caused great harm to the German economy and created much ill will. Since World War II, and especially in the last decades, North America has experienced an unparalleled economic boom. What will happen when times turn bad and families must choose between grandma's care and a child's college tuition?

Most patients and families are shielded from the true costs of long-term coverage at the end of life. The great exceptions are people who lack medical coverage, working people in their 50s and early 60s. What might be truly dangerous is to give physicians incentives to curtail care at the end of life while ethical bulwarks against physician-assisted dying are weakened. That could easily become not just a wave but a tsunami, especially during a major depression and intergenerational war over who should pay the medical costs of an aging population.

The Roles of Physicians

Some doctors argue that "Physicians should not kill" and should be healers only. This statement assumes incorrectly that physicians can always heal. That is false. The mortality rate is 100 percent among humans. No human has ever been "healed" of death. Eventually, each human must confront death with his or her physician.

Second, to simplistically assert that, "Physicians should not kill" begs the key question of this chapter. It is like saying that, "Physicians should do not what is wrong," while assuming without argument that such-and-such is wrong.

More than one way exists to be a compassionate physician to dying patients; for example Quill's method versus Kevorkian's. A good physician makes sure his patient isn't depressed, choosing death because of lack of relief of symptoms that can be treated, or a victim of social prejudice. The short interviews by Dr. Kevorkian and his layperson sister of out-of-state patients who arrived in town the day before they were killed, did not meet the highest standards of humanism in medicine.

As for Ana Pou, her role drew mixed reactions. On one hand, if it was a triage situation, she acted mercifully. But what if it wasn't a true situation of triage, because unknown to her, help was on the way? This is like the movie when a ship captain makes people jump from the lifeboat to drown, and the next morning, the captain sees a ship that will rescue them.

Mistakes and Abuses

Physicians make mistakes. Surgeon Christiaan Barnard recalled a young woman with ovarian cancer who repeatedly begged him to kill her painlessly with morphine.[47] Aware that she was terminal, Barnard decided to help her. When he came into her room with a syringe loaded with morphine, she was quiet, and he thought at first that she was in too much pain even to scream. Then he realized that she was semiconscious, beyond pain, and he changed his mind. The next morning, she felt better; soon she was in remission, and then lived another few months. Stories like this abound in medicine.

What if Ana Pou had hesitated? Waited one more day? Rescue would have come and some of her patients would have lived.

In Holland, some critics claim that physicians often misdiagnosis "intractable and unbearable" suffering. In Janet Adkins's case, many people were quick to say that physicians aren't infallible diagnosticians and that patients sometimes defy a dire prognosis.

Let us put this point differently. In bioethics, many discussions begin with a phrase like, "If a patient has a terminal illness. . . ." Notice the word "if." In presumably terminal illnesses, few claims are absolute until the patient's last days. Before then, how "terminal"—how close to death—the patient is may depend on many factors that are not easy to assess: the patient's attitude, the family's attitude, the attitude of staff members, the quality and level of care, and so on. Moreover, some terminal patients are misdiagnosed and they recover. Physician-assisted dying allows a mistaken diagnosis to become a death sentence. Once physician-assisted death occurs, there is no appeal.

Israeli physician Seymour Glick also reveals a dirty little secret of medicine: every physician has some patients that he or she really strongly dislikes. Some deaths are messy, some families are intolerable, and sometimes, physicians make mistakes and harm patients. In all these cases, physicians want the cases to "go away." The easiest way to make them go away is for the patients to die. But we should never open this door.

Anna Pou, Again

According to statements Anna Pou made to *Newsweek*, on Thursday, September 1, the remaining staff met and believed that no further evacuation or help was coming to them. They were stranded with nine critically ill patients and 2,000 dirty citizens roaming their halls without security. The staff then decided to euthanize the remaining nine patients by sedation; Dr. Pou would administer the drugs.

Unknown to her, the parent organization of LifeCare had hired private contractors to remove the nine patients. In addition, all other critically ill patients had been successfully removed from Memorial, including two 400-pound men who could not walk, patients from intensive care units, and tiny, premature babies.

Pou herself likens her situation to battlefield conditions and notes that physicians receive no training in ethics or medicine about how to act in such situations. Bioethicist Alto Charo notes, "From her perspective, these patients are now terminal . . . and they're terminal under particularly terrifying conditions: extreme discomfort, [probably] panic, and the prospect of being abandoned while helpless. [If Pou could not save them] her next obligation would seem to be . . . to give them enough medicine that they're not in any pain and they're not in any panic and it may or may not hasten their deaths."[48]

Dr. Timothy Quill said the drugs Dr. Pou gave are typically used to relieve pain and anxiety, not for euthanasia. For the latter, she would have used, like Kevorkian's Mercitron, barbituates and paralytics, but instead she used morphine, which both eases pain and decreases respiration, and midazolam (Versed), a very powerful, fast-acting drug used before major surgery and which evaporates anxiety and pain.

At her trial, like Kevorkian, Dr. Pou insisted she did not intend to kill her patients but only to relieve their pain. The grand jury concluded that not enough evidence existed to conclude otherwise, and, as said, probably believed that extenuating circumstances should be considered in judging Pou.

CONCLUSION

With the *Quinlan* decision in 1976, critics predicted that euthanasia would sweep North America. In the 30-plus years since, two states have legalized physician-assisted dying, where less than 100 patients a year use the law. Holland continues to accept its liberalization, and Belgium and Switzerland have liberalized their laws, too.

Nevertheless, physician-assisted dying remains contentious in American medicine. Perhaps the most heartfelt concern is among disability advocates, who fear that lack of resources will push people with disabilities into premature deaths. Certainly the experience of the patients at Memorial Hospital in New Orleans after Hurricane Katrina should give us pause about what might happen to similar patients under an unexpected, national, financial "hurricane."

Adequate screening for depression in patients with terminal cancer continues to be a concern. One review of patients requesting assistance in dying in Oregon questioned whether such patients had received such screening.[49]

FURTHER READING AND RESOURCES

Gerald Dworkin, Ray Frey, and Sissela Bok, eds., *Euthanasia and Physician-Assisted Suicide: For and Against,* New York, Cambridge University Press, 1998.

Kathleen M. Foley and Herbert Hendin, eds., *The Case against Assisted Suicide: For the Right to End-of-Life Care*, Baltimore, Johns Hopkins University Press, 2002.

Tom Beauchamp, ed., *Intending Death: The Ethics of Assisted Suicide and Euthanasia,* Upper Saddle River, NJ, Prentice-Hall, 1996.

Timothy Quill and Margaret Pabst Battin, eds. *Physician-Assisted Dying: The Case for Palliative Care and Patient Choice*, Baltimore, Johns Hopkins University Press, 20.

R. Steinbrook, "Physician-Assisted Death—From Oregon to Washington State," *New England Journal of Medicine* 359:24, 11 December 2008, pp. 2513–2515.

Susan Okie, "Dr. Pou and the Hurricane: Implications for Patient Care During Disasters," *New England Journal of Medicine*, 358:1, 3 January 2008.

DISCUSSION QUESTIONS

1. If you were Anna Pou and believed no rescue was coming for your nine patients, would you have done the same as she did?
2. Almost all the patients who died in Oregon and Washington have been white and educated. Why do you think other types of people didn't use the law?
3. If physicians were on salary rather than being paid per procedures, would more terminal patients be killed quicker?
4. Do views about physician-assisted killing depend on whether you think humans are basically selfish and sinful or good and compassionate?
5. Does the doctrine of terminal sedation (double effect) make sense? Can anyone really know what is in someone else's mind?

CHAPTER 4

Abortion

The Trial of Kenneth Edelin

This chapter discusses abortion and its history prior to its legalization by the U.S. Supreme Court in 1973, the controversial case of Kenneth Edelin who aborted a late-term fetus the same year, subsequent legal developments, and ethical issues about abortion. It also discusses the 1973 *Roe v. Wade* and 1992 *Casey* decisions, as well as controversial fetal experiments in the 1970s, fetal and fetal-tissue research, and emergency contraception (Plan B).

The essential question for this chapter concerns the morality of abortion.

KENNETH EDELIN'S CONTROVERSIAL ABORTION

The case of Kenneth Edelin began in Boston in October 1973. To understand it, we must understand events that happened several months earlier that year, in January, when the U.S. Supreme Court legalized abortion in *Roe v. Wade*.

Researchers had earlier performed experiments on to-be-aborted fetuses at Boston City Hospital, where Edelin served as chief resident in obstetrics. Some physicians reasoned this way: Since aborted fetuses were going to die anyway, why not use them in experiments to help other fetuses?

This reasoning creates controversy in many quarters in ethics. If unclaimed, runaway pets will be killed after three days in the pound, why not use them in medical experiments to help humans and other dogs? If terminal patients are going to die anyway, why not enlist their consent in testing new drugs or procedures? Most infamously, Nazi physicians reasoned that if Jews were going to die anyway in concentration camps, why not use them in medical experiments? (See Chapter 8, Research on Animals and Chapter 9, Research on Human Subjects.)

This research studied substances ingested by the mother that might harm the fetus. To determine which drugs crossed the placenta, physicians gave women undergoing abortions the antibiotics clindamycin and erythromycin and also examined aborted fetuses. They discovered that these antibiotics crossed the placenta and concentrated in fetal livers.

In another study in 1973, researchers tried to develop an artificial placenta. They obtained eight fetuses by hysterotomy weighing between 300 and 1,000 grams. When researchers placed the largest of them in a warm saline solution that mimicked the amniotic sac, it gasped frantically and moved its limbs as it died.[1] In another experiment on lack of glucose to the brain, researchers severed heads of 12 nonviable fetuses after stopping their hearts but before anoxia damaged their brains. The researchers successfully maintained the fetal brains with artificial replacements for glucose.[2]

An article describing the first experiment appeared in June 1973 in the *New England Journal of Medicine*, a publication edited in Boston.[3] Boston Catholics received copies of it in the mail.

Protestant theologian Paul Ramsey called such experimentation "unconsented-to research on unborn babies" and exploitation of a "tragic case of dying" babies.[4] These experiments outraged Americans. After publicity about them in 1975, Congress banned all federally funded research involving fetuses, and because it did not know where to draw a line, also banned funding of research involving human embryos.

A councilman held a hearing in September 1973 to investigate the experiments on fetuses. During it, antiabortionists packed the auditorium to hear Mildred Jefferson, an African-American assistant professor of surgery at Boston University, who opposed abortion. At his trial, she testified against Edelin.

Jefferson testified that some women undergoing abortion in a study at Boston City Hospital were too young to consent legally and had not consented in writing. If the researchers had failed to obtain legal consent, they could be charged with grave robbing, illegally procuring bodies for medical experimentation.

As a result of these hearings, nothing happened to the researchers or to Boston City Hospital, who continued to experiment on fetuses. But Catholic Bostonians festered about legalized abortion. In this milieu in late 1973, Edelin performed a controversial abortion at Boston City Hospital.

Kenneth Edelin was 35 years old and the son of a postman. He grew up poor in Washington, D.C. After undergraduate work at Columbia University, he received his M.D. from Meharry Medical College, interned in Ohio, and then served for three years as a U.S. Air Force physician. In 1971, he began his residency at Boston City Hospital, known as a public hospital for poor people and the model for the television show *St. Elsewhere*. When the case occurred, he had just become the first black chief resident in OB/GYN in the hospital's history.

"Alice Roe" is a pseudonym for a 17-year-old black West Indian student from Roxbury, a poor suburb of Boston, who decades later Edelin called "Evonne." Edelin's faculty supervisor, Hugh Holtrop, examined Evonne, estimating her to be 22 weeks pregnant. Enrique Giminez, a first-year resident from Mexico, estimated her to be 24 weeks pregnant (Giminez later testified against Edelin); a third-year medical student, Steve Teich, who assisted during the abortion, agreed with Giminez's estimate. At the time, the underfunded hospital had no ultrasound machine and could not make a more precise estimate.

Even though Holtrop had admitted Evonne, and although a late second trimester fetus was involved, he delegated third-year resident Edelin to perform the abortion. Like most attending physicians at this hospital, Holtrop had a private practice and spent little time at the hospital, so third-year residents normally did this kind of surgery.

To complicate matters, Holtrop had obtained Evonne's and her mother's permission for another fetal experiment, this time to see if aminoglutethamide increased the hormone output of the placenta. Accordingly, Holtrop gave Evonne aminoglutethamide intravenously and analyzed her urine over the next 24 hours. His study took place on October 1–2, 1973.

Edelin planned to abort the fetus by injecting saline solution into the amniotic sac, but the next day, when he inserted a needle to sample her amniotic fluid, he drew blood. This indicated that Evonne had an anterior placenta, one attached to the front wall of her uterus. Saline injected into the placenta could travel into her bloodstream, where it could be lethal.

So Edelin rescheduled the abortion as a hysterotomy for the next day. A hysterotomy is abortion by caesarean surgery and involves cutting through the lower abdominal wall. Instead of Giminez, Edelin chose as his assistant the third-year medical student Teich. However, Giminez watched the hysterotomy anyway, uninvited, from a distance.

What happened next is controversial. Giminez later testified that Edelin made the cesarean section, reached in, cut the placenta from the abdominal wall, waited three minutes, and then removed a dead fetus. If such a wait took place, it is important, because a baby cannot breathe on its own inside the uterus: it begins breathing only when it is brought outside. Edelin would soon be charged with neglecting the baby by not removing it immediately, causing it to suffocate.

Afterward, someone took the fetus to the morgue, and—as required by hospital policy for aborted fetuses weighing more than 600 grams—preserved it in formalin. This meant that the district attorney had a body for the crime and photographs of it to show a jury.

THE CASE IN THE COURTS

A grand jury decided that enough evidence existed to indict Edelin. Newman Flanagan, the prosecuting district attorney, was known as a competent, tough showman; Edelin's trial lawyer, William Perkins Homans, Jr., a rich Bostonian, often defended unpopular causes. Judge James McGuire presided.

Flanagan charged Edelin with manslaughter, defined in Massachusetts as "wanton, reckless" omission or commission of an act which causes death; Massachusetts law further defined "wanton, reckless" conduct as "the legal equivalent of intentional conduct" and as "disregard of the probable consequences to the rights of others." Judge McGuire told the jury: "The essence of wanton or reckless conduct is the doing of an act or the omission to act where there is a duty to act, which commission or omission involves a high degree of likelihood that substantial harm will result to another."[5]

Massachusetts did not pass an abortion law until August 1974 (19 months after *Roe v. Wade*), and in the absence of a specific state law, Judge McGuire instructed the jury that *Roe v. Wade* was "absolutely controlling." Since *Roe v. Wade* emphasized with viability, the jury thought it had to determine whether Evonne's fetus had been viable (whether this is true will be discussed later).

The Supreme Court had said only that viability is "usually" placed at 24 to 28 weeks, not that viability necessarily falls within that range. It had not specified how to determine whether a late-term fetus was viable. In Evonne's case, if the fetus was not viable, no person had been killed; and if no person had been killed, a manslaughter charge could not be brought.

Edelin testified that the procedure he performed on Evonne had seemed long to Giminez because at this stage of pregnancy, the thick abdominal wall had not yet stretched enough to be easily cut. Because he considered it safer than a vertical incision and because it would leave less of a scar, Edelin said he had made a Pfannenstiel ("bikini") incision. One surgeon commenting on the case wrote that making such an incision would take a while, especially for a resident who had never done one before, but not three minutes.[6] Edelin testified that Giminez had confused the initial abdominal incision with the second incision detaching the placenta.

Over the angry objection of defense attorney Homans, district attorney Flanagan introduced a picture of the fetus as evidence. Homans argued that the picture would be inflammatory and would tell laypersons nothing about fetal viability. Judge McGuire allowed one picture to be shown, but charged the jury with not viewing it "from any emotional point of view."[7]

When Flanagan summed up, he argued that when Edelin cut the placenta, the fetus had been viable and hence a person; that Edelin had waited three minutes; that this delay constituted "wanton, reckless conduct"; that legal abortion was not intended to produce a dead fetus, but merely to end a pregnancy, and therefore that Edelin should have saved the viable fetus (which Flanagan said had been live-born) before cutting its placenta.

Judge McGuire instructed the jury that an unborn fetus was not a person and could not be the subject of a manslaughter indictment. Such an indictment could refer only to a person, which Massachusetts law defined as a fetus that has been born, *a baby*. Birth was the key event, and the judge instructed the jury: "You must be satisfied beyond a reasonable doubt . . . that the defendant caused the death of a person who had been alive outside the body of his or her mother."

So the jury had to decide: (1) Had Evonne's fetus been alive outside her body? (2) If so, did the baby die as a result of "wanton, reckless conduct" by Edelin? The jurors said "yes" to both points and convicted Edelin of manslaughter.

Judge McGuire sentenced Edelin to a year of probation. If this conviction and sentence had stuck, he would have lost his medical license.

The Massachusetts Supreme Court heard Edlelin's appeal on direct review. Meanwhile, Boston City Hospital offered him a permanent position.

In 1976, more than three years after Edelin had aborted Evonne's fetus, the top Massachusetts court overturned his conviction, declaring that no evidence of criminal negligence had been presented at his trial. The high court said, "In the comparative calm of appellate review, the essential proposition emerges that the defendant had no evil frame of mind, was actuated by no criminal purpose, and committed no wanton or reckless act in carrying out the medical procedures on Oct. 3, 1973."[8] Because its judges split about abortion and the case, the Court did not require a new trial but simply acquitted Edelin.

Upon hearing of his acquittal, Edelin was "jubilant." He said, "It's great to be able to smile again after two-and-a-half years."[9] In his television news program that evening, anchor Walter Cronkite triumphantly announced that Edelin had been acquitted of "manslaughter by abortion."[10]

William Nolen, a surgeon-writer who carefully examined the evidence in the case, concluded that the fetus had not been outside the womb, had not been born, and thus there should have been no manslaughter charge.[11] Nolen's concluded so not only as a surgeon but also as someone who opposed abortion.

For the ethics of abortion, Nolen believed that Edelin had intended to abort a late fetus and once he had opened Evonne, had been surprised to find her fetus viable. Nolen doesn't say that Edelin suffocated the fetus, but he does say that whether a newborn has a will to live can be known only if the physician takes it out of the womb, slaps it, and helps it to breathe:

> What is disturbing in the Roe case is that, by his own admission, Edelin made no attempt to see if the child had that spark. As [Jeffrey] Gould [another physician who testified] said, the will to live isn't always immediately apparent; it becomes obvious only if "the physician will try to stimulate, will try to give a little bit of oxygen, and look for a favorable response. . . ."
>
> The Roe baby wasn't given this bit of provocation that might—just might—have shown it had the will to live. Why? The answer is distressingly simple. No one wanted the Roe baby to live.[12]

Interestingly, both Newman Flanagan and Kenneth Edelin worked in Boston for the next three decades. Newman was one of the longest-serving district attorneys in America. Edelin chaired both OB/GYN at Boston City Hospital and the same department at Boston University School of Medicine. He later became Chairman of the Board of Planned Parenthood Federation of America. (A 2008 tribute to him by Planned Parenthood can be seen on YouTube, as can the famous anti-abortion video, "The Silent Scream.")

BACKGROUND: PERSPECTIVES ON ABORTION

The Language of Abortion

This book uses medically accepted terms for the stages of a human life; after sperm meets egg and conception occurs, an *embryo* results, which after nine months until birth is called a *fetus*, which at birth is called a *baby*.

Definitions of these terms have legal and ethical consequences. For example, a baby can be the subject of a homicide charge, but not a fetus. Critics of abortion object to the connotation of "fetus" as a being containing less value than a baby and refer to the growing fetus as a "baby."

Abortion and the Bible

Without interpretation, the Bible or the Torah do not explicitly forbid abortion. In this regard, Paul Badham, a British professor of church history, writes:

> The Bible certainly teaches the value of human life, and forbids the murder of any human being (Psalm 8). But life, in biblical terms, commences only when the breath enters the nostrils and the man or woman becomes a "living being" (Genesis 2:7). . . . Consequently in biblical terms the fetus is not a person. This is brought out clearly in the laws relating to murder. . . . For whereas "whoever hits a man and kills him shall be put to death" (Exodus 21:12), ". . . if some men are fighting and hurt a

> woman so that she loses her child, but is not injured in any other way, the one who hurt her is to be fined." . . . And this absence of concern for the fetus is also implied by the imposition of the death penalty on women who conceive out of wedlock, without any consideration being given to the fact that this killed both the fetus and the woman (Deuteronomy 22:21, Leviticus 21:9, Genesis 38:24).[13]

Nor does Jesus explicitly speak about abortion anywhere in the Gospels.[14]

If the Old Testament or Gospels do not explicitly condemn abortion, why do some Christians reject it? The answer takes us through history.

The Old Testament took its final form during the fifth century before the Common Era (BCE) and the New Testament was finalized around the year 200 of the Common Era (CE) when Christianity began as an organized religion. Christianity has always opposed abortion, but its view of what constitutes an abortion has changed over 2,000 years.

By the fourth century CE, Christian teaching about sex was in crisis. Christianity idealized celibacy, but if too many Christians took it seriously, Christianity would die out (as the later Christian Shakers did). Practically, most people could not uphold lifelong celibacy. Consequently, Augustine revised Christian teaching to allow sexual intercourse in marriage, but only if the couple intended to have children.[15] It follows for Augustine that abortion is sinful because it thwarts the only justification for having sex: to produce a child.

In the twelfth century, Christian doctrine began to separate abortion from homicide by distinguishing between "formed" and "unformed" embryos. The concept had to do with the soul rather than with physical development.

In the thirteenth century, St. Thomas Aquinas held that God ensouled male embryos at 40 days of gestation, female embryos at 90 days. Aborting a male embryo at 40 days was punished more severely than aborting a female embryo at the same age, since the male was formed but the female was not. Although abortion at any time was sinful, penalties increased when the fetus was formed.[16]

During the nineteenth century, scientific evidence discredited the Thomistic concept of ensoulment. Microscopes revealed life at tiny stages, including human life.

In 1870, Pope Pius IX resisted the growing power of science by convening the First Vatican Council. It declared that his edicts and those of future popes would be infallible.[17] From 1869 to 1900, the Church encouraged veneration of Mary (which had been neglected), supported Creationism against geological explanations of the origins of the Earth, emphasized miracles (Fatima was recognized shortly afterwards), and vigorously attacked Darwinism.

Around 1850, popes denounced abortion in increasingly absolutistic terms. During this time, Catholicism came close to teaching that personhood began at conception, a view called *immediate animation*.[18]

The *doctrine of double effect* allowed two exceptions: ectopic pregnancy and uterine cancer (in which uterus and fetus must be removed together). According to this doctrine, an action having two effects, one good and the other evil, is morally permissible under four conditions: (1) if the action is good in itself or not evil, (2) if the good follows as immediately from the cause as from the evil effect, (3) if only the good effect is intended, and (4) if there is a proportionately grave cause for performing the action as for allowing the evil effect.

Historical Catholic doctrine was stricter than the law. During the seventeenth century, European common law did not indict women for aborting even a quickened fetus. Finally, in 1803, an English statute made abortion of a quickened fetus a capital crime.

From the seventeenth through the nineteenth centuries, American law followed English common law: Abortion before quickening was only a misdemeanor. In 1973 in its *Roe v. Wade* decision, the United States Supreme Court reviewed the legal background of abortion and concluded:

> It is thus apparent that at common law, at the time of the adopting of our Constitution, and throughout the major portion of the 19th century, . . . a woman enjoyed a substantially broader right to terminate a pregnancy than she does in most States today. At least with respect to the early stage of pregnancy, and very possibly without such a limitation, the opportunity to make this choice was present in this country well into the 19th century.[19]

In America, this leniency changed after the Civil War, when most states criminalized abortion. From 1870 to 1970, the American medical profession opposed abortion.

Feminist historians in particular argue that this opposition stemmed from paternalism, misogyny, and protecting professional turf by male physicians and men. "Anti-abortion legislation was part of an anti-feminist backlash to the growing movement for suffrage, voluntary motherhood, and other women's rights in the nineteenth century."[20]

Before the Civil War, midwives delivered most babies, and in doing so, competed with physicians over birth. After this war, physicians took over birth, and most physicians were men. So bans on abortions helped men drive midwives out of obstetrics and helped medicalize birth.

The Experience of Illegal Abortions

Before the Supreme Court legalized abortion in 1973, women who had abortions often had horrible experiences. Physicians who performed abortions often did so only for the money, and some demanded sex. Others lectured women on their promiscuity.

Though abortion is painful, abortionists didn't use anesthesia. Beforehand, physicians didn't explain to women what would happen or why. If damage occurred, women had no legal recourse. Women frequently did not know the name of the abortionist, who forbade them to contact him again. Illegal abortions were very expensive and were beyond the reach of poor women and teenagers. (And still may be: a legal abortion at 10 weeks of gestation costs on average $523 in 2009.)[21]

Despite these conditions, during the 1950s and 1960s, hundreds of thousands of American women had illegal abortions. Some died as a result: 193 died in 1965 alone, and during the 1960s, over 1,000 died.[22]

Because what they had done was illegal, victims of botched abortions came into emergency rooms only at the last moment. Some died of widespread abdominal infection, and those who recovered often were sterile. Poor women of color ran the greatest risks; in 1965, 55 percent of abortion-related deaths were among them.

1962: Sherri Finkbine

Living with her husband and their four children in Phoenix, Arizona, in 1962, Sherri Finkbine became pregnant with a fifth child.[23] During her fifth month of pregnancy, she took thalidomide, an anti-nausea drug. It was just becoming apparent then that thalidomide is a teratogen ("monster former") that produces babies with missing arms or legs. Thalidomide had been tested on animals, but not on *pregnant* animals. The tragedies it caused made the FDA test all future drugs on pregnant animals.

Sherri Finkbine requested an abortion at a local hospital, ostensibly for her health, but really to abort a fetus that would be born missing its arms and legs. However, if she had the abortion, the district attorney threatened to prosecute her, so the Finkbines flew to Sweden, where therapeutic abortion had been legal since 1940. Swedish physicians then aborted her severely deformed fetus.

1968: Humanae Vitae

In 1968, five years before *Roe v. Wade*, Pope Paul VI issued his encyclical *Humanae Vitae*, which declared use of birth control to be a sin. The edict startled liberal Catholics and drove them to defy church teachings. A quarter of a century later in 1993, Pope John Paul II vigorously defended *Humanae Vitae* and its ban on birth control.[24]

The 1968 encyclical had an unintended effect: when they were not allowed to teach both sides of the moral issues about contraception at Catholic University in Washington, D.C., which as a *magisterium*, taught only official Catholic views, Catholic priests such as Warren Reich, Albert Jonsen, William Curren, and Paul Tong left the priesthood and Catholic universities. These apostates became founders of the new field of bioethics, a field that tries to teach all sides of moral issues in medicine.

1973: *Roe v. Wade*

In the years preceding *Roe v. Wade*, 18 states liberalized laws about abortion. Hawaii began in 1970, followed by Colorado, North Carolina, and California. Governor of California Ronald Reagan signed its bill into law.

The decision of the United States Supreme Court in *Roe v. Wade* (1973) concerned Jane Roe, a woman from Dallas, Texas, whose real name was Norma McCorvey. Wade was Henry Wade, district attorney of Dallas County. When this case began in 1970, Norma McCorvey wanted a safe, legal abortion and could not get one there, so she challenged the Texas law.[25] (She later recanted and became an antiabortion advocate.)

The Supreme Court had already decided in *Griswold v. Connecticut* (1965) that the Constitution's implied right to privacy or liberty allowed couples to receive birth control pills. *Griswold* noted this kind of right in 1942 in *Oklahoma v. Skinner,* which noted a fundamental right to reproduction and control of one's body to block a law allowing involuntary sterilization of habitual criminals.

In *Roe v. Wade,* it decided that the same liberty included the right of a woman to decide whether she wanted to stay pregnant or to abort her fetus, or put differently, whether a state could pass a law prohibiting such abortions, which most had previously done.

This new right was not unqualified. A woman's right to abort her fetus was balanced against the rights of the fetus to live, which increased as its gestational age increased. The Court decided that the State's interest in protecting unborn life becomes compelling at viability, such that after that point, its interest in protecting unborn life allows states to pass laws banning most abortions.

In 1973 in *Roe v. Wade*, the Court used a trimester system to mark viability, where viability divided the second from the third trimester of fetal development. The Court defined viability as the point when a fetus is able to live outside the mother's womb. It placed viability between 24 and 28 weeks. A later decision by the same Court ignored the trimester system but retained viability as the key marker for the above purpose.

Note two things: first, a state *may* forbid abortion, but need not, in the third trimester. Second, even if states pass laws forbidding abortions in that trimester, exceptions must be allowed to preserve the *life* or *health* of the mother.

Antiabortionists argue that this permission constitutes a loophole justifying any abortion. Two physicians can almost always be found who will say that continuing the pregnancy would endanger the mother's health.

Abortion Statistics

After abortion became legal, American women had about 1.5 million abortions per year, a figure that remained steady for a decade.[26] During the last decades, the number has steadily dropped. The exact number of abortions per year is controversial. The Centers for Disease Control are required by federal law to track this number, but they rely on voluntary reporting by county and state clinics, some of which don't cooperate. The Alan Guttmacher Institute, which tracks abortion providers, has the most accurate figures. It says that in 2007, 1.2 million American women had abortions.

ETHICAL ISSUES

Edelin's Actions

Edelin waited three minutes before he removed Evonne's fetus. Even if he was innocent of any legal charge, was his behavior ethical? As Nolen said, all he had to do was remove it, slap it on the fanny, and it would have lived. If it had trouble breathing, he could have given it oxygen or technical assistance.

The baby may have been healthy and someone may have adopted it. If Evonne had wanted the baby and the baby had been born premature at this time, Edelin certainly would have done everything to keep it alive. Should a life be so precariously valued merely because a teenage mother doesn't want it?

Personhood

What is a person? With abortion, some philosophers draw a distinction between a person and a human being. They argue that although a fetus is human, it does not meet certain criteria of personhood; and that since a fetus is not a person, it does not have a right to life. In this sense, *human* is a factual term, whereas *person* is an evaluative term.

Mary Ann Warren famously defends *a cognitive criterion of personhood* and holds that a fetus does not meet this criterion.[27] According to her, to be a person is to be able to think, to be capable of cognition. What separates a person from a rat is certain capacities—for advanced reasoning, reflective self-awareness, use of language, agency, and consciousness of the external world. Warren does not think that any one of these capacities alone is sufficient for cognition; rather, these capacities define as a group the core criterion. A being lacking *all* of these capacities fails to meet the cognitive criterion and cannot be a person. So a first trimester fetus (when most abortions are done) for Warren is not a person.

Let us examine some issues concerning this cognitive criterion. To begin, the definition may be both too broad and too narrow, because it includes some nonpersons and excludes some persons. The cognitive criterion does seem to admit to personhood some beings that we don't traditionally regard as persons; for instance, some chimpanzees communicate, are conscious, may reason and may be self-aware, yet we don't ordinarily consider them persons. Perhaps, however, we are prejudiced against chimpanzees and the cognitive criterion should make us reconsider our views.

The cognitive criterion may imply that society should not protect human beings whose cognitive capacities are absent, have been lost, or that are merely potential, such as patients in the late stages of Alzheimer's disease, permanently comatose patients, or newborn babies.

A major objection to this criterion is that, if a fetus can be killed because it fails to meet the cognitive criterion, why shouldn't other beings also be killed who fail to meet it? America has thousands of patients in long-term persistent vegetative state and hundreds of thousands of elderly humans in end-stage dementia. If their cognition is gone, can they all be killed? The cognitive criterion in itself seems to say they can.

Personhood as a Gradient

Why does personhood have to be all or nothing? In practical reasoning, the all-or-nothing fallacy consists of treating complex issues as if they have only two simplistic, extreme answers when in fact there are many compromises in between. Often, practical solutions reside not on black or white poles but in gray areas in the middle.

Biologically, we know that the human embryo develops by degrees during the first trimester into a fetus, and then over the next trimester, the fetus grows into viability, and finally, during the last trimester, into a baby. No one event or day along this nine-month journey marks *the* day of personhood. The most accurate view is that personhood accumulates by degrees over time.

According to this view, a two-year-old is more of a person than a newborn baby, and a 26-year-old at the height of his powers and health is more of a person than a two-year-old. If personhood depends on capacities, then a human at maximal capacities is more of a person than a human with few capacities.

At the end of life, people lose personhood by degrees, especially with diseases that rob them of their minds. A 90-year-old man who once had an I.Q. of 140 is only "half the man he once was" with initial Alzheimer's and an I.Q. of 70.

We think of personhood as all or nothing for two reasons. First, some people believe that a metaphysical event occurs in which human bodies get ensouled or where a soul departs. Before that event, there is no personhood and no moral value, and after that event, it is there.

Second, people confuse personhood with moral concern. If granddad with Alzheimer's at 90 is only half the person he once was, that does not mean that his caretakers owe him only half the concern given to a complete person. Just the opposite: humans who have lost their former capacities need *more* concern and care than persons at maximal capacity. Who a full person is differs from whom we care about.

That's true for nonhuman animals, too. Some of them may be half-persons, especially as they function in our family. Some family pets may be as high on a family's scale of concern as its children.

In biology, the gradient view expresses human evolution by degrees from other primates, and primates in turn from lesser organisms. All life is an evolving continuum, connected by common ancestors and by degrees, not huge leaps.

Nevertheless, the gradient doesn't solve all problems at the margins of personhood. If humans at end-stage Alzheimer's have lost 99 percent of their cognition, can they be killed? If baboons share 99 percent of genes with humans, are they also persons? If not, why not?

Marquis and Quinn on Potentiality

If we accept the cognitive criterion, a problem arises. If what makes people valuable is cognition, is it wrong to deprive beings of potential cognition? And wouldn't deprivation of potential cognition make abortion wrong?

Philosophers Don Marquis and Warren Quinn offer a powerful argument against abortion. They start with two premises: first, what is wrong about killing a person—a college student, for example—is depriving him or her of future cognitive experiences; second, what is wrong about killing an adult person is also what is wrong about killing a human fetus.[28]

Their argument is an interesting one, and many people accept their first premise. Other explanations of why it is wrong to kill a person—that killing violates a person's rights, for instance, or that killing is against God's will—beg the question: phrases such as "violation of rights" and "against the will of God" are simply other ways of saying that an act is wrong.

As for the second premise, it does seem that what is wrong with killing a competent, adult human is that such an adult strongly desires to go on living, and his family strongly desires this too, and when he is killed, all these people have their desires thwarted. Moreover, because almost everyone in society wants to continue living, the murder of anyone threatens us all and makes us skeptical of society's ability to protect us.

But can a being like an early fetus, without an already existing self or personal identity, have a personal future of which to be deprived? Marquis's and Quinn's second premise may be vulnerable to attack.

Consider an analogy: Imagine an omnipotent deity—God—who creates a universe, then considers creating a second parallel universe but decides against it. Now imagine a powerful evil force—Satan—who wants to destroy the existing universe. It seems that destruction of the existing world by Satan would be wrong; but it does not seem wrong for God to refrain from creating a second world. Although God has disallowed a vast amount of cognitive experiences in the parallel universe, he has neither done any wrong nor wronged any person in not creating it. In the same way, failing to allow the potential cognition of a human fetus to come into existence wrongs no existing person.

Still, it is easy to imagine oneself as a fetus and grieving if one had been aborted and not come into existence. But is this fair? Doesn't it put one's "self" erroneously into the picture when, by definition, that self never existed?

What about contraception or masturbation? This objection is intended as a *reductio ad absurdum* of the idea that we should bring into existence beings with future cognitive experiences. As either of these prevents potential persons from coming into existence, are they wrong? Probably not. They seem to be a straw man—a false opponent, too easily refuted. No antiabortionist wants to produce billions of extra people and once conception occurs, things do seem different as a distinct human life has started.

Indeed, pro-life champions see each particular person as valuable from conception. Federal judge John Noonan advocates a genetic criterion, and argues that when sperm and egg meet and merge genes, a genetically unique individual is created. The resulting embryo has all the potential in its DNA to be a full person, provided that it finds a nurturing uterus.[29] This seems to be the root idea behind the objection to using human embryos in medical research, or using them as little factories to make embryonic stem cells.

But is *potential* to become a person the same as being a person? What about the thousands of frozen embryos stored around the world? If some woman doesn't adopt them and implant them in her uterus, they will eventually deteriorate and die. Are we thus allowing thousands of "persons" to die by lack of adoption?

Another problem with the genetic criterion is that it collapses the distinction between being human and being a person as we realize when we consider that a brain-dead human has a unique set of genes. Moreover, through human cloning, 99.9 percent of his genes could be replicated one day, and would that imply that he has been 99.9 percent resurrected? That's unlikely, because what most of us want by immortality is not for our genes to continue but for ourselves to do so, i.e., our memories and our present desires that exist in that bundle of perceptions we call "ourselves." So these implications seem to be a *reductio ad absurdum* of the genetic criterion.

A third possible criterion for personhood might be called the *neurological criterion*. This minimal version of the cognitive criterion defines a person as a human being with a detectable brain wave. This simple standard applies to many issues of medical ethics; it recognizes as persons both quasi-anencephalic babies and adults in persistent vegetative states. With regard to abortion, the neurological criterion would consider a fetus a person when it developed brain waves, but not before (a fetus develops brain waves at about 25 weeks).

Viability

The concept of viability is vague. A vague concept is one with no sharp boundaries, e.g., baldness. When does viability begin? In *Roe v. Wade*, the Supreme Court said only that viability is "usually placed" at about 28 weeks, but "may occur earlier, even at 24 weeks."

In Edelin's trial, district attorney Newman Flanagan seized on this vagueness and tried to establish that Evonne's fetus had been viable. One antiabortion physician testified that a baby could live outside the womb after as little as 12 weeks of gestation. But for how long? Only a few minutes, the physician testified, though maybe for longer. However, the defense attorney, William Homans, counterpunched by asking the physician how he defined viability; the physician said that viability was "capacity to survive [outside the womb] even for a second after birth." As Homans questioned several other physicians who were testifying as expert witnesses for the prosecution, he got each of them to admit that he had never known a fetus to survive for even a few days outside the womb before 24 weeks of gestation.

Remember that legally, viability didn't ultimately matter in this case. Even if the fetus was viable, if it didn't exist outside the womb, there could be no legitimate charge of manslaughter.

On the other hand, legality isn't ethics. Viability matters a lot more to ethics. It's one thing to abort at 13 weeks a tiny fetus with no chance of living on its own; it's quite another at 24 or 26 weeks when continued life is possible. That's one reason why many physicians who do abortions don't perform such late-stage ones.

Edelin's critics knew exactly what was meant by viability: ability to survive independently of the mother. In reality, some fetuses that are born early are not viable: They will die no matter how hard physicians try to keep them alive. Others will survive and will do only if given the chance to live.

To Edelin's opponents, the point was that he had never tried to determine viability. His supporters replied that of course he had not tried because *the whole point* of abortion is to kill a fetus. The point is not to look inside the uterus, see if the fetus is viable, and if it is, rescue it. No, the goal of abortion is to produce a dead fetus.

The Argument from Marginal Cases

In the Edelin case, one question that arose was, "Where do you draw the line?"—that is, the line between fetuses which may and may not be aborted. Reasoning based on this kind of question is called the *argument from marginal cases*, and it is one of the most widely used ideas in ethics.

With abortion, the argument from marginal cases is as follows: Beings at the margins of personhood cannot be nonarbitrarily distinguished from those at the core. If it's wrong to kill a newborn baby, it's wrong to kill it the day before it's born, and so on, being wrong to kill the growing being any time after conception.

This argument can appeal to a gradient of personhood. Where pro-choice advocates say an embryo is not a baby, antiabortionists point to the smooth continuum and say there is no place to draw the line. No matter what week of gestation we consider, it is arbitrary to make that week the marker of personhood, because the fetus of a week earlier has almost the same qualities. Whatever time or marker is chosen, someone can always ask: Why not choose a day before?

Is the argument from marginal cases a good one? Consider an analogy with the color spectrum: although each shade in the spectrum resembles the shades next to it, we can distinguish colors from widely separated colors. Similarly, a full-grown oak tree differs from an acorn, even though an acorn becomes an oak by continuous growth. Similarly, we can distinguish an eight-cell human embryo from a newborn baby. Marginal cases do not make distinctions impossible.

In *Roe v. Wade*, the Court said that in the first two trimesters, the interests of competent adults to control their bodies outweigh the growing interests of the fetus to live. But it could have equally stressed a continuum of development for the fetus, back from birth to embryo, such that the fetus has some rights in the second trimester, as only very strong reasons justify abortions then. Especially with abortions available now in the first trimester, and with genetic screening available for many common conditions, second semester abortions seem less justified, as the fetus then has more of those qualities that make it somewhat of a person under the cognitive criterion or gradient.

Thomson: A Limited Pro-Choice View

Suppose we admit that the fetus in the Edelin case was a person. Does it follow that killing it was immoral? Philosopher Judith Jarvis Thomson argues that it was not.[30]

Imagine you have been admitted to a hospital for an operation, and awaken to find yourself hooked up to a famous violinist. His kidneys have failed and his blood is entering and leaving your body through tubes. Without your permission, your kidneys have been used to keep the violinist alive.

Thomson argues that it is immoral for the hospital to force you to keep the violinist alive. Although it would be saintly of you to agree, you are not *obligated* to do so. Why? Because you did not consent to have your body burdened this way and no one else has a right to make you use your body to keep another person alive.

Just as the violinist cannot demand as a right that you keep him alive by allowing your kidneys to be used, so too, a fetus has no right that a woman keep it alive. For Thomson, the most telling case is rape, because a rape victim has not consented to sexual intercourse or conceiving a child. She thinks a similar argument applies when a woman has used contraception responsibly but it fails.

Thomson's argument is an example of reasoning by analogy. The violinist's dependence on the other patient is analogous to the fetus's dependence on the mother. In analogical reasoning, the closer the fit between the two things compared, the stronger the inferred conclusion is supported.

Critics such as philosopher Francis Kamm object to Thomson's analogy. They argue that the patient who is being involuntarily used can simply unhook herself, and that detaching tubes from your body is not like killing a fetus. Since something active must be done to end a fetus's life, for a proper analogy, the violinist would have to be blocking the patient's way out of the room, so that the patient could escape only by cutting up the violinist.[31] (Better: imagine a gigantic baby blocking the way out.)

The above arguments suggest abortion as self-defense. In the sixteenth century, theologian Thomas Sanchez used Augustine's doctrine of just war to identify an embryo growing in a fallopian tube as an unjust aggressor against the mother's life. So Sanchez maintained that a mother could kill such a lethal embryo in self-defense.[32]

Feminist Views

One feminist writer argues that the key question about abortion is whether women should be forced to bear children in a way in which men are not. If an embryo is a person who has a right to life at the mother's expense, then women will always be potential slaves of biological reproduction:

> With all the imperfections of our present-day attitudes, I'm still a lot better off in terms of the sexual choices I have than women of my mother's generation. I was a lot better off after the sixties than I was before then. What sexual freedom I now have has been very hard-won. I wouldn't give it up for anything. . . . There is a larger crisis, one that has to do with the tensions between feminism and the backlash against it. On the one hand, society is encouraging sexual freedom; on the other hand, it's punishing people for indulging in it and not emotionally preparing them for it. Both women in general and teenagers in particular are caught in the middle.[33]

"God Must Mean for Me to Be Pregnant, Else I Wouldn't Be"

Some people believe that each human pregnancy happens for a reason. Each human embryo that has been conceived and survived to implant itself in the uterine wall was meant by God to have been created at this place and time. Any interference with the growth of that embryo would thwart God's plans. As one sometimes hears, "God must mean for me to be pregnant, else I wouldn't be."

Two replies can be made to this view. First, how does a woman know God's will about a particular pregnancy? Unless God speaks to her directly, how can she just assume that planning when to have children is not God's will for her? How does she know that God does not want her to do what she believes will be best for her, now and in the future?

Second, such a view is fatalistic in one's personal relation to God. It seems reasonable to ask, "Why must I accept everything that happens? If everything comes from God, doesn't the choice to have an abortion also come from Him? Why make the fatalistic assumption that one can follow God's will only by accepting pregnancy? Why can't a reasoned choice to have an abortion also reflect God's will?"

A Culture of Life or a Culture of Death?

By 2008, after 35 years of legalized abortion, and with at least 1.2 million abortions a year, American women aborted at least 40 million human fetuses. Pro-life champions argue that such easy access to abortion has started to create a "culture of death," one that has increased with the legalization of assisted suicide for terminally ill patients in Oregon and Washington.

As we noted in Chapters 1 and 3, it is easy to push a false notion of autonomy that masks underlying prejudicial structures and scarcities of resources for the disabled, or lack of treatment of symptoms for the dying, especially depression and boredom. Too often, death seems the easy way out.

Take the Edelin case. He did not have to produce a dead baby. He could have saved the viable fetus and Evonne could have given it up for adoption. She had a right to have the fetus removed from her body, not to a dead fetus.

Since World War II and the Great Depression, America has had no great crisis, but that could always change in the future. Is our culture ready? If millions of baby boomers need long-term care, will the culture provide for them or urge them to take an early "final exit"? Society's pendulum has moved too much toward Death; it needs to swing back toward Life.

Suppose that for the last 35 years, no opposition to abortion had existed. What might have happened? Abortion would be much more easily available, with perhaps every small city having a clinic and competition bringing down prices. Instead of 40 million abortions, we might have had 400 million. Would that have been a good thing?

Catholicism, conservative Protestanism, Islam, and Orthodox Judaism oppose the easy availability of abortion as accelerating a culture of death. Are they not right to say, "This involves who we are and we must oppose this?" Aren't hospitals affiliated with such religions within their rights not to provide abortions? As such, shouldn't they witness as good citizens for their core values? Just as Jews are horrified that so many stood by passively when 6,000,000 Jews were killed in concentration camps, shouldn't others be horrified that 40,000,000 fetuses never got a chance to live?

Abortion as a Three-Sided Issue

Many people living in a tolerant democracy where individual liberties are respected fail to understand how they got where they are or to understand the larger, worldwide picture. In the United States, they forget that our modern policy of individual rights and personal liberty represents a hard-won victory that citizens of many other countries never achieved.

For instance, if they became pregnant before their midtwenties or after they already had a child, beginning in 1979—when the government imposed a limit of one child per family—thousands of women in China underwent forced abortions—a practice that continues today in rural China. In Romania, the dictator Nicolae Ceaucescau denied millions of women contraception or abortions because he wanted a larger population.

Perhaps this ignorance explains why the media frame abortion as an issue with only two sides: antiabortion versus pro-choice. In fact, the global picture of abortion is three-sided, with two extremes and a compromise: *forced birth* versus *forced abortion,* with individual choice as the middle ground.

Antiabortion Protests and Violence

During the 1980s, two Texans attacked several abortion clinics in Florida. In 1984, protestors bombed or burned 24 abortion clinics, including one in Pensacola, Florida, that took place on Christmas morning and was described by one conspirator as a "birthday present to Jesus."[34]

By 1990, public opinion had turned against antiabortion violence. As a result, the antiabortion movement turned to *Operation Rescue*, an organization founded by Randall Terry in 1988. Modeling themselves on the nonviolent demonstrations in the South during the Civil Rights Movement, protesters practiced civil disobedience in front of abortion clinics. Police jailed some for blocking traffic. During the 1990s, the movement also targeted physicians who performed abortions, often picketing their homes.

Yet some still killed in the name of stopping abortions. Physician David Gunn was killed in 1993 as he left an abortion clinic in Pensacola, Florida. In 1994, antiabortionist Paul Hill, a former minister, killed physician John Britton and his security escort as they left another abortion clinic in Pensacola. In 2003, Florida executed Hill for the murder.

In January 1998, an explosion rocked the campus at the University of Alabama at Birmingham. Across the street at the Ronald McDonald House and a block away at a dorm, windows shook from the blast. When he touched the package outside the small abortion clinic, Robert Sanderson, an off-duty Birmingham policeman, was killed. When the dynamite inside exploded, hundreds of nails ricocheted off a steel plate inside into the face, torso, and legs of Emily Lyons, a nurse at the clinic, and into Sanderson. Due to intense efforts a few blocks away at the UAB hospital, Lyons survived.

An alert UAB student spotted Eric Rudolph leaving the scene and police searched for him for five years in the hills of North Carolina. Arrested in 2003, he confessed in 2005 to bombing abortion clinics in Birmingham and Atlanta, to bombing gay/lesbian nightclubs, and to bombing the Centennial Olympic Park during the 1996 Olympics, where he killed 3 people and injured 111 others.

In 1998, antiabortionist James Koop crouched behind the backyard fence with a high-powered rifle and shot Dr. Barnett Slepian through his kitchen window. During the previous four years, snipers also shot and wounded three Canadian physicians. In 2009, physician George Tiller was killed in his church in Wichita, Kansas. Both Slepian and Tiller had been targeted by antiabortion groups for decades and had vowed to continue providing abortions.

Live Birth Abortions and How Abortions Are Done

Attempts to abort late-term fetuses have sometimes resulted in live births. In 1977, physician Ronald Cornelson testified in a California criminal court that after a botched saline abortion resulted in a live-born 2 1/2-pound baby, his colleague William Waddill had choked the infant and suggested injecting it with potassium chloride to kill it.[35] Waddill was tried twice for murder, but both juries deadlocked. In 1979, at the University of Nebraska Medical Center, after an attempted abortion, another 2 1/2-pound baby was born alive; it was purposefully left unattended and died after a few hours.

Because of such cases, physicians today rarely abort a fetus after 23 weeks. Today, physicians doing abortions rarely use prostaglandins to induce abortion because, although safer than suction or surgical techniques, they result in 30 times more live births.

For first trimester abortions, the most typical technique was formerly injection of saline or urea, followed by dilatation and curettage (scraping, a technique called D & C); a process now replaced by suction curettage or uterine aspiration. Most abortions are done in the first trimester.

For late-term abortions, dilatation and evacuation (D & E) is used: The fetus is cut into parts and removed piecewise. To ensure that all the pieces have been removed—since any fragments left behind would produce infection in the mother—the dismembered fetus must be reassembled outside the womb. Late second trimester or third trimester abortions use hysterotomy, as in the Edelin case.

Because abortion is controversial, residency programs in obstetrics sometimes offer no training in performing abortion. Some residents in obstetrics have demanded such training.[36]

In 2005, a review of several hundred scientific papers concluded that nerve connections in the fetal brain are not developed enough before 29 weeks for the fetus to feel pain.[37] As such, the authors concluded, aborting a fetus before this point caused it no pain and no anesthesia need be used to spare the fetus pain.

Fetal Tissue Research

Tissue from aborted fetuses may help patients with neurological disorders such as Parkinson's disease. The tissue required for such neurological research must be adrenal tissue producing dopamine, and it must be obtained from fetuses whose gestational age is 8 to 11 weeks, since after 12 weeks the tissue begins to differentiate into the normal cells of the brain and loses its elasticity. Treatment consists of dopamine delivered as fetal cells: In the operation, a small hole is drilled through the patient's skull and fetal cells are dripped directly into the devastated area of the brain.

A panel of the National Institutes of Health studied this issue and concluded that even if abortion were immoral, fetal tissue obtained from abortions could be used for research if the woman's decision to donate tissue was separated from, and came after, her decision to abort.[38] In 1993, President Clinton lifted the four-year ban on fetal tissue research.

Emergency Contraception

In America, the traditional approach to preventing pregnancy has been either abstinence or contraception, with abortion as a backup for failures. A middle ground exists between these extremes.

Emergency contraception has been used without publicity for 35 years in America. It consists of taking a double dose of birth-control pills within 72 hours after an act of unprotected sex, followed by a second dose 12 hours later.[39] When the first dose is taken within 72 hours after unprotected sex, emergency contraception reduces the risk of pregnancy by 75–90 percent.

Such pills contain estrogen and/or progesterone and block the release of the egg from the ovary, block the movement of the embryo down the fallopian tube, or prevent implantation of the embryo in the endometrium.

Emergency contraception either requires a woman to have birth control pills on hand or to be able to obtain them within 72 hours after unprotected sex. A woman cannot wait for a pregnancy test because her urine changes chemically only after embryonic implantation.

In 2006, the FDA approved Plan B, a progestin-only form of emergency contraception, for over-the-counter sales to women over 18. In the year after this change, sales of Plan B surged. In 2009, a federal judge ordered the FDA to approve the same for 17-year-old women.

The American Medical Association defines pregnancy as beginning when the embryo implants on the uterine wall, but not all physicians accept that definition. Some believe that pregnancy begins with conception in the fallopian tubes, and as such, refuse to prescribe IUDs, which interfere with implantation.

In 2005, pharmacists at a Walgreens in Illinois refused to fill prescriptions for Plan B, as did some employees at Wal-Mart pharmacies. Since Plan B blocks implantation of a fertilized embryo, these pharmacists considered Plan B to be an abortion agent.

Women physicians successfully sued Walgreens and Wal-Mart to make Plan B available by prescription at all of its pharmacies. Walgreens then fired pharmacists who refused to fill prescriptions for Plan B, igniting a debate about conscientious refusal of pharmacists to fill prescriptions.

Maternal versus Fetal Rights

Nancy Klein was in her 20s in 1989 when she went into a coma at an early stage of her pregnancy. Her physicians wanted to abort her fetus to increase her cerebral blood volume and to awaken her. They were also reluctant to give Nancy certain drugs that might injure a fetus brought to term. Antiabortionists went to court to block the abortion, while Nancy Klein's husband, Martin, pressed for it. Martin prevailed and the abortion was performed while people protested outside. After 11 months, Nancy emerged from the coma and now lives a normal life.

In 1985, Angela Carder in Washington, D.C., was dying of a rare form of cancer and had requested chemotherapy and resisted a cesarean section to save her 26-week-old fetus. The baby was delivered alive anyway, but died two hours later. Angela died two days later.[40]

Both cases raised the issue of who the patient was, the mother or the fetus. Legally, the answer is clear. A fetus inside the womb is not a baby and not a person, but the mother is, so her wishes and her health trump the good of the fetus. But ethically, things become murky *if* either the mother is going to die or *if* the fetus is going to be born. But both cases above show that these "ifs" are often difficult to know.

A flashpoint for maternal-child conflict concerns pregnant mothers using alcohol or illegal drugs. Fetal alcohol syndrome causes the most mental retardation in children.[41] Between 1987 and 1992, 160 women in 24 states were charged with injuring a fetus during pregnancy by taking drugs such as cocaine.[42]

In 1993, the law tried to force Comelia Whitner to stop using drugs for the good of her fetus, forcing her to choose between mandatory drug rehabilitation and jail. The South Carolina Supreme Court upheld the law in *Whitner v. South Carolina*.

Critics said the law prosecuted pregnant black women using cocaine, but not pregnant white women drinking alcohol, and claimed that prosecutors exaggerated harm to the fetus during gestation from cocaine. Defenders of the law estimated that 70,000 American women used cocaine while pregnant and agreed that pregnant women abusing alcohol, white or black, should also be prosecuted. Some wanted to prosecute smoking during pregnancy.

Viability

In 1983, Justice Sandra Day O'Connor predicted that medicine would push viability "further back toward conception" and that the trimester system established in *Roe v. Wade* would be on a collision course with itself. Her prediction has not come true.

Although medicine has made intense efforts to treat premature babies more effectively, the consensus in neonatology is that "before 23 or 24 weeks, [the fetus] simply cannot survive. And nothing that medical science can do will budge that boundary in the foreseeable future."[43] The unsolvable problem is that even with a respirator, the lungs are too immature to function earlier than after 23 or 24 weeks of gestation, and certain essential organs, such as the kidneys, do not develop early in pregnancy.

This recently acknowledged fact weakens one argument against abortion. Clearly, the argument from marginal cases must lose some of its force, since lung viability has served for over 30 years as a practical indicator of viability and as a mark of when a state can outlaw abortion.

In 1979, in *Colautti v. Franklin*, the Supreme Court made its major decision about viability. It said that "the determination of whether a particular fetus is viable is, and must be, a matter for the judgment of the responsible attending physician," thus precluding another case like Kenneth Edelin's.

The Supreme Court Adjusts *Roe v. Wade*

In the decades since *Roe v. Wade*, abortion-rights advocates have pressed for broader protection and antiabortion forces have mounted legal challenges to the original decision. All of this came to a head in 1992 with the Supreme Court's decision in *Planned Parenthood v. Casey*. The Court reaffirmed the "essential holding" of *Roe v. Wade*, including "the right of a woman to choose to have an abortion before viability and to obtain it without undue interference from the State."[44] This decision appeared to say, "Here we stand on abortion, and we will hear no more cases challenging it." Since then, the Court turned down cases aimed at challenging *Roe v. Wade*; however, over the last decades, it has fine-tuned this legal decision.

In 1976, in *Planned Parenthood v. Danforth*, the Court invalidated state laws requiring a woman to get consent for an abortion from either a matrimonial or a biological father. The Court held that such consent amounted to giving these men a veto over the woman's decision.

The *Danforth* decision also said that a state cannot pass a law giving parents of teenage girls an absolute veto over a decision to have an abortion. Two later decisions allowed a state, before a teenager's abortion, to require the minor to obtain the *consent* of one or both parents, or required the clinic to *notify* one or both parents. By 2006, 44 states had laws requiring a parent's consent or notification when minors sought abortions, although nine of those states did not enforce their laws.[45] Such laws had to have an escape clause where the minor could appeal to a judge for an exception to parental notification or consent.

In *Harris v. McRae* (1980), the Court held that, although a woman has a right to an abortion, she does not have a right to one at government expense. Congress passed laws banning use of public funds for abortions for women unable to afford them, and many states followed suit. *Webster* (1989) said that states may ban public employees or public hospitals from performing abortions.

In *Casey*, 1992, the Court ruled that informed consent and a 24-hour waiting period did not constitute an "undue burden" on women seeking abortions. Antiabortionists said this change brought abortion into line with informed-consent requirements for other surgical procedures. Pro-choice advocates pointed out that many surgical procedures would not occur if hospitals enforced a similar 24-hour waiting period.

As said, *Casey* signaled a pivotal affirmation of "the essential holding" of *Roe v. Wade*, that the right to abortion is grounded in the Constitution. A majority of justices repeated what a previous Court had said in *Eisenstadt v. Baird*: "If the right of privacy means anything, it is the right of the individual, married or single, to be free from unwarranted governmental intrusion into matters so fundamentally affecting a person as the decision whether to bear or beget a child."

Partial Birth Abortions

Critics define as a "partial birth abortion" one that is performed in the third trimester or especially, just before birth. The phrase connotes the advanced state of the fetus, and how, even on the gradient view, it is almost a person.

The rights of late-term fetuses arise in murders of pregnant mothers (Lacy Peterson) and abortions in the late third trimester. Killing a pregnant woman and her child is a heinous crime, and to inflict greater punishments, people push for a charge of double homicide. Similarly, few reasons justify killing a fetus after eight months of gestation, and the methods to do so are grim and surgical.

Opponents of abortion hope that everyone can agree to protect fetuses from such acts and push for changes in the law to do so. Pro-choice advocates oppose such legal changes, fearing a slippery slope to protecting the fetus from abortion at earlier stages.

State legislatures frequently have passed bills making such changes, but federal courts have struck them down 18 out of 19 times.[46] Why? Because a long legal tradition has defined a baby as created at birth, not before, with a criminal charge only being capable of being made against a baby, and courts have been reluctant to overturn that tradition. To do so would be to go into territory where there is no logical stopping point until before viability.

FURTHER READING AND RESOURCES

Kenneth Edelin, *Broken Justice*, Peterborough, U.K., Pond View Press, 2007.
Francis M. Kamm, *Creation and Abortion*, New York, Oxford University Press, 1992.
Don Marquis, "Why Abortion Is Immoral," *Journal of Philosophy* 86, 1989, pp. 183–202.

Warren Quinn, "Abortion: Identity and Loss," *Philosophy and Public Affairs* 13, 1984, pp. 24–54.
Michael Tooley, *Abortion and Infanticide*, Oxford, Oxford University Press, 1983.
Mary Ann Warren, "On the Moral and Legal Status of the Fetus," *The Monist* 57, 1973, pp. 43–61.

DISCUSSION QUESTIONS

1. If the fetus had slipped out during Edelin's procedure and been outside the womb, even attached to an umbilical cord, would it have been illegal to kill it? Should that matter *ethically*?
2. How should "pregnancy" be defined? By formation of a unique embryo in the fallopian tubes or by implantation of an embryo in the uterus?
3. How can anyone ever truly know what's in the mind of another to judge someone by the doctrine of double effect? Someone may say he's trying to save the life (or health!) of a pregnant mother, not desiring to end the life of a fetus, but who can tell? Isn't this a fault of the doctrine?
4. Fetal sonograms are now being used to give pregnant women vivid pictures of their fetuses in the first and second trimesters. Some women viewing such pictures reverse their decisions to have abortions. Given that fact, should all women planning abortions be required to view such live images?
5. Some women regret having abortions. What weight should we give such regrets in public policy about abortion?
6. Is a fetus necessarily a person at birth? What's so magical about birth? Maybe, even on a gradient view, we should not declare personhood until much later, say, six months.
7. "God must want me to be pregnant or I wouldn't be." Is this a fair view?

CHAPTER 5

Assisted Reproduction, Multiple Births, and Elderly Parents—Time to Regulate?

Between 1978, which saw the world's first "test-tube baby," and 2008, which saw "Octamom" Nadya Suleman adding eight to her brood of test-tube produced children, assisted reproduction has raised many ethical issues. This chapter discusses Louise Brown's birth, surrogate mothers, buying eggs of younger women, the McCaughey septuplets, and older women having children, such as Carmen Bousada, who died at age 69 after giving birth at 66.

The essential question for discussion is: should we regulate American fertility doctors to limit multiple babies and older women gestating babies?

ASSISTED REPRODUCTION

The Octamom and the Gosselins

Nadya Suleman, 32 years old in 2009, of Whittier, California, had six embryos left over from previous in vitro fertilization (IVF) treatments with fertility physician Michael Kamrava. She did not want the remaining embryos destroyed and underwent another cycle of IVF to have all of them implanted. Two of the six embryos split into twins, resulting in a total of eight embryos. When sonograms in the first trimester revealed at least five fetuses, Suleman refused reduction and at birth on January 26, physicians delivered eight babies.

Much criticism focused on Michael Kamrava, the physician who implanted Suleman not once but twice with six embryos. The American Society for Reproductive Medicine recommends implantation of just one embryo and permissibly, two. Since Nadya already had children from previous cycles of IVF, and since two of these children were disabled, for Kamrava to implant six more embryos was wrong and likely created even more disabled children.

The year 2009 also saw a lot of attention given to the family of Kate and Jon Gosselin. The Gosselins had deliberately created a family of twin girls (born from artificial insemination by husband [AIH] in 2000) and sextuplets (three girls and three boys) in suburban Pennsylvania. Fertility doctors started the sextuplets by injecting Kate with drugs to stimulate her ovaries (as in the McCaughey case) and afterwards introduced Jon's sperm. Informed of six pregnancies, the Gosselins chose not to reduce and all six babies were delivered by caesarean in 2004.

Jon & Kate Plus 8 filmed the controlled chaos of this family of ten and became a hit show in 2007 on cable television. Putting the kids on television also glamorized having multiple babies. Shortly after birth, a plastic surgeon did free plastic surgery to correct the distortion of Kate's stomach after gestating six babies.

In April 2009, when both had extramarital affairs, the Gosselins headed for divorce, for which they filed in June. Thereafter, Jon seemed to abandon his responsibilities as a father. Both parents seemed immature and not focused on the best interests of their eight children.

Meanwhile, Nadya Suleman wanted her own reality show and in 2009, signed papers for one. To protect her children, a California judge appointed a guardian for the children, making sure all money went for them.

Background: Louise Brown, the First Test-Tube Baby

"Test tube" conception is called IVF. ("In vitro" means "in glass.") It involves fertilization outside the womb, in a Petri dish.

Lesley Brown, the mother of the first child conceived in vitro, had damaged Fallopian tubes from ectopic pregnancies. For her IVF, one of her eggs was removed and put in a Petri dish, where doctors mixed Brown's sperm to form an embryo. Doctors then returned the embryo to Lesley's uterus and, like normal conception, Lesley gestated the embryo to birth.

For normal conception, sperm move up the vagina, through the uterus, and into one of the narrow Fallopian tubes. The two tubes, the size of the lead in a mechanical pencil, each can carry an egg from an ovary to the uterus.

A woman has all her eggs at birth, but only one egg is normally primed each month for conception. Drugs such as Clomid and Pergonal stimulate the ovaries to release more than one egg, a process called *superovulation*.

In at least 40 percent of pregnancies, and possibly as many as 70 percent, the embryo fails to implant on the wall of the uterus, often because of genetic irregularities. More commonly, the mix of hormones is not quite correct.

After one year of trying, about one married couple in 11 cannot conceive a child. Infertility stems from many factors, including a woman's age, damage from pelvic inflammatory disease, previous abortions, uterine abnormalities, and low sperm count or low sperm motility. Infertility is often blamed on the woman, but men account for 50 percent of it.

Two decades of research by Robert Edwards, a physiologist at Cambridge University, preceded the first IVF birth. Edwards worked with mice in the 1950s and learned how to precisely balance hormones to induce ovulation.

In 1965, 13 years before the birth of Louise Brown, Edwards created a human embryo one night after adding his own semen to a ripe human egg in a Petri dish.[1] Edwards thereby fulfilled one of the great fears about scientists: lone scientist late at night in his lab artificially creates human life, stealing mystery from it. Perhaps Edwards realized people would be frightened by his feat, so he destroyed the embryo. Later, he tried to repeat it, but could not. Nor did he announce to others what he had done.

In his research, Edwards needed to create many embryos and return only the healthiest to the uterus. To do so, he needed eggs and such eggs had to be removed from female volunteers. Enter Patrick Steptoe, an obscure gynecologic surgeon practicing in a small hospital near the industrial city of Manchester, who in the 1960s became Edwards's partner. Steptoe used a newly created laparascope (a long thin tube containing a lens with a light) to remove the eggs.

Over the next decade, the duo attempted IVF to create a pregnancy. In the first phase, they implanted an embryo 41 times in a Fallopian tube, but each time, it failed to go farther. In the next phase, they recruited 100 infertile female volunteers and implanted an embryo directly into the uterus of each. Their 102nd attempt resulted in the birth of Louise Brown.

In 1977, Dr. Steptoe told Lesley she was pregnant and waited to see if she would keep her fetus. Before this, a few women had had eggs successfully fertilized in vitro, but each had lost the embryo during gestation. Lesley made it to five months, and her amniocentesis showed a normal pregnancy (if it had been abnormal, Steptoe would have aborted it). She spent the last month of her pregnancy at Oldham Hospital, by then under siege by the media.

Steptoe delivered the baby, a girl, by cesarean section on July 25, 1978. In order to avoid reporters, he operated around midnight with only a few people present.

The Browns called the normal, 5 pound 12 ounce girl "Louise Joy," who the father said was "beautiful, with a marvelous complexion, not red and wrinkly at all."[2] Immediately after the birth, John Brown said, "For a person who's been told he and his wife can never have children, the pregnancy was 'like a miracle.' I felt 12 feet high."

For Louise Brown's birth, London newspapers ran huge banner headlines, "IT'S A GIRL!" "THE LOVELY LOUISE!" "BABY OF THE CENTURY! JOY TO THE WORLD!"

Some competitors, who had hoped to be first, dismissed Steptoe's achievement as a "cheap stunt." Richard Blandau, a well-known fertility researcher and a competitor, criticized Steptoe for not revealing how many failures had preceded his success and for giving "false hope to millions of women."[3] But Blandau missed the point: Louise's birth mattered not because of its improbability, but because it could be done at all.

Patrick Steptoe died at age 74 in 1988, a week before Queen Elizabeth II was to have knighted him at Buckingham Place. The same week, Robert Edwards became a Fellow of the Royal Society, a great honor in the English scientific community.

Louise Brown's mother chose to have a second child, Natalie, by IVF in 1982. In 1993, the three female Browns appeared on American television to support research in assisted reproduction. At age 15, Louise was a chubby girl whose friends teased, "How did you ever fit into a test tube?" In 2004, she married, with Edwards attending her wedding. Her naturally conceived son was born on December 20, 2006.

Harm to Research from Alarmist Media

New ways of making babies have always fascinated the media. Approaches by the media to such babies range from alarmist to naively uncritical.

Warren Kornberg, editor of *Science News*, wrote in a 1969 op-ed in the *Los Angles Times* that issues about assisted reproduction, cloning, and human genetics raised questions "more important" than those raised by nuclear weapons.[4]

In his early years, Robert Edwards worked on infertility at the National Institute for Medical Research in London. After an alarmist television show on IVF that opened with pictures of an exploding atomic bomb, the institute suspended his funding. Edwards claims that his scientific supervisor, who had also frozen sperm, flatly told him his work was "unethical"; when asked "Why?" she would say only, "Because it is."[5]

Edwards left for Cambridge University, where he worked on a Ford Foundation grant to study population control and fertility. Because his work offended some, the Ford Foundation stopped funding him in 1974.

The press incorrectly called Louise Brown a "test-tube baby." This term implied something bizarre—that a baby had been created without egg or sperm. When Lesley later took her baby outside, neighbors expected to see a little monster.

The press equated means of overcoming infertility with genetic manipulation and, as with cloning later, predicted creation of mindless slaves or dangerous superhumans. The *London Times* equated IVF with state-controlled eugenics. In contrast, John Brown saw IVF as merely "helping nature along a bit."

Newspapers and television shows constantly compared IVF to Aldous Huxley's 1932 novel *Brave New World*. Yet they were muddled: The controls that Huxley feared stemmed from psychological conditioning. *Brave New World* worries about behaviorism, a school of psychology then poorly understood as IVF was in 1978. Although *Brave New World* opposed taking away choice from citizens, people cited it to justify taking away reproductive choice from citizens.

Later Developments in Assisted Reproduction

The first IVF baby in America, Elizabeth Carr, was born in 1981. In 500 clinics, American fertility physicians now deliver about 50,000 babies a year from IVF.[6] The worldwide total is probably over a million.

Only 5 percent of babies today conceived by assisted reproductive technology (ART) result from IVF. Less dramatic techniques create most ART babies, such as egg stimulation and injection of concentrated sperm.

Unfortunately, for most of the last three decades and today, about 75 percent of couples who pay for cycles of IVF and who spend from $13,000 to $100,000 go home without a baby. In 2002, fertility clinics claimed that about 23 percent of attempts at IVF allowed couples to take home a baby, although the actual figure may be more like 20 percent.[7] Chances worsen for women over 40 and drop with each unsuccessful attempt, from 13 percent on the first to 4 percent on the fourth.[8] At age 47, chances drop to almost zero.

Sperm and Egg Transfer

Sperm Around 1850, physician J. Marion Sims, while practicing in Montgomery, Alabama, artificially inseminated 55 infertile women with their husbands' sperm (AIH).[9] He produced one pregnancy, though it later miscarried. He was forced to stop because of strident condemnation of his work.

Later in the 1890s in America, Dr. Robert Latou Dickinson was vilified for practicing AIH, although he persevered. Dickinson was accused of abetting "adultery."[10]

It took a century after Sims's first inseminations for people to accept artificial insemination (AI) of sperm. Had Sims *paid* his first sperm donors, his critics would have been legion. The net result? Hundreds, maybe thousands, of couples in America and Europe remained infertile, blaming each other for being barren, going childless not by choice but by fate, and not having heirs.

Today, most people accept insemination of sperm. Indeed, Americans have gone from accepting: (1) AIH to (2) artificial insemination of another donor's (AID) sperm into a woman's womb to (3) paying a man for use of his sperm to create a pregnancy, to (4) insemination of anonymous donor sperm into unmarried women wishing to become pregnant, to (5) selection of sperm from a catalog of pictures of men listing their achievements. Today, couples and single women can select sperm from men at about 400 sperm banks, where sperm donors receive between $50 and $75 per visit or where they have donated their sperm free.

Notice that for decades, critics rarely noted that men were paid to donate sperm, even though genetically, sperm do not differ as gametes from eggs (cells of males and females, each contain half the chromosomes necessary for sexual reproduction).

Egg Transfer Australia's Carl Woods in 1983 created the first human pregnancy from an egg transfer. In the next 15 years, 6,000 middle-aged women gave birth using eggs from young women.[11] In the 1980s, scientists began *gamete intra-Fallopian transfer (GIFT),* which unites sperm and egg not in a Petri dish but inside a Fallopian tube, approximately where normal conception takes place. A Belgian group in 1993 succeeded in using a single sperm to fertilize an egg, a process called *intracytoplasmic sperm injection (ICSI),* making it possible for one sperm to be used to achieve a pregnancy.[12]

By the 1990s, egg retrieval no longer required surgery—it could be done by tubal aspiration using ultrasound imaging.

Because of assisted conception of twins to celebrities such as Geena Davis at 48, Jane Seymour at 44, Holly Hunter at 47, and singletons in their 30s as Christie Brinkley, Angelina Jolie, and Celine Dion, today's young women too often believe they can wait to become mothers until their 30s. Most celebrities don't disclose their use of egg donors. For the average woman, only 7.8 percent at them of age 42 will have children with their own eggs because 90 percent of their eggs will be abnormal.

But a woman over 40 can gestate embryos created from eggs of younger women, giving the older woman a biological connection to the baby, creating a *biogenetic child,* one connected biologically and genetically to two different females. About 10 percent of IVF attempts today use such eggs. This works for women who have severe genetic diseases in their families, who have eggs damaged by chemotherapy or poisoning, who have had several miscarriages, or who suffer from premature menopause.

The world's first IVF child conceived with a younger woman's egg occurred in California in 1984; then the eggs had to be removed cumbersomely under anesthesia. The end of that decade saw another technological breakthrough when a thin needle guided by ultrasound retrieved the eggs by going through a vaginal wall.[13] That 10-minute procedure under light anesthesia could be done in a doctor's office, not in a hospital operating room, and it changed the industry. By 1990, with a new, steady supply of young eggs, fertility doctors showed that many older women could gestate embryos.[14]

This key fact makes us consider the need for regulation of the fertility industry, which has lacked such oversight since its inception. Only the conscience of fertility physicians counters the torrents of older, childless couples wanting to create biogenetic children, and perhaps that is not enough.

Scientists once thought age of sperm or age of gestational mothers caused infertility, but these can be overcome. The absolute barrier to successful gestation is age of the egg, with rapid drop-offs as eggs deteriorate in women over age 27.

As said, young eggs in older surrogates make a big difference. Using egg transfer, the success rate for taking a baby home jumps to 30 percent, and more important, 30 percent *regardless of the age of the female gestator,* making egg donation the great hope for many infertile couples.

Freezing Gametic Material

In 1997, the first birth occurred using previously frozen human embryos at an Atlanta clinic run by Bruce Tucker.[15] In 1990, two embryos were created from different eggs at a California clinic.[16] One was implanted and became a baby; the other remained frozen. Seven-and-a-half years later, doctors implanted the second embryo and it became a male fraternal twin to his 7-year-old brother. Emma Davis was an IVF baby born in Britain in 1989; her sister, Niamh, also created as an embryo in 1989, was born 16 years later in 2006.[17] The record for such siblings created together by IVF but born apart is 21 years.

In 2002, a California clinic began to freeze eggs of young women about to undergo hysterectomy but who wanted to later bear children.[18] In 2007, other clinics similarly froze ovarian tissue for women who wanted to preserve or delay childbearing.[19] However, after thawing, it remains to be proven how viable these eggs/tissue will be.

Embryos are screened (selected for good and bad qualities) during assisted reproduction in several ways. As with freezing and thawing of sperm for insemination, freezing and thawing screens because embryos incapable of successful implantation do not survive. As explained previously, sexual reproduction also screens because 40 to 60 percent of embryos, half because of abnormalities, fail to implant.

When embryos and sperm are stored and frozen, mishaps occur. In the 1990s, a white Dutch couple had nonidentical twins, one of whom was black (the black couple who created the embryo decided to adopt the baby). In 2002, a white couple in London had black twins because the wrong embryos had been implanted in the woman. (We'll never know how many embryos get mixed up between same ethnicity-couples.)

Keeping embryos frozen costs couples $200 a year and creates ethical dilemmas for originating couples.[20] Some couples do not want their embryos destroyed but also do not want them donated to other couples or used for research.

On the criminal side, IVF pioneer physician Cecil Jacobsen of Fairfax, Virginia, used his own sperm instead of the intended fathers' to create as many as 75 embryos throughout the 1980s. He went to jail for it in 1992. In the mid-1990s, Dr. Ricardo Asch at UC Irvine was caught switching donor eggs without women's consent and fled the country to avoid prosecution.

Payment for Assisted Reproduction: Adoption

Because roughly 1 out of 11 couples in North America is infertile after a year of trying to conceive, and because IVF works for only 23 couples out of 100, demand is high for healthy, adoptable babies. Because most couples in North America are white and want a white child, demand for healthy, white babies has skyrocketed.

Because of such demand, the average couple in 2002 seeking to adopt a baby paid agencies $20,000. In their quest for a healthy toddler, some couples paid $100,000. Other couples paid on average $22,000 for a Vietnamese baby, $17,000 for a Chinese baby, and $8,000 or less for a black baby.[21]

Like transfer of eggs or organs, agencies do not technically sell babies, which is illegal. But a new industry has sprung up that connects couples to pregnant women who might put their babies up for adoption. According to one investigative journalist, "That has left only the thinnest line between buying a child and buying adoption services that lead to a child."[22] The doubling of licensed child placement has increased adoptions in North America in the last few years to nearly 2,000.

In 1993, Russia had no foreign adoptions, but in 1997, it placed more children in America than any other country. Many adoptions also come from Romania, the Balkans, Vietnam, and China.

Although black critics have recently decried the differential payments that seem to demean black babies, virtually no one has condemned payment. Virtually no one has criticized "pregnancy counseling centers" that encourage pregnant girls to give up their babies for adoption, while charging lucrative fees to couples who adopt those babies.

Paid Surrogacy: The Baby M and Jaycee Cases

Fertilization of embryos outside the womb made it possible for another woman to gestate that embryo to birth, creating so-called surrogate mothers, either for pay or altruistically. For short, we'll call them surrogates.

By 1986, several hundred women had helped infertile women gestate babies when biochemist Bill Stern and pediatrician Elizabeth Stern hired Mary Beth Whitehead for $10,000 to bear a child created by his sperm and Whitehead's egg through AI. At birth on March 27, 1986, in Monmouth County Medical Center in Long Branch, New Jersey, Mrs. Whitehead claimed to have bonded with Baby M, aka Melissa Stern, and refused to give her to the Sterns. When Mr. Stern threatened legal action, Mrs. Whitehead fled to Florida with Melissa, but she was discovered and returned to New Jersey.

At the lower court trial in 1987, Judge Harvey Sorkow upheld the contract, said it did not constitute baby selling, required Whitehead to hand over the baby, awarded her $10,000, and decided it would be best for the baby never to see Mrs. Whitehead again. On appeal in 1998, the New Jersey Supreme Court unanimously reversed his decision, declared Mrs. Whitehead the legal mother with full visiting rights, and invalidated surrogacy contracts. Mrs. Whitehead later became a well-known critic of surrogacy. By 2008, Melissa was a senior at George Washington University in Washington, D.C.

Several states reacted to the Baby M case by criminalizing commercial surrogacy, laws still in effect in 2010. Arkansas, Florida, Ohio, Virginia, Nevada, and New Hampshire legally recognized paid surrogacy. At least 26 states have no law about surrogacy. California, which has many paid surrogates, recognizes a series of decisions in case law as regulating paid surrogacy.[23]

Jaycee Buzzanca, aka "the child with five parents," was born in March 1995 from a paid surrogate and became embroiled in a divorce between the parents who hired the surrogate. Jaycee was also conceived from sperm and egg other than from the parents who hired the surrogate. A California Appeals court ruled in 1998 that the parents who had hired the surrogate were legally responsible for him.

A common objection to paid surrogacy is that it's not best for the child. Paying for gestation creates a confused identity for a child who has at least three, and maybe five, parents. On the other hand, most cases of surrogacy seem to turn out fine.

Is it better not to exist than to have been borne by a surrogate? It's obviously ideal to be gestated by the owner of the egg that was fertilized for your conception, but what if that's not possible? We'll discuss this more below.

In the Gujarat State in southeast India, the Akanksha Infertility Clinic offers many willing surrogates for Indian and foreign couples at $5,000 instead of the $50,000 fee common in America. Is this not a reductio ad absurdum of a field that cries out for regulation?

Payment for Assisted Reproduction: Egg Donors

Originally, young volunteers supplied eggs for older women, but altruism didn't meet the demand. Paying for eggs is euphemistically called "egg donation," and in America in 2006 egg donors earned on average $4,217.[24]

Egg retrieval is more complicated than obtaining sperm. A woman takes drugs daily for a month or more to induce superovulation, after which eggs are aspirated as previously explained. Some people claim that the drugs increase risk of some cancers over the life of the woman, but no long-term data support this claim.

In 1999, a famous ad ran in newspapers at Princeton and Yale Universities stating that an anonymous couple would pay $50,000 for the eggs of a "woman over six feet tall and with SAT scores over 1,450."[25] Payment also runs high for donors of Jewish or Asian background, because they donate less frequently.

Multiple Births: Before the Octamom and the Gosselins

Although the Octamom and the Gosselins made news in 2009, multiples and their problems have a sad history.

Births of multiples has been growing steadily since the birth of Louise Brown in 1978. For most couples without reimbursement for IVF, the easiest way to overcome infertility is to take the drug Clomid, and if that doesn't work, Pergonal or Metrodin to stimulate the ovaries to release many eggs at the same time. The problem then is that introduction of sperm can fertilize one, two, or eight eggs.

IVF, in contrast, allows physicians to control how many embryos are introduced.

In a multiple pregnancy, nutrients and oxygenated blood in the womb become scarce. To prevent disabilities resulting from deprivation in utero, physicians recommend selective reduction (abort) of all but one or two fetuses.

In 1985, a Mormon couple, Patti and Sam Frustaci, conceived septuplets but refused to have such a reduction, so four of their seven babies died; the three survivors had severe disabilities, including cerebral palsy.

In 1987, and with the help of Pergonal, Ron and Roz Helms of Peoria, Illinois, had quintuplets. One child spent a year in a neonatal intensive care unit (NICU), another had seizures, and a third has cerebral palsy. The quints' medical bills for their first decade topped $3 million.

Multiple birth babies are often premature, are three times as likely as single babies to be severely handicapped, six times as likely to have cerebral palsy (which may not show up for two years), and may have to spend many months in NICUs.

In 1996 in England, after taking the fertility drugs Merton and Pregnyl for two days, Mandy Allwood released seven eggs and had sex. All of her eggs were fertilized. Four months later, a London tabloid offered her a large payment for exclusive rights to her story if, and only if, all her embryos made it to term. This began a pattern of new mutual exploitation of mothers of multiples and the media. Mandy announced she would not reduce any and would go for maximal births. As a result, she lost all seven.

In 1997, Denise Amen and her husband were offered the chance to reduce five growing embryos but refused. One of their quintuplets was born blind and others are "developmentally slow."[26]

In 1997, an Iowa couple, Bobbi and Kenny McCaughey, used Pergonal to superovulate Bobbi and introduced Kenny's sperm, conceiving seven embryos, refused to reduce any, and chose to risk having disabled babies. They said that the results were God's will.

At their fourth birthday in 2001, Joel suffered seizures. Nathan and Alexis have cerebral palsy.[27] During the first years, Natalie required a feeding tube. Although Bobbi and Kenny McCaughey homeschool their children, they send Nathan and Alexis to a special public school for developmentally challenged children.

In 1997, Jacqueline Thompson had sextuplets in Washington, D.C. After the death of one, the mother today struggles to raise five teenagers.[28] Unlike the McCaughey's, this single black mother's story drew scant media attention, no offers of television appearances or reality shows, and few donations by volunteers or companies.

In 1998, octuplets—six girls and two boys—were born to the Nigerian-born American citizens, Nkem Chukwu, age 27, and Iyke Louis Udobi, 41. In 2009, the Chukwus tried to tour the world with their eight, 10-year-old children under their self-chosen theme, "Promote Healthy Families," but it was unclear how successful the tour would be.

The probability of an impaired baby varies directly with the number of embryos allowed to gestate. In other words, if six are implanted, one is almost certain to be born with cerebral palsy or blind. Unfortunately, the chance of having any baby at all also varies directly with the number of embryos implanted—hence, the ethical dilemma of how many embryos *should* be implanted.

Older Parents

As said, by using eggs of younger women and ICSI, older people can create their own children. In 1980, Carl Woods accepted a 42-year-old woman as his first IVF candidate because of her increased chances of birth defects. She had a normal baby.

In 1993, a 59-year-old Englishwoman gestated twins from embryos fertilized by her husband's sperm and eggs donated by a young woman. In 1998, at age 57, American Judy Cates did the same.[29]

In 1990, one-third of American assisted reproduction clinics excluded women over 40. By 1998, the practice of using eggs of younger women had moved such limits to age 55.

Several births pushed this debate into public consciousness. In 1997, after lying about her age, 63-year-old Arceh Keh gave birth to a healthy baby girl. In 2005, 66-year-old Adriana Iliescu gave birth to a healthy baby daughter in Romania. In 2004, two 57-year-old women, Aleta Saint James, an unmarried woman, and Rosee Swain, a great-grandmother, gave birth to twins using IVF and eggs of younger women.

In 2007, at age 67 and after having lied about her age at a fertility clinic in Los Angeles, Maria Carmen del Bousada gave birth to twins in Barcelona, Spain. Two years later, she died of cancer, leaving two orphans.

Should society encourage seniors to have children when they may be dead when their children reach 18? In 1968, Senator Strom Thurmond at age 66 married a 22-year-old former Miss South Carolina and had four children with her (he died at age 100 in 2003). Actor Tony Randall fathered a daughter in 1997 at age 77 (he died at age 89 in 2005). Should fertility clinics place restrictions on women that they don't place on men?

One answer focuses on the best interests of the children. Regardless of whether it's a man or a woman, is it in a child's best interest to be a newborn of a parent approaching 70? How likely is it that the elderly parent will be around for the child's senior prom? Certainly being orphaned at age two is not ideal for the Bousada twins, and Adriana Iliescu will be unlikely to see her daughter's 18th birthday. Moreover, raising children takes energy and vigor, qualities that diminish rapidly in the senior years.

Given these facts, are 70-year-old seniors vain in having children? Or selfish, in wanting something to cherish, carry on one's name, or possibly, take care of one in old age? Shouldn't we make it illegal for them to have children so late?

Gender Selection

Because X chromosomes weigh more than Y chromosomes, a modified flow cytometer called Microsort can separate heavier from lighter sperm, producing accurate results 90 percent of the time.[30] Although intended for use in preimplantation genetic diagnosis, MicroSort may be used to select male babies.

Gender selection has been a problem in countries such as China, the Republic of Korea, and India. For centuries there, parents have seen females as less desirable than males. Using sonograms, many families aborted female fetuses to try again for a male child.

Despite laws that ban testing for sex in India and China, at least 60 million females there are missing. After decades of such practices in China, in 2001, 20- to 44-year-old never-married men outnumber two-to-one their female counterparts, who are sometimes kidnapped and sold into marriage. By 2020, one million excess Chinese males will seek to marry.[31]

Sex selection is sexist and leads to imbalances of the sexes in the population, as happened in China. Perhaps it, too, should be banned.

ETHICAL ISSUES

Unnatural

In 1978, the year of Louise Brown's birth, the Vatican condemned IVF and since then, has not changed its position. Its *Instructions* of 1987 equated IVF with "domination" and "manipulation of nature."[32] In 2008, in "Dignity of the Person," it emphasized that children should be created only through sexual intercourse by a married couple.[33] The document bans IVF, freezing embryos, and genetic screening of them.

Paul Ramsey, a famous, socially conservative Protestant theologian at Princeton University, in 1970 equated IVF with genetic manipulation and predicted societal horrors from it. He implied that if physicians could find a tiny egg and fertilize it, why couldn't they alter its genes?[34] He predicted that if they could, they would; and he held that if they did, it would be sinful.

Ramsey came up with some provocative phrases suggesting vague but disturbing harms to society: "test-tube babies," "dial-a-baby," "playing God." He was especially good at creating neologisms for rhetorical effect: "mercenary gestation," "supermarket of embryos," "spare-parts man" (a hypothetical cloned twin grown for this purpose and kept unconscious), "celebrity seed" (sperm banks), "human species suicide" (eliminating genetic diseases).

When Lesley Brown was several months pregnant and at the invitation of Sargent Shriver, Robert Edwards attended a symposium on the ethics of IVF at Washington's Kennedy Institute for Bioethics. While senators, national columnists, and other scientists listened, Ramsey condemned IVF and Edwards. As Edwards described it:

> He had to be seen and heard to be believed. I had to endure a denunciation of our work as if from some nineteenth-century pulpit. It was delivered with a Gale 8 force, and written in a similar vein a year later in the *Journal of the American Medical Association.* He doubted that our patients had given their fully understanding consent. We ignored the sanctity of life. We carried out immoral experiments on the unborn. Our work was, he thundered, "unethical medical experimentation on possible future human beings and therefore it is subject to absolute moral prohibition." I was as much surprised as made wrathful by this impertinent scorching attack. He abused everything I stood for.[35]

Ramsey's view of IVF was not based on its presumed consequences to the child, to the parents, or even to society. Rather, in a view that resurfaced 20 years later in debates about research on embryos, it stemmed from the idea of an embryo as a person. IVF is wrong in itself, Ramsey held, because it is "unconsented-to experimentation" on a person, the "embryo."[36]

During the 1970s, then Episcopal priest Joseph Fletcher defended IVF against the claim that it was unnatural:

> It is depressing, not comforting, to realize that most people are accidents. Their conception was at best unintended, at worst unwanted. There are those who are so bemused and befuddled by a fatalist mystique about nature with a capital N (or "God's will") that they want us to accept passively whatever comes along. Talk of "not tinkering" and "not playing God" and snide remarks about "artificial" and "technological" policies is a vote against both humanness and humaneness.[37]

For Fletcher, each kind of case should be considered on its own merits to see if it would help or hurt humanity; society must not be locked into antiquated religious prohibitions that take no account of consequences. Religion is best when it is "pro people," not when it worships abstract "thou shall not's":

> The real choice is between accidental or random reproduction and rationally willed or chosen reproduction. . . . Laboratory reproduction is radically human compared to conception by ordinary heterosexual intercourse. It is willed, chosen, purposed and controlled, and surely those are among the traits that distinguish Homo sapiens from others in the animal genus, from the primates down.[38]

In part because he disagreed so much with the views of conservative Christianity, Fletcher gave up the priesthood and became a secular thinker, becoming in some ways the first such bioethicist.

Physical Harm to Babies Created in New Ways

Many people predicted that the first baby born after IVF might be defective. This is understandable because in the 1940s, an Italian researcher named Petrucci had claimed to have fertilized a human egg in vitro, grown it for 29 days, and then destroyed it because it was "monstrous." Petrucci's story fueled fears about monsters, though he had never given evidence for his claims.[39]

At Louise Brown's birth, one obstetrician emphasized that severely defective babies could be created, and that "the potential is there for serious anomalies should an unqualified scientist mishandle an embryo."[40] Another obstetrician said, "What if we got a cyclops? Who is responsible? The parents? Is the government obligated to take care of it?"[41]

Leon Kass, later chair in 2002 of George W. Bush Bioethics Commission, warned, "It doesn't matter how many times the baby is tested while in the mother's womb," he averred, "they will never be certain the baby won't be born without defect."[42] Without the certainty of a normal baby, Kass condemned experimental conception.

Some Nobel Prize winners surprisingly condemned experimental methods of conception. James Watson feared that deformed babies would be born and they would need to be raised in custodial homes or killed.[43] (Watson later recanted.)

Max Perutz, who won the Nobel for work in chemistry, also condemned IVF research:

> I agree entirely with Dr. Watson that this is far too great a risk. Even if only a single abnormal baby is born and has to be kept alive as an invalid for the rest of its life, Dr. Edwards would have a terrible guilt upon his shoulders. The idea that this might happen on a larger scale—new thalidomide catastrophe—is horrifying.[44]

In 1977, in *Who Shall Play God?* the alarmist Jeremy Rifkin began three decades of opposition to new reproductive techniques. Rifkin decried assisted reproduction as evil "genetic engineering," which he defined as "artificial manipulation of life."

Socially conservative, pioneering bioethicist Dan Callahan argued like Kass that the first case of IVF was "probably unethical" because there was no possible guarantee that Louise Brown would be normal, though it would be ethical to proceed with IVF after a healthy birth. He added that many medical breakthroughs are "unethical" because we cannot guarantee that the first patients will not be harmed—implying an odd criterion of ethics for medical experiments.[45]

These general arguments do not seem compelling. What these critics overlooked was that no reasonable approach to life should avoid all risks. A highly unlikely result, even if that result is bad, still represents a small risk.

Over the last 30 years, we learned a few things about actual physical harm to IVF babies. Babies conceived through it have approximately twice the normal rate of birth defects, around 4 percent overall—instead of the norm of 2 percent.[46] IVF children are at greater risk for Beckwith-Wiedemann syndrome, which causes enlarged organs and cancer in children, and five to seven times more likely to develop retinoblastoma, a rare cancer of the eye.[47] Another study found that 9 percent of babies conceived through IVF or ICSI had birth defects versus 4.2 percent of those naturally conceived. Another American study found that babies conceived through IVF were three times more likely to be born underweight and premature than babies naturally conceived.

The figures above exclude the greatly increased risk of implanting multiple embryos conceived by IVF. One possible cause of these defects may be a subtle change in expression of genes caused by IVF that in turn may cause serious genetic damage.[48] Researchers have suggested an IVF registry to track such problems.[49]

The concept of absolute versus relative risk matters here. Given that the *absolute risk* of an abnormal child overall is small, a slightly increased *relative risk* from IVF conception doesn't matter that much, as couples having IVF babies still have small risks of serious problems.

Psychological Harm to Babies Created in New Ways

Jeremy Rifkin first raised the issue not of physical harm but of *psychological harm* by having a new kind of origin:

> What are the psychological implications of growing up as a specimen, sheltered not by a warm womb but by steel and glass, belonging to no one but the lab technician who joined together sperm and egg? In a world already populated with people with identity crises, what's the personal identity of a test-tube baby?[50]

Psychological trauma could also come from badly motivated or immature parents, an issue discussed below in connection with children of Nadya Suleman and the Gosselins.

Paradoxes about Harm and Reproduction

Can children be harmed by in vitro conception? Theologian Hans Tiefel wrote, "No one has the moral right to endanger a child while there is yet the option of whether the child shall come into existence."[51] But can a "being" be harmed who may not exist?

Call this the *paradox of harm,* the seemingly self-contradictory idea that someone can be harmed by being born. This idea appears to be paradoxical because, first, it seems queer to say that we can harm a being by bringing it into existence; second, it seems equally odd to say that a mother, who could have prevented harm to her child but did not, did anything wrong.

A *paradox* results when two different meanings of a key term are used simultaneously. Paradoxical statements can be dissolved by carefully specifying the different meanings in each part of the statement and deciding which meaning applies to each. With the paradox of harm, any approach to dissolving it must distinguish between different meanings of "harm." Like "good," "harm" covers a broad range of meanings. In law school, such meanings are covered in one of the major courses, *torts*.

Let's distinguish two ways of thinking about harm. In the first, both a baseline and a temporal component are necessary, so that a change occurs which makes someone worse off. In this *baseline harm,* an adverse change in someone's condition is required. With the baseline concept, someone who doesn't yet exist cannot be harmed, because there is no baseline from which change can occur. (Consider the old Yiddish joke: 1st—Life is so terrible! Better to have never existed. 2nd—True, but who is so lucky? Not one in a thousand.)

In the second way, harm involves comparing a present deficient condition with what normally would have been. In this *abnormal harm,* someone can be harmed by being brought into existence with some defect that could have been avoided by taking reasonable precautions. With abnormal harm, the event or omission that causes the defect is the cause of harm. The abnormality concept underlies the belief that women should do everything possible to have healthy, unimpaired babies: That anything less than the maximal effort is blameworthy, and that it is wrong for a woman to take risks with a future person's intelligence or health. To sum up these two concepts of harm:

Baseline Harm. Requires a starting point (baseline) from which an adverse change is plotted; that is, it requires an existing being who is made worse off.

Abnormal Harm. Requires a norm of development that is not met, for example, because of a doctor's actions or omissions while a woman is carrying a fetus.

In *wrongful life* cases in the courts, it is claimed that the lives of some children are so miserable that their very existence is a tort. In *wrongful birth* cases, the claim is not that the child's life is totally miserable, but simply that the child has been damaged by being born less than normal. Wrongful birth suits appeal to the normality concept. The courts have rejected wrongful life suits by assuming the baseline concept; that is, they have assumed that preventing a birth or killing a baby cannot possibly be a benefit, even to prevent or end a life of total harm.

These two concepts of harm can be applied to IVF. According to baseline harm, a person created by IVF cannot thereby be harmed because otherwise that person wouldn't have existed. According to abnormal harm, IVF could harm a baby if it caused some defect or deficiency that a normal baby would not have had.

Wronging versus Harming

For utilitarians or consequentialists, what matters about new kinds of human creation is that babies are not harmed. On the other hand, virtue theories or deontologists such as Kantians focus on the motives of prospective parents. Whether it is AID, IVF, surrogacy, or cloning, they ask, "What would a good mother do? What kinds of risk would she take?"

This deontological approach emphasizes that, even though a child might not be harmed by being brought into existence, a mother can still be wrong in bringing the child into existence. That's because "wrong" here is divorced from consequences to the child and instead married to the motives of the mother in conceiving a child. To take a mundane example, if a mother conceives a child not because she wants a child but to try to force a wealthy man to marry her, then the child who comes into existence is not harmed, but the mother is wrong to bring the child into existence for this motive.

In a Scottish study in 2005 of women trying to conceive at an infertility clinic, most of the 81 women would, if given an either-or choice, rather have a child with cerebral palsy or partially blind than no child at all.[52] But is this the right motive for approaching childbearing? This issue intensifies with dilemmas raised by implanting multiple embryos, where couples face choices between risks of no child and risks of several children with disabilities.

Let us distinguish between the ideal and the permissible regarding traditional conception and assisted reproduction.

Best Interests. What methods of conception are best for children brought into the world? What methods are permissible?

Best Motives. What motives are best for parents to have in creating children? What motives are permissible?

Using this distinction, some motives might be allowable, e.g., the motive of having kids so "someone will take care of me in my old age," even though we acknowledge they are not ideal. Similarly, it is probably in the best interests of children to be created by traditional sex by a married couple.

Harm by Not Knowing One's Biological Parents?

Can a child be harmed by not knowing his genetic ancestors? Yes, if he later needs to find out specific genetic information or to discover who his biological parents were. Even if a donor of sperm or egg wishes to be anonymous, there are ways of giving the child this information.

One compromise solves this problem by allowing gametic donors (either sperm or egg is used as reproductive material) or surrogates to be *confidential* but not *anonymous*. In this practice, agencies keep from children created the names and identities of donor gametes, but these donors can update their files every few years so that their biological children can know about their genetic diseases and lives. This practice protects the desire of some donors and some surrogates not to have contact with children created from their gametes, while also giving them the chance to change their minds.

It is mainly the adoptive parents who don't want their children to know such donors.[53] Surprisingly, many sperm and egg donors, or surrogates, do not mind maintaining such records and want to know about the lives of such children.[54]

Pediatrician/internist Matthew Neidner registered online in 2006 with the Donor Sibling Registry and discovered that his sperm over ten years had helped create nine children, who can see his picture on-line and follow his career.[55] Single women in San Diego selected his sperm from his profile at the Fertility Center of California.

Is Commercialization of Assisted Reproduction Wrong?

Sale of gametes either could be intrinsically wrong—just wrong in itself—or indirectly wrong, because of associated negative consequences. The first belief stems from religious or Kantian premises about the inherent value of humans being incompatible with aspects of their conception being priced in the market.

> Valuing human life is incompatible with paying someone a price for sperm, eggs, embryos, or gestation, making the resulting baby a commodity.

Someone may also look at the larger structure of society and claim, emphasizing a view of justice, that reproductive relationships between people should not be subjected to money or that such transactions violate natural law. In other words, reproduction should be natural and free, not something bought through a contract.

So this statement opposes payment for sperm, eggs, surrogacy, and presumably physicians working in fertility clinics.

Defenders of payment ask whether enough young women will go through egg donation for altruistic reasons. Altruism hasn't worked in other areas of medicine. Voluntary donation has failed to meet the need for blood for operations, organs for transplantation, or bone marrow for leukemia patients.

So if we don't permit compensation, we will not get enough eggs from young women and hence, infertile couples will not get the babies they want. If we regulate compensation and ban a real market, other problems arise, such as trying to set the right fee for everyone. Finally, if payment for assisted reproduction is wrong, why isn't payment for adoption? If payment for assisted reproduction is not for babies but merely for services, why isn't payment also banned for adoption?

Sometimes objections about payment to women imply that men are exploiting women. From reading interviews with paid surrogates, this does not seem to be true.[56] Paid surrogacy empowers many women who do it, making them special and allowing them to contribute to their family's income. A surprisingly large number of women become surrogates despite objections from husbands, or they battle husbands who want to keep the gestated baby.

A Need for Regulation?

Faced with the many problems of assisted reproduction, one wonders whether it's time to regulate this process, specifically, in banning implantation of sperm or embryos where more than two births are possible, and banning implantation of embryos in women over age 55, with rigorous proof required of age.

Given that the ART industry generates $1 billion in fees per year, given what critics call "the wild west of medicine" where almost anything goes, some minimal regulation of assisted reproduction might be good for the process, and especially for the children it creates.[57]

If we are going to continue allowing payment for assisted reproduction—for sperm, eggs, surrogates, and the services of physicians—perhaps it is now time to regulate the field. We return to this question later.

Screening for Genetic Disease: A New Eugenics?

At some clinics and with permission, researchers store extra eggs or embryos for later use with infertile couples.[58] Other agencies store sperm. Prospective couples can screen for future traits of children in two ways: by scrutinizing the background of the egg or sperm donors, or by testing actual embryos for genetic conditions such as Down syndrome. Is such expanded choice good for couples and children or a new eugenics?

Some critics oppose any selection by prospective parents and argue that parents should be forced to accept the first available embryo, or that embryos should be randomly assigned. Similar critics once argued that all adoptable babies should be placed before couples were allowed to try IVF.

Some prospective couples, e.g., Japanese-American, want an embryo from parents who will be ethnically as close to them as possible. They also desire to maintain, as much as possible, the illusion that the child came from their gametes. For them, choice of skin color or ethnicity matters a lot.

Other couples want to avoid a child with disabilities, such as a Down child or a child with fragile X syndrome (a condition leading to retardation). If couples are allowed to do some screening for genetic diseases, will this lead to them wanting only perfect babies or to a new eugenics?

Perhaps not. One reason it is not is the cost of screening: for a single disease, it can be as much as $20,000, which most insurance companies will not pay.[59] It is unlikely that a couple will screen out hundreds of embryos and implant only the perfect ones because few couples have the millions of dollars to pay for so many screening tests. Should an inexpensive screening test be available where a couple could screen an embryo for hundreds of genetic diseases, this objection might carry some moral weight.

Even if such a test becomes available, we need to ask, what's wrong with couples wanting a baby that's as healthy as possible at birth? Isn't this what properly motivated parents should desire? Isn't this why pregnant mothers should avoid alcohol, tobacco, or other harmful drugs during pregnancy?

Designer Babies?

This is a large question, connected in part to questions about eugenics and controls on biotechnology. Note that many people believe that it is permissible to use such techniques to let infertile couples choose *against* diseases that embryos might carry. Sensationalistic stories imply that preimplantation diagnosis will lead to eugenics, but is this leap realistic?

When a young woman is paid for her eggs, the clinics remove the eggs and fertilize them with a variety of different sperm, keeping records of each embryo created. Couples may then select an embryo from this woman's eggs (seeing a picture and description of her) that will be fertilized by sperm from a man whose picture they see and whose life they read about.

What worries critics is that if couples already want to try to influence traits of their future babies, and if there is a market for sperm and egg sellers, then couples will select traits in ways the critics don't like. That is, they will select traits of men and women that the purchasing couple deems desirable. As one such critic said in discussing a market for egg donors, "this approach is harmful not only because it serves to reinforce social prejudice but also because it fragments women as persons by commodifying their characteristics, which seems at least as harmful as commodifying their eggs."[60]

But critics who decry selection of traits in embryos always ignore adoption. Why is selection by ethnicity or race bad in one case but permissible in the other? Why is selection by ethnicity and race plus large payment permissible for adoption but not for eggs or embryos or surrogates?

In other areas of life, people decide what they value in others in joining fraternities, sororities, and country clubs, in hiring and firing, in dating, in choosing a person to marry and to create children with, in making friends, in deciding where to live, and in choosing whom to mentor. Many of these choices reinforce existing attitudes and the government does not ban them.

The media and advertising shape the way millions of young people dress and wear their clothes, and could easily sway them similarly about the kind of children they should want. Maybe we should be worried.

Arguments for Regulation of Fertility Clinics

Three decades have passed since Louise Brown's birth and society has matured. We have gone beyond the alarmism of early critics and few people, except the Vatican and Leon Kass, think that new techniques of assisted reproduction are inherently wrong. People have even become accustomed to the unnatural sight of a woman pregnant with five, six, or even seven growing fetuses.

But what we all now know is that being a multiple is not good for the child, who runs a high risk of later having a lifelong disability. Nor is it good to be born to a single, nearly 70-year-old woman, who will likely die relatively soon and leave the child an orphan. Even if the woman is wealthy, this is not good for the emotional health of the child.

So yes, it's time for government to regulate American fertility clinics in four ways: (a) No assisted reproduction for women over age 55, and real testing must be enforced (seriously, in America it's easier for the elderly to buy reproductive services than it is for teenagers to buy alcohol); (b) No implantation of more than two embryos and no introduction of sperm when ovaries mature more than two eggs. This will reduce the number of multiple births, and attendant disabled children, by 99 percent; (c) No selection of gender of embryos except for sex-linked genetic disorders. As explained, it violates the dignity of women and is sexist to allow people to use assisted reproduction to get a first-born male child. (d) No selection of a child to match the disability of existing parents with a disability, e.g., deaf parents who want a deaf child. It is not in the best interests of any child to be born deaf, and parents who want such disabilities in their children are not properly motivated.

To insure a baby, especially when a couple lacks insurance to cover IVF, American physicians and infertile couples want to implant more than one embryo or multiples. In 2009, Missouri and Georgia proposed laws to limit implanting to two embryos. Such laws would limit multiples and babies with disabilities.

Arguments against Regulation of Fertility Clinics

During the 1970s, American banned use of federal funds for experimentation on embryos. This ban hoped to stop assisted reproduction research, but fertility clinics subsidized their research from fees paid by clients.

At the time, critics doubted that couples would pay much for assisted reproduction, especially given such low chances of having a baby. But critics erred. Over a million American couples paid for some form of assistance in ART clinics.

An unintended but foreseeable by-product of the ban was that neither National Institute of Health nor Institutional Review Boards could regulate assisted reproduction research in private clinics. That lack of regulation led to many breakthroughs, fueled in part by competition between ART clinics for success in creating babies. It also created a $1 billion industry for American medicine as patients fly to this country from allover the globe to get what they can't get in their home countries.

So, if it's not broke, don't fix it. A few aberrant cases should not bring down the whole system. Physician Michael Kamrava can be sued on behalf of the disabled babies for breach of the standard of care, sending a message to other physicians in fertility medicine.

Another problem is that reproductive medicine, with its research on human embryos, fires passions in social conservatives, who believe such research attacks the dignity of humans. Once politics controls who can buy assisted reproductive services, will a slippery slope occur? If we make it illegal for a physician to help a couple have a firstborn male child, or a 60-year-old woman to gestate a child, what's next? Banning assisted reproduction altogether, the way the Vatican advocates?

The Missouri and Georgia laws, although limiting multiples and babies with disabilities, would also limit the number of babies born. Isn't it better to exist, even with a disability, than not to exist? Especially to parents who want you?

CONCLUSION

Given that Nadya Suleman already had six children, Dr. Sharma's acceptance of her as a fertility patient certainly was "a huge ethical failure."[61] And for him then to implant all six of Suleman's remaining embryos moved the case from ethical failure to ethical tragedy—tragedy for the 14 children to be parented by this immature, single woman.

Assisted reproduction is a special kind of medicine, wrapped in the joys of creating wanted babies, but also rife with controversies. As older women bear such babies, and as more embryos are implanted creating more multiple births, we need to think more about harms to new children and less about the desires of infertile parents.

FURTHER READING AND RESEARCH

Cynthia Cohen, ed., *Oocyte Donation,* Baltimore, MD, Johns Hopkins University Press, 1997.

Joseph Fletcher, *Ethics of Genetic Control: Enduring Reproductive Roulette,* New York, Doubleday Anchor, reprinted by Prometheus, Buffalo, NY, 1984.

Elaine Tyler, *Barren in the Promised Land: Childless Americans and the Pursuit of Happiness,* Cambridge, MA, Harvard University Press, 1995.

Paul Ramsey, *The Ethics of Fetal Experimentation,* New Haven, CT, Yale University Press, 1975.

Stephanie Coontz, *The Way We Never Were,* New York, Basic Books, 1992.

RESOLVE: The National Infertility Association http://www.resolve.org/main/national/advocacy/insurance/facts/history.jsp?name=advocacy&tag=insurance

DISCUSSION QUESTIONS

1. If fertility clinics are regulated, shouldn't adoption agencies also be regulated? Shouldn't there be age limits on who can adopt? Shouldn't couples also be banned from saying they want a baby of a certain sex?
2. Is it better to be born with a 65-year-old single mother than not to exist at all? Is this a fair question? What's wrong, if anything, with the way this question is asked?
3. Why should there be any restrictions at all on choices of parents about babies with assisted reproduction? What's different about this process that gives governments the right to impose such restrictions? We don't impose any tests at all on who can have a baby and we even let people have babies who use tobacco and alcohol during pregnancy. Given such low standards, isn't it contradictory to impose higher standards on assisted reproduction?
4. Isn't selling one's eggs to the highest bidder like prostitution? Kant would object to both because both treat one's body as "a mere means." Is it wrong to so commodify one's body and be paid for doing so?
5. IVF may not be unnatural but gestating eight fetuses is. Nature extracts a terrible price on the resulting children. The same thing happens when an elderly woman gestates a baby with artificial hormones. Aren't both processes thwarting nature, unnatural, and hence, "just wrong?"

6. Is assisted reproduction "pro-life?" Since 1 in 11 couples in America can't conceive after 1 year of trying, and if they want to have babies (versus abortion), what's wrong with their using assisted reproduction to have babies? Even if some tiny embryos are lost in the process of trying to conceive—which also occurs for 50 percent of embryos conceived through normal sexual relations—what's wrong with couples wanting their own children and using medical science to try to have them? How can such desires not be "pro-life?"

CHAPTER 6

Embryos, Stem Cells, and Cloning

Since the announcement of the cloning of Dolly the sheep in 1997, controversy has surrounded using human embryos in research and cloning anything human, whether to create embryos, stem cells, or babies. This chapter discusses such controversies including one of the greatest frauds in science. At its end, it discusses cloning to produce children, or *reproductive cloning.*

This chapter's essential question for discussion is: does cloning embryos or humans raise *special* ethical issues or do these issues mirror those in research and assisted reproduction?

EMBRYOS

Historical Background of Embryonic Research

Roe v. Wade in 1973 made abortion legal in all states (see Chapter 4). As soon as laws permitted abortions, researchers *legally* experimented on 20 live-born fetuses, seemingly degrading nascent human life.[1]

Five years later, physicians reversed infertility by creating "test-tube" baby Louise Brown, without cultural agreement or approval of an ethics committee. As discussed in Chapter 5, Steptoe and Edwards created and destroyed about 100 human embryos to perfect their techniques of in vitro fertilization (IVF). Then, as today, the creation of babies by IVF had the foreseen but unintended by-product of sacrificing human embryos that did not implant. Again, human life at its beginnings seemed under attack by technicians far removed from the natural wombs of motherhood. And unbeknownst to critics, Edwards had himself actually once created a human embryo from a human egg in a lab late one night.

In 1979, obstetricians Howard and Georgeanna Jones established the first American IVF clinic at Eastern Virginia Medical School (EVMS). In 1981, they achieved the first American baby born with IVF, Elizabeth Carr. While the embryo that became Elizabeth Carr was being created, opponents protested outside. Conservative Christians saw IVF as alien, suspect, and as violating principles of natural law because humans were being created in artificial ways, outside of sexual intercourse and the womb.

So began the politics of the embryo, which have intensified over the last 25 years. Three different advisory boards created by Congress recommended allowing research on embryos, but such research never got funding.

In 1977, the Ethics Advisory Board concluded that some research with embryos should be permitted, but Congress never accepted its conclusions. This board never took up the separate issue of what kinds of research with embryos could be federally funded.

In 1981, Mario and Elsa Rios, a wealthy American couple, died childless. Their IVF-created embryos then existed in frozen limbo. Because neither the Rios nor their infertility clinic in Australia had provided for their deaths, the question arose whether the embryos could be destroyed. If implanted in surrogates, the embryos could result in children who could later sue for support.

An ad hoc committee of the Australian government required scientists to preserve the embryos until they were adopted. They never were, and over the years, the freezing made them deteriorate (as will happen to all frozen embryos eventually), making the issue moot.

In England and Australia, governments allowed public monies to fund medical research that used embryos up to day 14 of life. Australian infertility companies soon began to license their breakthroughs to American physicians.

The Davis Case In 1990, another case about embryos occurred. Mary Sue and Junior Davis of Tennessee divorced and fought for custody of seven embryos frozen in an IVF clinic. Both had remarried. After her remarriage, Mary Sue Davis wanted to donate their embryos to an infertile couple. In 1992, the Tennessee Supreme Court decided that Junior needn't become a father against his will. After that, a lower Tennessee court ruled that he could destroy the embryos, which he did.[2]

In 1994, the *Human Embryo Research Panel* concluded that federal funding of research with embryos would improve the success and safety of procedures to reduce infertility, and that prohibiting federal funding would harm the quality of such research.

It called those embryos *research embryos* and those leftover after successful IVF, *spare embryos*. The panel rejected the compromise that research could be done only on spare embryos. Why? It said that embryos from unsuccessful couples attempting IVF had higher rates of genetic abnormalities, so basic research on their embryos needed to be done also.

Politically savvy members of the panel thought Congress would accept their modest recommendations, but, preoccupied with partial-birth abortions in 1995, Congress rejected them.

In 1996, Congress added *the Dickey-Warner Amendment* to the National Institute of Health's (NIH) NIH's appropriations bill: "None of the funds made available in this act may be used for . . . research in which a human embryo or embryos are destroyed, discarded, or knowingly subjected to risk of injury or death greater than allowed for research on fetuses in utero."

Geneticist Marl Hughes had once made *Science* magazine's list of top breakthroughs for his technique of taking DNA from a single cell of a human embryo and testing it for cystic fibrosis. Taking the cell did not damage healthy embryos, but such testing did mean that embryos with cystic fibrosis would be destroyed.

Although the ban on federal funds had stayed in effect, scientists such as Hughes could work on embryos that were *privately funded,* such as that which Hughes obtained from Planned Parenthood. In 1997, Hughes had private funds to pursue embryonic screening and much larger federal funds to pursue other genetic research that did not involve human embryos. Yet Hughes lost all federal funding because such funds had paid for a small refrigerator mistakenly placed in the private lab where he stored his embryos.

Dolly Is Announced, 1997

On February 24, 1997, every newspaper in the world screamed that a lamb named Dolly had been created by cloning (she had actually been born previously on July 5, 1996, but patents on the techniques didn't come through until February). Cloning, a technique previously thought impossible to create mammals, conjured scary scenarios from science fiction. Dolly's birth galvanized interest in cloned human embryos, especially embryos that might be created through cloning, implanted in a woman, and gestated to a human baby.

Where they had felt ambushed by *Roe v. Wade,* the birth of Louise Brown, and the unanticipated success of IVF clinics, social conservatives vowed this time to resist. It is as if they said to scientists, "At cloning, we draw the line and beyond, You shall not pass!"

The Science of Cloning

"Cloning" is an ambiguous term, even in science, as it may refer to molecular cloning, cellular cloning, embryo twinning, and somatic cell nuclear transfer (SCNT). The latter is what occurred in Dolly and what most people care about. It takes the nucleus of an adult cell and implants it in an egg cell where the nucleus has been removed.

A variant of this process called fusion (which was actually done to produce Dolly) puts the donor cells next to an enucleated egg and fuses the two with a tiny electric current. Because the pulse that produces fusion also activates egg development, a blastocyst—an embryo of about 100 cells—starts to develop. In fusion, mitochondria from both the donor and the egg recipient mix, whereas in strict transfer of a nucleus, mitochondria are present only in the enucleated egg.[3]

At a 1997 conference on mammalian cloning, Wilmut stressed that his techniques were inefficient: he started with 277 sheep eggs and got only one live lamb. Nevertheless, his statement has been widely misunderstood, partly because he has emphasized how many eggs he started with and not how many fetuses resulted in live births. The actual statistics were: 277 eggs fused in oviducts with sperm, 247 recovered from oviducts, 29 of which were transferred at the stage of morula or blastocysts, which created 13 pregnancies in lambs, three of which came to birth, and one of which, Dolly, was healthy and lived.[4]

Immortalized Human Stem Cell Lines Created, 1998

What are stem cells and why are they important? Found in embryos, bone marrow, and the umbilical cord, stem cells help the injured body grow new cells. If the body loses blood, it activates stem cells to make new blood. As primordial cells, stem cells can develop into any kind of differentiated cellular tissue: bone, muscle, nerve, etc. In theory they could be directed to form new bones, neural cells, and cardiac tissue, and to cure diseases.

Physicians already knew that the human body had stem cells, but they had no easy way to grow them. Then in 1998 John Gearhart of Johns Hopkins University and James Thomson of the University of Wisconsin discovered how to continually produce stem cells—create immortalized stem cell lines—rather than tediously derive them from minute amounts of tissue from embryos or fetuses.

In effect, Gearhart and Thompson discovered how to make human embryos into tiny "stem cell factories." Just such objectification and commodification of human life really bothered critics, who felt that using human embryos for such purposes demeaned the dignity of human life and led down a slippery slope to demeaning all human life.

Gearhart and Thompson made their discoveries using private funds. Given that NIH funding was the world's treasure, should it bankroll these scientists and their new findings?

ACT Uses Cow Eggs to Grow Human Embryos

In 1998, Advanced Cell Technology (ACT) of Massachusetts announced that it had made differentiated human cells revert to a primordial state by fusing them with cow eggs. Although the cow egg was just the medium for the nucleus of the human cell (the nucleus of the cow egg had been removed), the procedure sounded alarms. Once again, biotechnology seemed out of control. President Clinton and his National Bioethics Advisory Commission (NBAC) condemned any attempts to create children out of such hybrids (although no one wanted to try to create such a being or was suggesting doing so).

NBAC Backs Research on Embryonic Stem Cells

Although it condemned reproductive cloning in 1998, the NBAC concluded in 2001 that the government should fund research on stem cells created from human embryos. Congress never accepted this recommendation, in part because cloning embryos connected to the larger, controversial issue of reproductive cloning.

Cloning soon took up more media time than any issue in the 35-year history of bioethics. With physicist Dick Seed wanting to clone himself, and the spiritual group Raelians, Pamayiotis Zavos, and Severino Antinori falsely claiming to have cloned a human fetus, cloning created one sensational story after another, scaring people about identical babies being produced like immortalized stem cell lines.

Adult Stem Cells Discovered, 2001

In 2001, scientists discovered stem cells not only in bone marrow but also throughout the human body. Researchers started using them in research rather than using stem cells derived from human embryos.

In the next five years, researchers discovered that many organs and tissues contain precursor cells that act like stem cells. These adult stem cells became specific kinds of cells more quickly than embryonic stem cells. One director of an institute for regenerative medicine says, "Brain stem cells can make almost all cell types in the brain, and that may be all we need if we want to treat Parkinson's disease or ALS. Embryonic stem cells might not be necessary in those cases."[5] Similar, specific adult stem cells can be obtained from the intestine, skin, liver, and bone marrow. With heart disease, the director of Harvard's Stem Cell Institute says, "If you could find a progenitor cell in the adult heart that has the ability to replicate, it's likely easier to start with that than begin with an embryonic stem cell, which has too many options."[6]

But most adult organs contain few stem cells, not nearly enough to use medically, and adult stem cells are even harder to grow than embryonic stem cells. More fundamentally, "Unlocking the secrets of self-renewal will most likely involve studying embryonic stem cells," says Harvard's director.

President Bush's First Press Conference, 2001

On August 11, 2001, President George W. Bush, in the first press conference on bioethics by an American president, announced his policy on federally funded research on human embryos. He rejected using such funds to create embryos for research, but allowed them for research on 60 stem cell lines created from spare embryos. Carried live on television in prime time, his press conference signaled that bioethics had arrived in American politics.

A year after that press conference, the number of stem cell lines appeared to be small, about 15. Scientists then questioned whether President Bush's policy would get them the biological material they needed. Three years later, scientists regarded the 15 stem cell lines as inadequate.[7]

Cloning and the Law

Senator Sam Brownback (R, Kansas) introduced his Human Cloning Prohibition Act of 2001, which stated: "It shall be unlawful for any person or entity, public or private, in or affecting interstate commerce, knowingly (1) to perform or attempt to perform human cloning; (2) to participate in an attempt to perform human cloning; or (3) to ship or receive for any purpose an embryo produced by human cloning." Also, "It shall be unlawful for any person or entity, public or private, knowingly to import for any purpose an embryo produced by human cloning, or any product derived from such embryo."

Because the Brownback bill pushed a total ban on cloning, including embryonic cloning, it failed.

A similar proposal to ban all forms of cloning worldwide, backed by the administration of George W. Bush, stalemated in the United Nations. Asian countries such as South Korea, Malaysia, and China, hoping to excel in biotechnology, aligned with European countries to resist the measure. Malaysia invested $26 million in its Bio-Valley to house 100 new biotech companies to work on stem cells and raise Malaysia to a world power in biotechnology.[8] China invested in cloning technology, hoping to gain where the West had stumbled.[9]

With Congress stalemated, action about cloning fell to the states. Californians in 2002 passed Proposition 71, giving $3 billion for stem cell research from human embryos. State legislatures across the land then battled to fund or to criminalize embryonic cloning. Wisconsin, New Jersey, Connecticut, Illinois, Washington, Ohio, and Maryland funded similar research, whereas Massachusetts, Missouri, Arkansas, Indiana, Iowa, Michigan, North and South Dakota voted to criminalize all cloning.[10]

By 2006, 13 states passed laws making attempts at reproductive cloning a crime, including Arkansas, California, Connecticut, Indiana, Iowa, Maryland, Massachusetts, Michigan, New Jersey, North Dakota, Rhode Island, South Dakota, and Virginia.[11]

Hwang Woo Suk Clones Embryos for Stem Cells, 2004

In 2004, seemingly out of nowhere, South Korean researcher Hwang Woo Suk announced that he had not only successfully cloned viable human embryos but had also derived viable stem cells from these embryos.[12] The South Korean team created 213 embryos and grew 30 of these to blastocysts. American researchers at Advanced Cell Technology had previously not been able to grow embryos to blastocysts, which contain an inner mass of stem cells. Hwang's achievement stunned American researchers.

Animal Cloning

In the eight years after Dolly's birth in 1996, scientists cloned animals important for food and research: two calves (1998), the lambs Molly and Polly to create Factor IX (1998), three generations of mice (1998), five pigs, (2002), a goat (2002), a rat (2003), many champion dairy cows and bulls (1998–2004), a horse named "Prometea" (2003), a mule named "Idaho Gem (2003)," and a deer named "Dewey" (2003).

They also cloned animals of endangered species such as the banteng (2003), a bovine native to Indonesia, and the African wildcat (2004). Critics feared that such cloning would lessen preservation of natural habitat for such species.

Scientists also cloned a cat named "Carbon Copy" or "CC" (2001). CC had a striped gray coat over a white base, unlike her ancestor, an orange calico. Critics claimed this showed that cloning didn't work, while CC's originator, Mark Westhusin, replied that of course CC's coat color differed, because random genetic reprogramming controls coat coloring and patterns.

In March 2005, the South Korean team of Hwang Woo Suk announced it had cloned an Afghan hound that it named "Snuppy." Because of their complex reproductive system, dogs had previously eluded cloning scientists, but Hwang's team did so, an achievement that remains undisputed. Later they produced five cloned "sniffer dogs" possessing an extraordinary ability to smell drugs at airports.

The Fraud of Hwang Woo Suk, 2005

Hwang Woo Suk stunned American researchers when he announced in May 2005 that he had cloned human embryos and stem cells from them. His account emphasized the Buddhist relaxed attention and skills of his team.[13] Importantly, he said these stem cell lines were genetic matches of cells of donors, opening doors to study cells of victims of particular diseases such as Alzheimer's or Lou Gehrig's disease.

The story received almost as much publicity as Dolly's birth. Carefully planned, it was announced at a meeting in Seattle of the American Association of Science. With his handsome face and Western suit, Dr. Hwang seemed to symbolize all that was progressive and therapeutic in medical science. And his successes seemed to be snowballing, showing American politicians the price of their hostility to funding research with cloned embryos.

Of course, controversy continued. Richard Doerflinger of the U.S. Conference of Catholic Bishops called the success a "clear and present danger" to the dignity of human life. Champions of victims of Parkinson's disease, such as the actor Michael J. Fox, hailed it as a major breakthrough.

Because federally funded American researchers could not perform similar research and because no major medical institution supplied researchers with eggs or human embryos, the Korean's research could not be easily verified.

Questions soon arose about the photos of embryos published in *Nature* and *Science* of Hwang's research, which did not seem to be of different embryos but the same ones. Pittsburgh scientist Gerald Schatten, listed as a coauthor on Hwang's paper, suddenly withdrew his name. Anonymous postings on the Internet from graduate students in Hwang's lab complained that Hwang had faked his results.

In 2005, Hwang's university and the South Korean government thoroughly investigated Hwang's work on cloned embryos. Assistants testified that Hwang had forced them to fabricate results and to alter pictures of embryos. The investigation concluded that Hwang had not in fact produced any stem cell lines from human embryos, had not discovered easy techniques for cloning embryos and had not produced matching stem cell lines to cells of donors. One of the biggest medical breakthroughs of the decade had been faked and became one of the most blatant frauds in the history of science.

Hwang went on trial in South Korea for misusing millions of dollars of funds specially given to him for his work and for violating Korean laws in bioethics. In this year, Hwang admitted to his fraud, but like Enron's Ken Lay and HealthSouth's Richard Scrushy, claimed that underlings had deceived him.

Like the Raelians, Hwang was a fake. Both stories received saturation coverage by the media and both damaged legitimate medical progress.

The Senate Vote and Presidential Veto, July 2006

On July 18, 2006, the U.S. Senate voted to expand federal funding of embryonic stem cell research, passing a bill that had passed in the House the year before. The next day President Bush, as he had promised to do, vetoed the bill, the first of his administration. At a news conference at the White House, the president explained his veto, saying the bill would be "crossing a moral line and would support the taking of innocent human life." He was surrounded by dozens of Snowflake children, who were born from an embryo-adoption program, and their parents. "These boys and girls are not spare parts," the president affirmed.[14]

Representative Nancy Pelosi of California, the House minority leader, retorted that Bush's veto was "saying 'no' to hope." Senator Orrin Hatch agreed, saying the veto "sets back embryonic stem cell research another year or so." In truth, during the eight years of George W. Bush's presidency, very little changed about federal funding of stem cells from human embryos.

Obama Administration Reverses Bush Policies

On July 7, 2009, federal regulators in the Obama administration set new rules for research with embryonic stem cells, effective immediately.[15] A new review panel composed of scientists and ethicists has been created. The main job of the panel is to make sure that the couple whose cells are used to create the embryonic stem cells give real informed consent to how their embryos will be used in medical research. Scientists and the American Medical Association were pleased with the results.

Induced Pluripotent Stem Cells Discovered

In 2007, researcher Shinya Yamanaka of Kyoto University discovered how to use four genes to tell skin cells how to revert back to pluripotent cells, called human iPS cells. Thus he learned how to use a few genes to tell a differentiated, somatic cell how to revert back to a primordial state and become an undifferentiated cell that could turn into anything. Now called induced pluripotent stem cells (iPSCs) or more simply, induced stem cells, these powerful cells appear to eliminate the need for human embryos to create embryonic stem cells.

This was a Nobel-Prize-worthy achievement. Yamanaka proved that IPSCs can be grown without creating human embryos and also bypassing the need for research embryos or eggs from female donors.

In July 2009, further progress occurred with induced stem cells.[16] Two Chinese teams created identical mice using embryonic stem cells created from iPSCs created from the skin of the ancestral mice. This achievement was considered the definitive test in proving that iPSCs can truly function as the equivalent of human embryonic cells.

Although this achievement appeared to end, or at least greatly diminish, the controversy over creating human research embryos, it started others. First, IPSCs can hasten the day when we could safely clone human babies. If the mice are normal, as they seem to be, then this is a gigantic step toward creating safe cloning of mammals. But then we must address the key question: is it evil to move toward cloning a human baby?

Second, iPSCs can move along the day when we could safely change the genetic traits of babies, then fears will arise about "designer babies." It's relatively easy to add or knock out an important gene in these created, embryonic cells, and hence, create special kinds of babies. Any IVF lab could do so one day. Is this another reason to start regulating such labs?

Third, the ethical issue arises of *stolen cloned babies.* If a scientist can use a skin cell from a mouse to grow an iPSC to grow a mouse embryo that is identical to its ancestor, then could he also use a skin cell from Brad Pitt to grow an iPSC to grow a human embryo that could be gestated by a woman over nine months for a baby identical to Brad Pitt? Should it be a crime, like identity theft, to steal Brad Pitt's unique genome?

In August 2009, a lab produced monkeys where researchers substituted the healthy mitochondrial DNA of mothers with DNA from mothers with terrible genetic diseases, then used the nucleus of the mother with the bad DNA to create the embryo that became the monkey.[17]

Recall the case from Chapter 5 of Jaycee Buzzanca, aka "the child with 5 parents," who was born in March 1995 from a paid surrogate and became embroiled in a divorce between the parents who hired the surrogate. Jaycee was also conceived from sperm and egg other than that of the parents who hired the surrogate. A California Appeals court ruled in 1998 that the parents who had hired the surrogate were legally responsible for him.

Could custody disputes arise involving swapped mitochondrial DNA? An infertile woman later wanting visitation rights to her "daughter" created with her genes, but a daughter with the nucleus of another woman, who gestated her as a fetus?

Finally, even though terrible diseases are inherited on mitochondrial DNA, including Alzheimer's disease, blindness, and muscle degeneration, changing the mitochondrial DNA in an embryo will not only affect the future adult but also affect the grandchildren and future progeny of that adult. This is germ-line, not somatic cell, gene therapy. Historically, such a change has been thought, correctly, to be a momentous move, one not to be taken lightly, because if anything unexpected happens, it cannot be reversed and will affect many people.

ETHICAL ISSUES INVOLVING EMBRYOS IN RESEARCH

Valuable from Conception

For Thomas Aquinas in the thirteenth century, ensoulment occurred at 40 and 90 days for male and female fetuses, respectively, and therefore nothing of value resided in the womb before those points. In 1869, Pius IX announced that abortion at any stage resulted in excommunication.[18] Since then, Catholic teaching has emphasized the value of human life "from the moment of conception." So it was no surprise that in 1982, Pope John Paul II said to a group of scientists,

> I condemn, in the most explicit and formal way, experimental manipulations of the human embryo, since the human being, from conception to death, cannot be exploited for any purpose whatsoever.[19]

Potential for Personhood

Many scientists say that before 14 days, the human embryo has no human form and cannot experience pain. Why then give it value? One reply is that, despite the facts that some zygotes become pathological tissue and some zygotes twin, the embryo is, as Jesuit priest Richard McCormick says, "powerfully on its way" to development as a person. Even though it may later twin or not implant, conservative believers see it as a member of the human family.

Why is that? As McCormick writes about the human embryo:

> . . . it remains [as having] potential for personhood and as such deserves profound respect. This is *a fortiori* weighty for the believer who sees the human person as

a member of God's family and the temple of the spirit. Interference with such a potential future cannot be a light undertaking.

Slippery Slopes

In addition to asserting the intrinsic value of the embryo, McCormick worries about what happens when human embryos are regarded as mere commodities for research. (In the following passage, "preembryo" refers to the embryo before implantation on the uterine wall.)

> If we concluded that preembryos need not be treated as persons, would we little by little extend this to embryos? Would we gradually trivialize the reasons justifying preembryo manipulation? . . . Furthermore, there is uncertainty about the effect of preembryo manipulation on personal and societal attitudes toward nascent human life in general. Will there be further erosion of our respect? I say "further" because of the widespread acceptance and practice of abortion.[20]

Here we first have a conceptual slippery slope argument, asserting that if trivial reasons justify experimenting on embryos before 14 days, then similarly, trivial reasons will justify experimenting on first trimester fetuses, and then on more developed fetuses. McCormick also has an empirical slippery slope argument here, predicting that acceptance of the deaths of embryos will generalize to acceptance of deaths of fetuses. (These two kinds of arguments about slippery slopes are discussed in Chapter 3.)

Reductio ad Absurdum

Many commentators think that treating the embryo as valuable because it is a potential person can be refuted by a reductio ad absurdum: a line of reasoning that shows that implications of an idea are absurd and thus cast doubt on the idea itself. In this instance, if a woman starts procreating in her teens and continues throughout her fertile years, she can produce a dozen or more children. If each potential person is valuable, then she ought to conceive as many children as possible. Given the consequences of overpopulation, this conclusion hardly makes sense.

If embryos are persons, the following involve killing persons: creating embryos for IVF and freezing them for later use, preimplantation genetic diagnosis, or medical research. Similarly, intrauterine devices (IUDs), which prevent implantation of embryos, also must kill persons.

If these implications are false, then the premise that generated these claims is false, and that premise was that human embryos are persons.

Of course, it might be possible, thinking of Judith Jarvis Thomson, to accept the premise that embryos are persons, but to deny a further premise that persons can never be killed. Also, when no particular woman has a duty to gestate them, there is clearly a philosophical difficulty in claiming a right to life for frozen embryos.

The Interest View

New York (Albany) philosopher Bonnie Steinbock argues that having moral status (that is, being the kind of being who must be considered from the moral point of view) is limited to beings who have "interests." Generally speaking, a necessary condition of having an interest is being able to desire something. One of the most basic desires is to avoid pain. We don't think vegetables feel pain, so we don't think they have desires. We do think cats and dogs feel pain, so we think they have an interest in avoiding pain.

The law makes a great deal of interests, conflicts among them, and how to resolve conflicts of interest. As such, the concept of interest covers a lot of intellectual territory.

As for embryos, it is commonly accepted that before the emergence of the primitive streak at 14 days, there is no possibility of any neural development such that any being could be "there" to feel pain. The human embryo at this stage is more like a blueberry than a tadpole.

As such, Professor Steinbock argues, the embryo has no desires about what happens to it, so it has no interests and no moral status. So it does not matter whether an embryo fails to implant in the uterine wall, whether it is dislodged by an IUD, or whether it is used in research. It only begins to matter when neurons form to create *sentience*, the ability to feel pain.

Steinbock distinguishes between moral status and moral value. Beings can have moral value, even if they lack moral status. For her to say that something has moral value is to say that there are moral reasons for protecting or being concerned about the thing. So wilderness and works of art can have moral value, even if they lack moral status.[21]

For Steinbock, embryos have moral value but no moral status, so there are reasons for protecting how they are used, for respecting them, and for not devaluing them as mere tissue.

Two-thirds of the human embryos stored at two fertility clinics in England had to be destroyed because the owners did not respond to a letter asking about their wishes.[22] Given that owners are the most affected by the destruction of the embryos, such couples do not put much value in the dignity of these embryos. At least, they do not when it comes to actually paying money to keep them alive or to writing a letter consenting to keep them alive in public clinics.

The fact that 400,000 embryos are now frozen and deteriorating over time and may become nonviable has also created a new kind of adoption. The *Snowflakes* program to date arranges adoptions of embryos, of which about 20 became babies.[23] The program charges up to $20,000 for this service, as it considers itself arranging an adoption.

England has allowed its scientists to create human embryos for research and to use them in such research for up to 14 days of development.[24] In the years in which that has been legal, no great changes in the fabric of English life seem to have occurred, nor has there been a massive slide down a slippery slope of loss of human dignity.

Potentiality and Cloning

The strongest argument of opponents of embryo research is the potential of the human embryo, given the right conditions, to become a person. But they have forgotten one thing: what cloning shows is that any cell of the body can become a person. The nucleus of a differentiated cell can be put into an enucleated human egg; a spark is applied; and a new embryo can be formed that is a near copy of the genetic ancestor.

The revolutionary aspect of cloning is that it makes not just embryos but *any human cell* special. The concept of the dignity of the embryo begins to collapse into the concept of the dignity of the cell.

Embryos and Respect

Bioethicist David Ozar once argued that although an embryo may not be a person, neither is it just a pebble or a tissue.[25] Embryos are not simply the property of an owner. They deserve respect in view of their potential as persons.

What does respecting an embryo mean? Well, for one thing, embryos should not be eaten, or be encased in plastic as earrings, or be bred into mixed-species hybrids. Gene Outka claims that respecting embryos also means that human embryos could not be substituted for the eyes of rabbits in testing cosmetics.[26]

Another way to state this point is to emphasize that a large amount of bodily products, such as bone, cartilage, blood, and tissue can be legally sold from cadavers. Some firms specialize in such sales and broker them to research institutions and medical schools. Respecting embryos would include banning them from being bought and sold this way.

It is possible to be a good scientist and treat human embryos with respect in medical research. One might make an analogy with animal experimentation. To test new forms of heart surgery or new kinds of lenses for human eyes, we harm animals. But in using animals for our benefit this way, we should minimize their pain and psychological terror and not make fun of them in any way.

Researchers who have the privilege of using human embryos should also be taught, required, and legally enjoined to treat them with the greatest respect. That respect prevents a slippery slope to devaluing other kinds of human life.

To make another analogy: physicians and medical students should treat the newly dead with respect and not practice intubation or spinal taps or surgery on them without the family's permission, for to do so is to offer no respect to the life just expired or to those who loved the patient. In the same way, one could argue that human embryos should be treated carefully in view of the persons that—under different circumstances—they could have become.

Indeterminacy Father Richard McCormick does not assert that human embryos are persons but thinks we should treat them as if they were. Why? Because we don't know exactly where personhood begins. To use his analogy, if the hunter is unsure whether something moving in the bushes is a deer or a human, he shouldn't shoot.

Similarly, at the other end of life, if we are unsure whether a patient will emerge from a coma, shouldn't we wait as long as possible before removing a feeding tube?

A subtler objection emphasizes the indeterminancy of the boundaries of sentience. When patients are under sedation for surgery, well-publicized stories have taught us that they can hear. Some patients have been declared dead and then awakened, recalling jokes made in their presence and procedures done on them (an important argument for not allowing medical students to train on the newly dead).

Similarly, we are not sure exactly when the embryo develops sentience. Perhaps the most rudimentary form is like phototropism when a plant bends toward light. Even so, when any doubt exists, we should be cautious and, under a general principle of respect, not subject embryos to any medical research, just as we would not subject patients in vegetative states to such research.

The Opportunity Cost of Missed Research

In any decade, few really major breakthroughs occur in medical research. The creation of immortalized stem cell lines from human embryonic was one such triumph. Not allowing this line of research to be federally funded is a major tragedy.

It is not enough to let private companies or other countries fund the research. American's NIH are the crown jewel of the world's scientific treasure, and it is a tragedy if such resources could not pursue this new area. Moreover, by allowing federally funded studies, we insure the highest level of peer-reviewed, objective research.

Banning use of embryos in federally funded projects, NIH deprives millions of people of new medicines that otherwise might not be discovered for another 100 years.

MY Tissue! One of the well-known problems of transplants of foreign organs, blood, and tissue into a patient's body is rejection of the foreign material when recognized by the immune system. Drugs that suppress the immune system to allow acceptance of foreign tissue may cause cancer after decades of use. It would be much better to grow bone, blood, organs, or particular masses of cells from one's own body for future use.

Creating embryos from one's own cells could be used to grow tissue for one's future medical needs. By using donor eggs, embryos could be created by embryonic clonings that were nearly identical, genetic copies of one's genome.

Libertarians argue that what an individual does with his or her body should be up to him or her. A federal ban on storing "self-made" medicine from one's own embryos allows Big Government to take away this personal liberty. By denying citizens such new medicines made from their own embryonic tissue, it takes away years from their lives.

Moot? The creation of IPSCs means that we can get the valuable stem cells we need for research without destroying human embryos. Whether you see this as a brilliant scientific discovery or a gift from God, or both, the fact is that the impasse of the last decade motivated scientists to seek a way around it, which they did.

Some researchers say we should keep all the tools on the table, and that human embryonic stem cells may be better for some purposes than IPSCs. Even so, with this new source of stem cells, some of the arguments above lose their punch.

REPRODUCTIVE CLONING

Reproductive cloning alarms many people, perhaps because of the way it's portrayed in movies and science fiction. As such, we first need to address some misconceptions about it.

Reproductive Cloning: Myths about Cloned Persons

Cloning Does Not Reproduce an Existing Person Reproductive cloning recreates the genes of the ancestor, not the ancestor himself. Cloning recreates the genetic base of a person, but a person's identity partly stems from nongenetic sources, such as his experiences growing up.

This means that you can't reproduce yourself. Of course, any resulting child would not have the memories of the adult ancestor. Narcissistic people who want to clone themselves will be disappointed. Cloning reproduces about 99.8 percent of the ancestor's genes (the other 0.2 percent come from mitochondrial genes in the host egg), but even 0.2 percent difference at conception can be significant. Identical twins have small differences in random inactivation of the X chromosome in embryonic development and this results in their different personalities and traits as adults.

Cloned Humans Would Not Be Drones but Persons A child created by reproductive cloning would, like any other fetus, need to be gestated by a woman for nine months. He would have no distinguishing marks on him to indicate his origins. He would feel, sense, think, and hurt like any other human child.

Would a cloned child's origins affect his status as a person? Critics once thought that IVF children might suffer discrimination, but that never happened. Most likely, children created by cloning would be persons with all the rights of other persons.

Leon Kass implied that prejudiced people might treat cloned children as less than human. If this were so, it might not be in their best interest to be originated this way.

But notice that the same logic implies that it might not be best to be created as a child of an interracial couple because "other people" might be prejudiced against such marriages and their children. The effect of such reasoning is to strengthen prejudice, not to weaken it, and to give prejudice too much weight in what, after all, is supposed to be *moral* reasoning. For this reason, we must be careful when we speak of children originated by cloning. To call them "clones" may be prejudicial if this term implies bad things about such children. Similarly, to imply that children created by cloning would be raised in batches connotes all kinds of bad, silly things, such as seeing them as zombies, as sources of organs for genetic ancestors, and in general, as less than human.

In short, babies created by cloning would not be *zombies*, but—legally and morally—*persons*.

Against the Will of God?

Many clergy believe that originating children by cloning is not God's will. God ordained in Genesis that humans should reproduce as did Adam and Eve, man and woman begetting children, and that is God's plan for humanity. To deviate from the plan is wrong. Just as gay men and lesbians were not meant in this plan to have children, so children were not meant to be created asexually.

Notice that this argument is an inference about God's will. Nowhere in any scripture does it say that medical science should not use reproductive cloning to produce children. Notice too that most advances in the history of medicine have been greeted by the same argument that a change is against God's will.

The Right to a Unique Genetic Identity

With Dolly's birth, the possibility emerged of cloning a human baby. Various people began to assert that what was wrong with cloning a human baby from a genetic ancestor's cells was that it would violate the right of each person to a "unique genetic identity." Some theologians at the Vatican made this claim (although they had never made it before Dolly's birth).

An initial problem about this argument concerns twins. Since so-called identical twins share 99.9 percent of their genes, is their right to a unique identity violated by being a twin? Certain techniques of assisted reproduction, such as implanting many embryos, drastically increase the likelihood of such twins. Are they wrong?

A bigger problem with this objection is the assumption that one's genes are one's identity. This reductionist line of thinking in modern genetics lies behind similar objections that a child created by cloning would not have a soul because it shared the same genes as the ancestor. Both objections assume that genes make the person, the self, the identity, and yet we know that is incorrect because environment also contributes to personhood (and possibly, so does free choice).

Unnatural and Perverse Many people also wonder about the motives behind cloning. They ask, why would anyone want to originate a child by cloning? Why not use the fun method of sex? If a couple is unable to have a child through sex, why not adopt?

Sexual reproduction is natural. Cloning, or asexual reproduction, is unnatural. What is good for plants or animals should not be used for humans.

Something is wrong with parents who want to clone a child. They are either narcissistic or so desperate—after all other methods of having children have failed—that they will subject their future child to a perverted experiment in which his personhood will be at risk when he later learns that he is "just a clone."

In reply, it should be noted that this objection begs a lot of questions. First it assumes that what is primitive or natural is always best. That is certainly not true for a man and a woman who are naturally infertile. Second, it assumes that the new way of making babies is perverse and therefore wrong, a charge that created many other new ways of making babies in the past. Finally, it assumes bad motives on the part of would-be parents.

The Right to an Open Future Critics claim that parents will choose to create a child with a certain genotype, say, that of an athlete, actor, or dad, with certain expectations. After their investment in IVF, they would expect the resulting child to have qualities similar to the ancestor.

But the future should be open to every child. It is wrong for tennis mothers to impose their wills on their children in their hell-bent determination to make them into tennis stars, wrong for East Asian parents to push their children from an early age into medical careers, and wrong for soccer dads and Little League coaches to push their children into athleticism.

Why is this so? The heart of the objection about a closed future lies in explaining this answer. At bottom is the premise that parents should not have children to fulfill their own needs, desires, or fantasies, but for the good of the child. In this sense, parenting should be Kantian, not egotistic.

If parents create children expecting specific traits (basketball skills, acting talent), then children can be damaged psychologically when they cannot, or choose not to, fulfill such expectations.

This argument lies behind the widely heard objection about "designer babies," i.e., that it is wrong for parents to try to create children with blue eyes and blonde hair and with a strong interest in music and tennis. Instead, parents should accept whatever God gives them as a gift.

The most dangerous idea of all is that parents should be free to reject, or not love, babies who lack the qualities they want. Already a dangerous tendency has started among some parents to not aggressively treat impaired babies suffering from genetic diseases at birth, followed by equally dangerous practices of death by abortion after a sonogram has determined a female fetus. If we add to this the possibility of using preimplantation diagnosis during IVF to not implant any embryo with cystic fibrosis or Down syndrome, we are already halfway to the bad place of parents rejecting children in the nursery when they emerge with the wrong genes.

Suppose a child is created from the genes of a girl who was an all-state champion in the breast stroke and who had ability in math, scoring in the top 1 percent of standardized tests and excelling in AP math classes in high school.

What is often overlooked is the role of supportive parents in such achievements. Now suppose that the child cloned never learns to swim and is never exposed to math and doesn't develop these abilities while she is young. In that case, we will learn, perhaps painfully, that parents of children cloned for certain abilities cannot just sit back and wait for the abilities to unfold, but will need to be just as involved as the ancestor's parents. If they are not, it will be easy to see where the blame should go.

Nevertheless, this argument emphasizes how bad parenting damages children and how society should not encourage bad parenting based on false expectations. This would be especially true if parents emotionally abandoned kids who did not meet their expectations.

On the other hand, this argument can go many places. Suppose the cloned child resembles the ancestor much more than expected and because the parents already know what the child can excel at, encourage her in that direction. Would that be bad for the parents or child?

Abnormalities

At present, a high rate of abnormalities plagues efforts to create primates by somatic cell nuclear transfer. Any such conception of a human baby by cloning would be an experiment on a child, and no such experiment is justified without a compensating benefit for the child. Such a benefit does not yet exist. As such, attempts to create a child by cloning the cells of a human ancestor and gestating it to birth are wrong.

Indeed, because a child is likely to be born with some genetic defect, conceiving a child from cloning might be a form of child abuse. If the motives of the parent were bad, then deliberately creating a child who was likely to be genetically defective would be like deliberately choosing to implant an embryo with cystic fibrosis rather than a healthy one.

Notice that this objection depends on the existing state of scientific knowledge. If scientists learn to originate baboons and chimpanzees by cloning without defects and learn how to originate all other mammals safely by cloning, then the chances of a defective cloned baby would drop drastically and the force of this objection would correspondingly diminish.

Notice that when we discuss abnormalities, we need a baseline for comparison. Over 50 percent of embryos created sexually, half of which are chromosomally abnormal, do not implant successfully in the human uterus and are lost. About 2 percent of live-born babies have some genetic defect. Millions of babies are born after the mother smoked or drank during their gestation, yet we do not criminalize such smoking and drinking during pregnancy. (Perhaps we should, but why should we focus on the sensationalistic, remote cases of cloning and ignore obvious harm to babies around us?)

Inequality

Some people start out life much better than others. Some children get two parents, four grandparents, lots of gifts at holidays and birthdays, special preschool and after-school tutoring, and the best private schools and universities. It seems unfair that some get so much but others, so little.

Over the last centuries, civilized societies have mitigated some of the more extreme effects of this *environmental inequality:* estate taxes have reduced how much can be inherited from parents, income taxes redistribute money from high earners to those on disability and public assistance, and expanding economies have created new opportunities for hard work and talent to get ahead.

Even so, the gap between rich and poor is astonishing, having widened over the last decade. Given that gap, reproductive cloning could start a new kind of *biological inequality,* much deeper than our existing, environmental inequality. Because reproductive cloning would normally involve a conscious choice to clone the genome of one person rather than another, it is likely that families would choose genomes with good qualities. If cloning could be done successfully, such families could create strong, clever, talented, energetic dynasties that outstripped normal humans. It would be a biological case of "the rich get richer, the poor get poorer." Princeton biologist Lee Silver calls the results the "GenRich" and the "Normals."[27]

This is something new in human evolution. Sexual reproduction randomly exchanges genetic material, and because of regression to the mean, makes sure that the great genetic norm of human nature never rises or falls too much. But in a single swoop, particular families single-mindedly devoted to raising their genetic stature could biologically out-distance normal humans over a few generations.

As such, reproductive cloning could endanger social justice. Moreover, because this danger is "written into biology," it would be much harder to undo. People without superior genes would find it much harder to compete against such superior people, even when competition was completely fair.

But is this the way we want the advanced countries of the world to go? Toward a deeply stratified society that divides into Superiors, whose genotypes were chosen by committed families bent on superiority, and Normals, whose genotypes were randomly assigned by the spin of the genetic roulette ball in sexual reproduction?

Good of the Child

Almost all ordinary discussions of cloning beg two important questions: they assume bad motives on the part of parents or scientists involved in creating a child by cloning, and they assume the child would be harmed by knowing he was created this way.

We can see just how much is begged when we counter these assumptions. First, a child created through cloning would know that he was wanted by his parents. After all, creation of such a child would require IVF, which at best is successful only 25 percent of the time. Thus, prospective parents probably would have to try several times to create the baby this way, and pay for their efforts.

In contrast, all that many people know about the wishes of their parents is that their parents had sex and did not abort. They have no clear evidence that their birth was planned. This fact especially applies to children created before *Griswold v. Connecticut* in 1965 made it legal for physicians to prescribe contraceptives.

To give this argument some play, assume that cloning children becomes safe. Besides knowing she was wanted, is there anything about origination by cloning that would be in the best interests of the future child?

Well, for one thing, few parents would knowingly re-create the genotype of an adult with a congenital disease. Insofar as possible, parents would choose children who would be healthy.

This in itself will be good for the child. Placing aside for the moment worries about eugenics, it is hard to ignore the good of a life where one is not constantly challenged by physical or mental disabilities.

Next, consider that certain traits might be genetically based. We already know that looks and physique are, because we see resemblances in a family. Suppose, too, that intelligence, wit, temperament, sociability, verbal ability, mathematical ability, and analytical ability are partly genetically based. To give the argument more rope, suppose that parents could choose children with some of these traits. Would doing so be good for the child?

It is hard to see why not. Although it may not be politically correct to say it, all other things being equal, it is better to live life as a beautiful, smart, healthy person than the reverse, and it is hard to see why such a life is not in the interests of the person created.

Of course, opponents will say that such a person has been created as a purchased "commodity" and is subject to the unrealistic expectations of the parent. We will consider the objection about expectations below, but for now, notice that this general line of objections applies to any service that parents buy for present children with the same goals in mind, such as sending children to elite private schools. Yet no one considers the latter to be bad for the children.

Finally, we should notice that there is a dilemma that proponents of reproductive cloning encounter in which either way, they lose. If cloning is unsafe, then it hurts the child, and therefore it's wrong to do. If cloning is safe, then it improves the child and is eugenic, and therefore wrong to do. Obviously, trapped in this false dilemma, proponents of cloning can never win.

At bottom, what may scare opponents of reproductive cloning the most is the possibility that it will work, be safe, and be in the best interests of the children created. Then some children will have more, biologically, than others, and some families may create biological dynasties. Be that as it may, these are not objections about the intrinsic evil of cloning, but indirect ones, focusing on harm to equality (and which we consider below).

Only Way to Have One's Own Baby

One of the main reasons to produce a child is to have a child with one's own genes. Whether it's to have one's family line continue or to have "a bit of me going into the future," no one questions the soundness of this parental motive.

Now in some rare cases, asexual reproduction will be the only method by which a parent can have a genetic connection to a resulting child. Men who are azoospermatic (producing no sperm) or women whose eggs are too old to conceive often still want a child who is genetically related. Reproductive cloning would allow each parent to have a child (assuming two children) with a strong (99.9 percent) genetic connection to the respective parent.

Although men with low sperm counts could reproduce sexually through intracytoplasmic sperm injection (ICSI) into a donated egg, there is no option for a man who lacks sperm and a woman who lacks good eggs and who also wants a genetic connection to a child. For either parent, the only route is the asexual one of using a cell from a nucleus of a differential cell, and using the genes inside it via cloning to create a human embryo.

The combination of two forces strengthens this argument in subtle ways. First, as they pursue careers, many women delay age of their first pregnancy, and when they marry so late that they cannot conceive, they are disappointed. At age 42, less than 10 percent of women carry healthy eggs; over 90 percent at this age will fail to bear a child with their own egg. Whatever child they adopt or create with donor eggs will have no genetic connection to them.

Second, it is easy to underestimate the urge to be genetically connected to a child. When government and private insurance refused to pay for IVF in the late 1970s, everyone thought that few parents would pay cash for the experimental procedures, much less that struggling college professors with little money would forsake cars and a house in attempts to have a genetically related baby. But they did, and a $1 billion industry was born.

Hence, the millions of couples with women in their 40s who are trying to conceive a child, and who strongly desire a genetic connection to a child or two, will be the prime movers in the quest to originate children by cloning. Hence, this argument will appeal to more people, and for different reasons, than might have been thought at first.

Stronger Genetic Connection

A child created by cloning would have *all* the parent's genes, not just half, right? So he or she would have not the usual 50 percent genetic connection to each parent, but nearly 100 percent to one parent. But if half a genetic connection is good, why is double not also good?

See this as an onus of proof argument. Since people and courts assume in public policy that a biological connection makes for a bond between parent and child, why would a stronger bond not be just as good or better? Whatever it is that makes genetic bonds good for children, is a stronger bond not also good? If not, why? If it's just the novelty of a stronger bond, that is not an argument against the bond, just a new item for empirical investigation.

Do our law and courts see the genetic connection this way? Indeed they do. In a dozen cases around the country, a baby who was adopted and had spent several years with an adopted family was returned to a biological parent with whom he shared a genetic connection after one of many disputes arose. The point here is not to judge the merits of the final resolution of custody of the child, but to emphasize how much weight the law puts on binding a parent to a child through shared genes.

In another context, countless talk shows feature unmarried women who have had sexual relations with more than one man, each of whom could be the father of their child. On these shows and often in life, the men say, "If it's mine, I'll support the child." And the law agrees, assigning paternity and requirements of child support if a DNA test identifies a particular man as the father. All of these cases point to the power we assume of the genetic connection to the child.

But those are sexual connections where only half a parent's genes are bequeathed to a child. Imagine a total, 100-percent genetic connection. Couldn't that be a good thing for a son, to have a father so tightly bound to him? Or for a daughter to have a mother so tightly bound?

Liberty

Those wishing to curtail reproductive cloning because it might increase social inequality need to put their cards on the table and not hide behind subterfuge. They rarely say exactly what they want to do and that is to decrease the liberty of the average person to have children and to create a family.

Now the liberty to create children and a family is not absolute and may be outweighed by a much greater social good. But in the rest of our lives, we prize liberty highly, especially when it comes to creating families and what goes on inside them.

In most areas of our personal lives, we are not willing to curtail our personal liberty to create more social-political-economic equality. For example, we could make private schools illegal and require all children to attend public schools. This would get the best parents involved in PTAs and community boards, which in turn would raise the level of all public schools, thereby helping equality. In the South, where private academies continue as the vestiges of racially segregated schools, and where elite preparatory schools create a class of highly privileged students, equality is not furthered by giving the best students the most resources.

But few people favor mandatory public schools because it would take away freedom from parents about how and where their children are educated. It is for this reason that some people hate busing, because it forces some children to be bused across the city in the name of equality.

The point is not about busing and public education but about how it is easy to pick on reproductive cloning, sacrificing it to equality, because so few people want to exercise this liberty. But the principle is the same: sacrifice liberty for equality. What justifies sacrifice in one area of reproductive life may be extended to another. For example, if only well-off people can afford IVF, shouldn't it be banned too?

A Rawlsian Argument for Cloning and Choice

John Rawls argued famously that the principles of justice would be chosen in a hypothetical social contract where parties choose under a veil of ignorance about their position in society when the veil rises.

Under this veil, it is in the interest of future children to possess as much natural talent as possible, with the best genes, and with the best chance at a long, healthy life. One could even argue, although this is controversial, that under this intra-generational veil of ignorance theory of justice, people are not just *permitted* to improve the genes of future children, but are *obligated* to do so. Why? Because it is wrong to choose lives for future people that make them much worse-off than they otherwise could have lived.

Links between Embryonic and Reproductive Cloning

Leon Kass wrote, "And yet, as a matter of policy and prudence, any opponent of the manufacture of cloned humans must, I think, in the end oppose also the creating of cloned human embryos."[28]

Because he fears that allowing cloning of human embryos will inevitably lead to implantation of a human embryo originated by cloning, he wants to test physicians and scientists who favor lifting the ban on embryo research by making them endorse "an absolute and effective ban on all attempts to implant into a uterus a cloned human embryo (cloned from an adult) to produce a living child."

To the criticism that the techniques of human asexual reproduction are not that complicated and that someone in the world will eventually originate a living child by cloning, Kass would put the onus of proof on those who would permit the "horror" of such origination: "Perhaps such a ban will prove ineffective; perhaps it will eventually be shown to have been a mistake. But it would at least place the burden of practical proof where it belongs: on the proponents of this horror."

If it is true that embryonic cloning cannot be divorced from reproductive cloning, then other things also follow. For one thing, if reproductive cloning is not intrinsically bad, then neither is embryonic cloning. If reproductive cloning is negative only because of abnormal results, then we should study how to prevent abnormalities by funding research in embryonic cloning.

In other words, the argument above says that because reproductive cloning is evil, we shouldn't fund anything that would help us do it. But if that is false and reproductive cloning is a tool—another way to make a baby and help start a family—then we should investigate all ways to create such a tool.

Not funding research on cloned embryos or on ways to prevent abnormalities in reproductive cloning in primates seems perverse. If abnormalities are the major reason for prohibiting reproductive cloning, then surely research to prevent them is justified. But if the real objection is the assumption of the intrinsic evil of reproductive cloning, then we should dispense with the cover argument about abnormalities and get to the real issue.

CONCLUSION

Cloning embryos has become less controversial because IPSCs provide new ways of making stem cells, yet using such embryos in medical research still raises the hackles of some. Reproductive cloning, still far off because of abnormalities, remains one of the controversial issues of our time.

FURTHER READING AND RESOURCES

Ronald M. Green, *The Human Embryos Research Debates: Bioethics in the Vortex of Controversy,* New York, Oxford University Press, 2001.

S. Holland et al., *The Human Embryonic Stem Cell Debate,* Cambridge, MA, Bradford/MIT Press, 2001.

In 1991, the *Kennedy Institute of Ethics Journal* published exchanges between Jesuit Richard McCormick and secular law professor John Robertson on the moral status of embryos in research. See Volume 1. In 2001 and 2002, Volumes 11 and 12 had several articles on the same topic.

Gregory Pence, *Who's Afraid of Human Cloning?* Lanham, MD, Rowman & Littlefield, 1998.

Gregory Pence, *Cloning after Dolly: Who's Still Afraid of Human Cloning?* Lanham, MD, Rowman & Littlefield, 2004.

Human Cloning Foundation, www.humancloning.org.

Francis Fukuyama, *Our Posthuman Future,* New York, Farrar, Straus & Giroux, 2002.

Leon Kass, *Human Cloning and Human Dignity: The Report of the President's Council on Bioethics,* New York, Public Affairs Press, 2002.

DISCUSSION QUESTIONS

1. Should cloning embryos be linked to reproductive cloning, or should the two issues be kept separate?
2. Is reproductive cloning now safe? How might it be made safer by studies of cloned nonhuman animals?
3. Should food from cloned animals be sold? Labeled as such?
4. Is a human embryo a person? A thing of value? Just tissue?
5. How has the discovery of induced pluripotent stem cells (iPSCs) altered the landscape of the debate about research on human embryos?
6. If cloning babies were safe, how might it create more inequality in society?

CHAPTER 7

The Ethics of Treating Impaired Babies

This chapter's essential question for discussion is: does it exhibit prejudice or compassion not to aggressively treat impaired babies at birth?

PREMATURE BIRTHS

The rate of premature births rose in America from 9.8 percent in 1985 to 12 percent in 2002,[1] reaching a half million births.[2] Although babies born at 28 weeks have a 90 percent chance of survival, extreme prematurity at 22 to 25 weeks causes many problems. About 80 percent of such babies will have neuromotor or mental disability.[3] Compared to only 2 percent of babies born full term, 41 percent of babies born extremely premature at age six had severe to moderate mental impairment.

Most obstetricians believe the Americans with Disabilities Act (ADA) (1992) requires them to aggressively treat all newborns. Whether that is correct will be discussed later, but notice that this view gives parents no say in what is decided.

Every issue in bioethics has a pedigree and aggressive treatment of impaired babies has a long one. That pedigree is the story of the Baby Doe cases, the Baby Doe rules, and the Baby Doe squads. *Baby Doe cases* arise when parents of impaired neonates forgo treatment to let their baby die. This chapter discusses the Infant Doe case in Indiana in 1982, the Baby Jane Doe case in New York in 1983, the Baby Doe rules, and the legal and ethical issues of these cases. At the end, the chapter returns to treatment of premies.

History

In ancient Athens, both Plato (in *The Republic*) and Aristotle (in his *Politics*) advocated killing impaired newborns. In ancient Sparta, a cyclops baby (that is, an infant born with a single eye or with both eyes fused) would be left to die in a country field. Ancient Romans also abandoned babies who looked grotesque by exposing them to the elements. During the next four centuries, exposure remained common: such letting die was legal and not considered infanticide. The Bedouin tribes of Arabia, the Chinese, and much of India practiced female infanticide for two millennia.[4]

Around the year 300, Roman emperor Constantine converted to Christianity and as such, forbade both abandonment and infanticide. However, the church had neither funds nor people to care for abandoned babies. Foundling hospitals for abandoned babies did not start until the eighth century in Milan.

During the Middle Ages, wet nurses acted as agents for parents wishing to rid themselves of children (a practice that would continue well into the nineteenth century). In the eighteenth century, when the population of Europe exploded, exposure-as-infanticide became a form of extreme birth control.

During the reign of Napoleon, women abandoned so many babies that Napoleon established his own foundling hospitals, where parents could deposit a baby on a turntable set into the front entrance, spin it to send the baby inside, and depart unseen. In France in 1833, mothers abandoned over 100,000 babies—20 to 30 percent of all births.[5]

Just as respirators and feeding tubes during the 1960s first allowed comatose patients to stay alive, so neonatal intensive care units (NICUs) during the same period allowed premature babies to live. During the 1970s, tiny respirators and feeding tubes also began to be used on such babies. They saved babies with congenital disabilities who otherwise would have died.

About a third of premature babies will suffer a significant lifelong disability.[6] Treating such infants creates an ethical dilemma. A similar dilemma arose in the McCaughey septuplet case, where implanting seven embryos resulted in several disabled children. Moreover, treatment in NICUs is expensive. Both the expense of NICU treatment and the low quality of life of some of its survivors began to raise questions in the 1980s about whether such babies should be treated at all. Such questions led to the events described below.

Cases and Controversies Preceding the Baby Doe Rules

By 1983, when the Baby Jane Doe case took place, and as a result of several earlier cases, a set of rules known as the *Baby Doe rules* had already been developed. These earlier cases are described below; the following section discusses the rules themselves.

The Johns Hopkins Cases, 1971 Down's syndrome is a genetic condition that always causes retardation and a characteristic facial appearance; it is often accompanied by cardiac or intestinal problems. In the early 1970s—at the time of the Johns Hopkins cases—physicians told parents that although the eventual IQ of a person with Down's could not be predicted at birth, it usually ranged between 25 and 60, with some severely impaired individuals below 25. (We will later discuss whether this information was correct.)

In 1971, when NICUs were new and physicians often omitted aggressive treatment from impaired newborns, three Down babies in the NICU at Johns Hopkins Hospital in Baltimore, Maryland, had life-threatening intestinal defects. Physicians and parents allowed two of them to die.[7]

One of the babies had *duodenal atresia,* a blockage between the higher duodenum and the lower stomach that prevents passage of food and water. The mother of this baby—a nurse who had worked with children with Down's syndrome—

knew that if she did not consent to surgery to open the atresia her infant would die. She refused to do so, as did her husband, a lawyer. Pediatric surgeons at Hopkins honored their decision and did not go to court to force them to operate.

Another mother who already had other children allowed her Down baby to die. According to theologian James Gustafson, she explained her decision to forgo treatment by saying, "It would be unfair to the other children of the household to raise them with a mongoloid."[8] (Because of the facial characteristics associated in Down's syndrome, it was at once called "mongolism," a term now considered prejudicial). Gustafson describes this mother's decision as "anguished," but notes that when she learned her baby had Down's syndrome, she "immediately indicated she did not want the child."

No one killed the two Down babies; they were simply allowed to die—physicians thought this course more acceptable morally and less likely to incur legal prosecution. One of these babies took 15 days to die; ordinarily, the baby would have died in about four days by dehydration, but some staff members surreptitiously gave the infant water.

The parents of the third baby eventually accepted treatment, and this baby lived. This baby's parents had originally been given a pessimistic prognosis for Down's syndrome by an obstetrician who referred them to Hopkins, which had allowed the other two babies to die. However—and perhaps significantly—the staff at Hopkins gave the third set of parents a more balanced view.

Pediatric Intensivists Go Public, 1970s

In the early 1970s, because of the increasing incidence of these cases, several well-known pediatricians went public. R. Duff and A. Campbell at Yale-New Haven Medical Center admitted they had forgone treatment for 43 impaired infants, who died early.[9] They caused a sensation and led to soul-searching by pediatricians at other NICUs, who wondered if they, too, were doing the right thing in aggressively treating all impaired newborns.

English physician John Lorber, a specialist in spina bifida, then argued that some babies suffer such extreme impairment that they are better off being allowed to die without treatment.[10] *Spina bifida* literally means "divided spine" and is a hernial protrusion through a defect in the vertebral column. It is the most common serious neural-tube defect, occurring in 1 in 1,000 live births. It may occur in the form of a *meningocele*, a protrusion of part of the meninges; or it may take the form of a *myelomeningocele*, a protrusion not only of part of the meninges, but also of the spinal cord (the nerve bundle).

A baby with spina bifida will almost always be paralyzed below the level of the opening and suffer bowel and bladder problems. The opening makes the baby vulnerable to infections such as meningitis. Quality of life depends on two factors: first, the level of the meningomyelocele; and second, the degree of associated problems such as hydrocephalus—a swelling of cranial tissue that commonly accompanies spina bifida.

A hydrocephalus often increases intracranial pressure and decreases blood flow to the brain, resulting in mental retardation. However, the probability of mental retardation can be reduced by aggressive surgical treatment involving tubes called *shunts*, which decrease the pressure.

Lorber developed criteria to predict which spina bifida babies, if left untreated, would die: the higher the meningomyelocele on the spine and the larger the affected area of the spine and its coverings, the greater the probability of attendant problems and of death. These criteria had risks and a dilemma: if left untreated, not all infants with spina bifida die, and for infants who live, nontreatment makes them worse off. Lorber's criteria seemed to make it possible to identify babies who would die: all those in his lowest category did die. During the 1970s, criteria like Lorber's were apparently used at Oklahoma Children's Hospital, where it was decided not to treat 24 babies with spina bifida who were in the lowest category and who all subsequently died.[11]

The Mueller Case: Conjoined Twins, 1981 In 1981, conjoined twins joined at the trunk and sharing three legs were born in Danville, Illinois, to Pamela and Robert Mueller.[12] Robert Mueller, a physician, was in the delivery room when their family physician, Petra Warren, delivered the babies, who were named Jeff and Scott. The Muellers and Warren decided together not to treat the twins aggressively, so they could die.

Other physicians in Danville divided deeply over the ethics of the Muellers's decision. An anonymous caller alerted Protective Child Services, which obtained a court order for temporary custody of the children.

Prosecutors charged the Muellers with neglect; later a judge dismissed that charge, but he did deny the Muellers custody. In September 1981, they regained custody after pediatric surgeons testified that they would be unlikely to successfully separate the twins and that they had a bleak prognosis.

Subsequent events in this case tell a different tale. The twins lived, still joined, for about a year, at which time they weighed 30 pounds.[13] Shortly thereafter, they were separated in a long operation. Scott, the weaker twin, died; but Jeff, the stronger twin, survived, and he later entered a regular school.

Some might also question the necessity of separating the conjoined twins in the first place. The desire for normality and to have singletons often creates an unstoppable force by parents and surgeons to turn all children into normal-looking singletons (a topic discussed in Chapter 12).

The Infant Doe Case, 1982 The Infant Doe case in Bloomington, Indiana, took place about one year after the Mueller case, but only over the course of a few days—from Infant Doe's birth on April 9, 1982, to its death on April 15. Infant Doe had Down's syndrome with tracheoesophageal fistula, and once again physicians split over forgoing treatment.[14]

The prognosis for tracheoesophageal fistula is more serious than for duodenal atresia and depends on the severity of the fistula, or gap. Infant Doe had a fairly small gap, and an early operation to close it would have had a 90 percent chance of success. However, in discussing the case with the parents, the referring obstetrician, Walter Owens, downplayed this fact and emphasized that some Down people are "mere blobs" and that the "lifetime cost" of caring for a Down child would "almost surely be close to $1 million." Infant Doe's parents decided not to allow the operation.

Hospital administrators and pediatricians disagreed with the parents' decision and contacted Monroe County judge John Baker. Owens testified before Baker that even if surgery were successful, "the possibility of a minimally adequate quality of life was nonexistent" because of "the child's severe and irreversible mental retardation."

Infant Doe's father, a public school teacher who had worked closely with Down children, agreed with Dr. Owens and felt that such children never had a "minimally acceptable quality of life." It is noteworthy that Judge Baker held this hearing late at night in a room at the hospital where no one recorded it and did not appoint a guardian *ad litem* for Infant Doe. The judge then ruled for the parents.

The county district attorney appealed to the County Circuit Court, and after losing there, to the Indiana Supreme Court. Both appeals failed: each time the court ruled for the parents. He then appealed to United States Supreme Court Justice Paul Stevens for an emergency intervention, but Infant Doe died, making the case moot.

Seven years later in 1989, the U.S. Civil Rights Commission cited the Infant Doe case as a landmark case of prejudice against disabled infants. Owens wrote about his role in the Infant Doe case, maintaining that he was "proud to have stood up for what I and a large percentage of people feel is right"; he also said he was glad that Infant Doe had died in only a few days and with little suffering, and glad that the parents were able to have another baby—a healthy child who, if the couple had been forced to treat Infant Doe, would not have been born. The commission concluded that Owens's evaluation was "strikingly out of touch with the contemporary evidence on the capabilities of people with Down's syndrome."[15]

The Baby Doe Rules, 1982–1986

National media extensively reported the Infant Doe case, which prompted President Ronald Reagan to direct the Justice Department and the Department of Health and Human Services (HHS) to mandate treatment in future cases. Reagan, who opposed abortion, had appointed C. Everett Koop as surgeon general. Koop had previously written a book opposing nontreatment of impaired newborns.[16]

Because states define crimes such as homicide and gross negligence and not the federal government, Reagan's Justice Department needed to find an indirect route to make nontreatment illegal. It created a way to do so but one revealing contradictions in the views of conservatives about government's role in personal life.

The executive branch can set social policy by reinterpreting prior Congressional legislation. In the 1960s, President Lyndon Johnson reinterpreted old laws to fight racial discrimination. Institutions violating the new interpretations risk losing all federal funds.

Through similar executive orders, lawyers for the Justice Department in 1982 interpreted nontreatment to violate Section 504 of the Rehabilitation Act of 1973, which forbade discrimination solely on the basis of handicap. This interpretation saw imperiled newborns as handicapped citizens who could suffer discrimination against their federal civil rights. Congress had originally meant this act to apply to adults and children with handicaps, not babies.

HHS then required large posters to be displayed on the outer glass walls of every NICU:

> DISCRIMINATORY FAILURE TO FEED AND CARE FOR HANDICAPPED INFANTS IN THIS FACILITY IS PROHIBITED BY FEDERAL LAW.

It also posted a toll-free 800 telephone number on the poster so anyone around an NICU could report abuses—including concerned nurses, disgruntled parents, ambulance-chasing lawyers, and anonymous cranks. New *Baby Doe squads,* composed of lawyers, government administrators, and physicians investigated complaints.

The contradictions in conservatism about the Baby Doe rules lay along two fronts. First, some conservatives claimed that politicians and judges should not interpret the Constitution and previous law, especially for their own evaluative agenda. When they attack such interpretation, conservatives cite abortion and *Roe v. Wade*. Clearly, the Baby Doe rules reinterpreted previous law. Second, political conservatives once believed that federal government should not intrude in a family's life, leaving such decisions to parents, but the new activism about abortion and infanticide signaled a new activism that pushed the government to enforce conservative social values on all American families through the power of law.

In 1983, the American Academy of Pediatrics successfully sued in a federal district court to block the Baby Doe rules. While this suit ran, the Baby Jane Doe case began.

Before we turn to it, we should describe the Baby Doe hotline and the Baby Doe squads. As long as they existed, the Baby Doe squads were ready on an hour's notice to rush to airports, fly across the country, and suddenly arrive—as a squad arrived one day at Vanderbilt University—like outside accountants doing a surprise bank audit. They seized records, took charts from attending physicians, and investigated all night. The squads thought they saved the lives of innocent babies.

Besides Vanderbilt, the University of Rochester also suffered (in the words used privately by some pediatricians) a "blitzkrieg by the Baby Doe Gestapo." Eventually, because of the objections by pediatricians and the national press, the squads were called off.

What was the ultimate effect of the hotline and the squads? One study discovered that Baby Doe squads did in fact *force* more treatment for six infants, who had operations they otherwise might not have had, but in no case did the squads *prove* a violation of the Baby Doe regulations.[17]

The Baby Jane Doe Case, 1983–1984

On October 11, 1983, physicians delivered Baby Jane Doe at St. Charles Hospital of Long Island, New York. Because she had several major defects, they transferred her to an NICU at University Hospital of the State University of New York (SUNY) campus at Stony Brook for care by neonatal specialists.

Her parents—known only as Linda and Dan—worked hard to improve their lives as lower-middle-class people. Linda, 23, and Dan, 30, had been married four months when she became pregnant. Dan had built two extra rooms onto what has been described as their "modest suburban home" in the "flatlands of eastern Long Island."

Baby Jane weighed six pounds and was 20 inches long. According to testimony, at birth she had spina bifida, hydrocephalus, a damaged kidney, and *microcephaly* (small head, implying a minimal brain or lack of most of the brain). Her spine was open with the meningocele protruding prominently. Her defects surely traumatized her parents.

At Stony Brook, surgeon Arjen Keuskamp recommended immediate surgery to minimize retardation by draining the hydrocephalus. After he examined Baby Jane, George Newman, a pediatric neurologist, told Dan that the baby would either die soon without surgery or could undergo surgery and be paralyzed, retarded, and vulnerable to continual infections in her bladder and bowels. According to Newman's later court testimony:

> The decision made by the parents is that it would be unkind to have surgery performed on this child. . . . On the basis of the combination of malformations that are present in this child, *she is not likely to ever achieve any meaningful interaction with her environment, nor ever achieve any interpersonal relationships*, the very qualities which we consider human.[18]

Keuskamp withdrew from the case and did not testify in court. About midnight on October 11, 14 hours after Baby Jane's birth, Newman probably told Dan something like his testimony in court.

After a good deal of soul-searching, Dan and Linda decided not to allow the operation to drain the hydrocephalus. They acted on their understanding of the distinction between extraordinary and ordinary treatment, disallowing surgery but allowing "comfort care": food, fluids, and antibiotics.

Based on what they had been told, they naively assumed that Baby Jane would soon die, but four days later she was still alive. A social worker wrote at this time that Dan was in "despair" because Baby Jane had not yet died; she also noted that Linda was determined to give Baby Jane "as much love as possible" while the infant was still alive. "We love her very much," Linda said, "and that's why we made the decision we did."[19]

Newsday reporter Kathleen Kerr broke the Baby Jane Doe story nationally on October 18, 1983. Kerr, who had numerous firsts on the story, was also the only reporter to interview the parents. She described the interview:

> Each time he began a sentence, Mr. A. let out a deep sigh, as though seeking strength to answer. Mrs. A. continually touched her husband's arm and rubbed it soothingly. Mr. A. shed his tears openly. . . . Mr. A. said, "We feel the conservative method of treatment is going to do her as much good as if surgery were to be performed. It's not a case of our not caring. We very much want this baby. . . ."
>
> "We're not being neglectful, and we're not relying on our religion [Catholicism] to give us the answer to what we're doing here."[20]

Baby Jane Doe continued to survive, and—as occurs naturally in some cases of spina bifida—her open spinal wound closed.

Baby Jane's Case in the Courts

On October 18, 1983 (the same day that Kerr broke the story), Lawrence Washburn, a municipal-bonds lawyer who lived in Vermont and who promoted right-to-life organizations, filed suit in a state court to force treatment for Baby Jane. Over the following weeks, the case speeded through the courts, because everyone wanted to avoid a repetition of the Infant Doe case, where the baby had died while appeals bogged down.

Judge Melvyn Tannenbaum held an emergency lower-court hearing on October 20. Because Washburn lacked legal standing to sue, Tannenbaum appointed another attorney, William Weber, as Baby Jane's guardian *ad litem* ("for this action or proceeding"), and empowered him temporarily to make decisions regarding Baby Jane's medical care.

At first, Weber supported the parents, but then an interesting fact surfaced. Having talked to Newman, Weber abruptly changed his mind when he read two items in Baby Jane's medical chart. First, he read that Newman had written that after surgery, Jane would be able to walk with braces.[21] Second, her chart said that the initial measurement of her skull was 31 centimeters (cm), which is within normal limits. A measurement of 31 cm would indicate that Baby Jane had a brain, perhaps even a normal brain.

Yet Newman had testified that the baby had microcephaly and would never be able to recognize her parents. Weber concluded that what Newman had written on the chart conflicted both with what he had told the parents and with his testimony in court. So dramatically, Weber decided that Newman's claim of microcephaly was "a lie" and on October 20, authorized surgery.

The case ended up in the appellate division of New York courts. The justices there decided that the law left decisions up to parents when a choice was available between two *medically reasonable options*. Interestingly, previous rulings of courts had required a "medically reasonable option" to be an option that was not only supported by evidence, but also in the interest of the child. The new judgment contradicted these precedents.

It is interesting to compare this decision in 1983 to the 2006 decision by the U.S. Supreme Court blocking Attorney General Ashcroft from enforcing a traditional definition of "legitimate medical purpose" in interpreting laws about terminal, competent adults (see Chapter 4). The 1983 interpretation clearly wants to let parents make important medical decisions in the nursery; the 2006 decision clearly wants to let physicians and Oregonians decide whether helping terminal patients die is a legitimate purpose of medicine.

These court hearings splashed across front pages of American newspapers. Perhaps this immense publicity created too much pressure. The courts seemed to forget about the traditional doctrine of *parens patria,* according to which the state protects helpless people against those who might neglect them.

After these court proceedings concluded, the parents said:

> I just want [all this] to end. Just to have a baby like this and deal with it is so much to go through right now. Just let us be with our daughter and leave us alone. . . . If there's hell, we've been through it.

By this point, however, the federal government had begun to act.

In October, the Justice Department informed Stony Brook Hospital that federal investigators wanted to see Baby Jane's medical records. This intrusion outraged the parents: "They're not doctors, they're not the parents, and they have no business in our lives right now."[22]

Stony Brook's lawyer then announced that the hospital would block the government from examining the records. HHS turned the case over to the Justice Department, which sued the hospital in federal court, charging possible discrimination against the handicapped. Attorney General Edwin Meese and Surgeon General Everett Koop personally led the suit.

Federal judge Leonard Wexler there ruled that the Justice Department could not have the medical record and that the parents had not decided against surgery for "discriminatory" reasons. (It is not clear if Judge Wexler had examined Baby Jane's hospital chart.)

The ruling pleased the parents. "I'm drained physically, mentally, and emotionally," Dan said; "I believed that you couldn't look at what we were doing and say we were wrong."

In 1984, the case reached the federal Court of Appeals for the Second Circuit, which again denied the government access to Baby Jane's records. This decision, which would presumably apply in similar cases, had the practical effect of making the Baby Doe rules useless: because the government could not obtain medical records from NICUs or hospitals, it could not enforce the Baby Doe rules. The Justice Department appealed to the United States Supreme Court, but two years later in 1986, in *Bowen v. American Hospital Association et al.*, the Supreme Court declared that no records needed to be released and, in effect, ended the Baby Doe rules, their national hotline, and their possible investigators.

Amazingly, during the court battles over Baby Jane, Linda and Dan actually changed their minds and permitted surgery to drain her hydrocephalus—a decision that became known only months later.[23] After contracting pneumonia, the baby had been given strong antibiotics (without these antibiotics, she might have died).

Baby Jane continued to live and went home on April 7, 1984, at age five-and-a-half months. At that time, one physician predicted that she would "probably always be bedridden."[24]

Five years later, Jane lived at home with her parents. According to Kathleen Kerr, whose stories about the case won a Pulitzer Prize for local reporting and who visited with the family over those years, Jane was:

> . . . doing better than anyone expected—talking, attending school for the handicapped, and learning to mix with her peers. She still can't walk and gets around in a wheelchair but her progress has defied the dire predictions.[25]

The reporting of Baby Jane's case in the print and visual media raised some disturbing questions, especially when we consider that Jane not only survived but also was able to live at home and even attend school. Recall that Dr. Newman had testified that Jane would never achieve any meaningful interaction with her environment or any interpersonal relationships. Why did Newman's opinion prevail? That should stimulate some thought.

During 1983, the momentum of the media in support of the parents—and with it the momentum of medicine and medical ethics—became so strong that the media portrayed dissenters as bigots. People read reports of the Baby Jane Doe case with their minds made up. In November, when Lesley Stahl grilled C. Everett Koop on *Face the Nation,* her tone painted him as a fundamentalist, parent-baiting Big Brother. Ed Bradley also did a similar hatchet job on Koop and the case on *60 Minutes.*

From today's perspective, Koop's answers during these interviews are impressive: He said that the medical chart had discrepancies and that he merely wanted to see it to learn what was best for the child.

One pediatric neurosurgeon who had treated over a thousand patients with spina bifida said that children whose heads measured 31 cm (as Baby Jane's did) are among "the very brightest" of such children, presumably implying that Baby Jane's IQ could be normal or better.[26] The public also did not learn that although hydrocephalus generally accompanies spina bifida, if shunted immediately, it may not cause retardation.

All the major media simply accepted George Newman's negative prognosis, and almost all dismissed William Weber, the child's court-appointed guardian, as a fanatic. The media's stance may have unduly influenced not only the general public, but even many physicians and medical ethicists, who took Newman's depressing prognosis as fact.

In retrospect, another astonishing aspect of the story escaped the public's notice. When Stony Brook Hospital resisted Koop's attempt to see Baby Jane's medical chart, the hospital's motives might not have been to protect the privacy of the family, but to protect itself from a court suit. Given that what Newman had written in the chart contradicted what the parents had heard him say, one can see that the hospital had a big problem.

Beyond a doubt, pediatricians disagreed about which treatment was best for Baby Jane, or about the "medically reasonable options" in this case. Unfortunately, the public never read about the two real sides of this medical controversy. As a result, the public came to believe that the case involved only moral questions about parental decisions and low quality of life, when in fact it raised questions about making decisions based on incomplete, biased information and a hospital protecting itself from a lawsuit.

It is astonishing that a story for which the journalist won a Pulitzer Prize has such major errors and omissions. It is astonishing that neither the *New York Times* nor the *Wall Street Journal* checked the story's facts independently. The media during this time so much favored the parents that perhaps it was politically impossible for any reporter to present another side.

Perhaps, too, that just shows how hard the story was to understand and how difficult it is for the public to get the real story. Physicians usually will not talk to reporters about a controversial case and will not criticize their colleagues to reporters. So the public finds out only in court what is really going on about the case.

In 1994, another reporter interviewed Jane Doe and her family:

> Now a 10-year-old, . . . Jane Doe is not only a self-aware little girl, who experiences and returns the love of her parents; she also attends a school for developmentally

> disabled children—once again proving that medicine is an art, not a science, and clinical decision making is best left in the clinic, to those who will have to live with the decision being made.[27]

In 1998, Paul Gianelli, who represented the parents in their legal battles, told reporters that Jane was 15 years old and still living with her parents, who guard her privacy and theirs. "It was a very sad case and yet satisfying," said Gianelli, who ultimately won in court for the parents.[28]

ETHICAL ISSUES

Selfishness

Theologian James Gustafson said Baby Jane Doe's parents selfishly did not want Baby Jane to live.[29] He said that Judaism and Christianity require us to live our lives for others. C. Everett Koop argued similarly: "Why not let the family find that deeper meaning of life by providing the love and the attention necessary to take care of an infant that has been given to them?"[30]

In contrast, the late John Fletcher, a former Episcopalian priest who later became a secular medical ethicist, said that he could "stand by the parents" in such cases and "would not want to come down real hard on them" for letting a baby die by forgoing treatment.[31] Others asked whether, if living for others was a religious value, nonreligious people should be forced to adhere to it.

Reluctance to raise a profoundly disabled child is not necessarily selfish and may be simply realistic. For a couple who both work, raising a severely disabled child usually means that one parent must give up a job and hence the couple will lose income. Moreover, caring for such a person is a lifelong job: people with Down's syndrome in 2002 had an average lifespan of 49, and some live into their 70s. Some Down children will outlive their parents. Is it really always selfish for parents to decide that they are not called to spend their own lives caring for such a person, especially if at birth they can choose a different life?

Disability advocates argue that disadvantaged children cannot be allowed to die merely because they don't fit into their parents' plans. Part of the responsibility of having sex, and accepting childbirth, is to accept whatever comes along. We can't let parents adopt the attitude of, "I'll only be a parent if my child is healthy and normal." They also stress that family values means that everyone in a family pulls together to help the least well-off member, whether that person is Baby Doe or Granny Doe. They reject the conceptualization of this case as parental autonomy versus Big Brother. Instead, they see the case as one of communitarian ethics, where "it takes a village" to see the potential of a Down child.

On the other hand, if we do not consider the family's good in some way, are we not implying that the every family must accept the birth of an impaired child, no matter what the hardships? As an institution, the family today seems shaky; how much can it take?

Newsday writer Fred Bruning urged everyone to leave the parents alone:

> Travelers familiar with Beirut claim it is a city lost to hope because consensus is impossible. Perhaps it can be said that parents of severely damaged children

> inhabit a Beirut of the spirit, a place where innocence has no armor, where there is no distinction between suffering and survival. The rest of us are strangers, and we ought to let the parents consult the doctors, reach their decisions, tend to their babies, grapple with their lives. We ought to respect their heartache and their wishes. We ought to leave them in peace.[32]

Abortion versus Infanticide

Today, many pregnant women undergo amniocentesis or sonograms, and if the results indicate a fetus with a chromosomal abnormality, many terminate the pregnancy and try for a healthy baby. Such abortions can take place legally late in the second trimester, when the fetus is large and perhaps at a stage of development where some premature babies are saved. This practice raises a significant ethical issue.

When amniocentesis indicates spina bifida, the fetus will almost always be aborted. But if spina bifida justifies abortion, why doesn't it also justify letting a newborn with spina bifida die? Similarly, if an abortion is permissible because the fetus has Down's syndrome, why shouldn't Down's syndrome justify allowing a baby to die?

Birth, after all, does not change the medical condition: in this sense, it can be argued that the significance of birth is merely symbolic or emotional. Note that this logic is neutral between opposed moral conclusions about nontreatment. That is, if there is no good reason why a neonate with, say, spina bifida should be allowed to die, then presumably there is no good reason why a fetus with spina bifida should be aborted.

If parents want to forgo treatment in these cases, then should they be required to justify the decision, or should they simply be left alone? When a woman decides to abort even a healthy fetus, she is not required to give good reasons. Why are we so much more concerned when an impaired newborn is involved?

Conceptually, the problem is to find a consistent position that includes accepting abortion but opposes letting parents decide to forgo treatment in Baby Doe case. If one accepts choice with regard to abortion because of a Down fetus, should one also accept choice about parents letting a Down newborn die? Or perhaps one should oppose both?

Killing versus Letting Die with Newborns

In a famous article, the late James Rachels asked whether it would not be more compassionate to simply kill impaired and imperiled newborns than to let them die slowly by forgoing treatment.[33] Rachels argued this way: In both forgoing and infanticide, the motive—the death of the baby—is the same, and so is the result: in both, the baby dies. If both decisions have the same motive, and if both decisions lead to death, how can the two decisions differ morally?

This might seem to be a matter of simple logic: whatever makes one decision good (or bad) should also make the other decision good (or bad). If so, the kind of action itself, as to its active or passive nature, should make no difference.

Some bioethicists disagree with Rachels, especially about nontreatment of newborns and infanticide. One reason they do is because people are not perfect and make mistakes; killing is too quick and too final. Merely allowing an infant to die leaves the door open for a while, in case parents or physicians have a change of heart. Another argument for forgoing treatment is that it shows more respect for the value of life: a quick end cheapens life, but when treatment is forgone, parents and professionals must suffer through the ordeal.

Personhood of Impaired Neonates

Before he became surgeon general, C. Everett Koop wrote that, "each newborn infant, perfect or deformed, is a human being with unique preciousness because he or she was created in the image of God."[34] On the other hand, Catholic theologian Richard McCormick argued that an infant can realize some "good" of its own only if it can potentially form human relationships.[35] So Koop assumed that any human newborn is a person, whereas McCormick's criterion would rule out anencephalic babies as persons.

McCormick's *potential-for-relationships standard* is a reasonable attempt to delimit personhood, but it has problems. It can be difficult to predict potential for relationships, which seems to depend on the attitude of parents. Associations of parents of babies with spina bifida hold that a person's potential cannot be known until his or her life is lived.

The *gradient view of personhood* asserts that the developmental stage of the fetus/baby really does matter morally. After all, a crying baby differs a lot from a two-day-old embryo. Several cognitive scientists and bioethicists believe that personhood develops along a gradient, such that the further along this continuum, the more the fetus is a person. This view rejects the all-or-nothing fallacy that an embryo or fetus is not a person one moment, but a person the next.

On the gradient view, it's worse to kill fetuses than embryos, and it's worse to kill fetuses just before birth than in the first trimester (which explains why many physicians are reluctant to perform so-called partial birth abortions). Similarly, a Down baby differs from a Down fetus: the former has more moral status and rights. The death of a baby requires more justification than the death of a fetus.

The distinctions of the gradient view drive some opponents to claim that no difference in personhood or moral status exists between human embryos and human babies. Both sides agree about the gradient and the continuum of development of personhood, but they disagree about the proper inferences to draw from this fact.

In Baby Doe cases, some bioethicists champion the *cognitive criterion of personhood.* It identifies certain characteristics, including reason, agency, memory, and self-awareness, and assumes that without them, personhood does not exist.

With regard to impaired infants, bioethicist Peter Singer once used the cognitive criterion to argue that children should not be regarded as persons until "a few months" after birth; physician and philosopher Tristam Engelhardt once held that infants are not persons until they form a self-concept, around the age of two (he has since given up this position). Philosopher Michael Tooley holds that they are not persons until they can use language.[36] For Singer, Engelhardt, and Tooley, newborns fail to meet the cognitive criterion.

As noted before, many families use the cognitive criterion in letting adult relatives die. However, its application to impaired newborns may be more questionable. Allowing parents to forgo treatment for an imperiled neonate is one thing; claiming that a child is not a person until age two seems to be quite another.

Personal versus Public Cases

Was Baby Jane's case a private, personal family decision or a case of neglect that public policy must not tolerate? One member of a group advocating recognition of the sanctity of life in public policy criticized the parents, maintaining that "private individuals and private groups of individuals don't have the right to make life or death decisions in private in an unaccountable manner."[37] On the other hand, many people argued that Baby Jane's parents should have been left alone to make decisions.

Do problems of personhood effectively prevent us from applying Mill's concept of harm in this context? Can we distinguish between private life and morality here? Mill's harm principle calls for government not to interfere with decisions that put no other person at risk of harm, but his principle may not help us in Baby Doe cases, if we think that impaired babies are persons.

If we decide that every impaired newborn is a person, it follows that no parent could decide to let such a child die, and this would severely limit a family's range of choices. But if we allow a wide range of choices, we allow each family to decide what personhood is. Can we allow that?

For example, the state of Tennessee intervened in 1983 over a father's religious objections to allow chemotherapy for 12-year-old leukemia patient Pamela Hamilton. Another such case occurred in Boston in 1988, when a young child became ill; the child's parents, who were Christian Scientists, called a practitioner instead of a physician; after apparently improving for a while, the child suddenly died five days later. Boston district attorney Newman Flanagan charged the parents with manslaughter.

Clearly society must strike a balance between allowing parents some choice about medical treatment of their children and protecting vulnerable children from misguided parents. But which parents are wise, which misguided? That is the question in what follows.

Conceptual Issue: Taxonomy in Ethics

Cases of treatment versus nontreatment are often grouped together and sometimes even lumped together with cases of assisted suicide and physician-assisted dying, as "euthanasia." This is confusing and possibly dangerous. As argued previously, we should differentiate physician-assisted dying, which involves terminally ill competent adults, from assisted suicide, which involves nonterminal competent adults. We should also distinguish these from nontreatment of incompetent adults in PVS and distinguish the above from allowing impaired newborns to die.

One reason why such distinctions matter has to do with criteria for forgoing treatment. Criteria for nontreatment of *never-competent* patients should presumably be much higher than the criteria for competent or formerly competent patients whose own wishes can be known or inferred. With never competent patients, the decision to forgo treatment must be based on evidence that is beyond a reasonable doubt, and this would also be true for babies who are presently incompetent but who later may be competent.

Degrees of Defect

In practice, criteria for nontreatment of impaired babies tend to be based on long-term prognoses and degrees of defectiveness in newborns.[38] Babies whose problems are "less serious" should be treated, whereas it would be permissible to let babies who are "most serious" or "gravely ill" die.

Cases between these two poles—cases such as spina bifida and Down's syndrome—create controversy because prognosis is far from absolute and may be influenced by moral frameworks.

Consider John Lorber's predictive criteria for spina bifida. One vocal critic of Lorber's approach is his colleague at the same hospital, pediatric surgeon R. B. Zachary. Zachary argues that the only options for babies with spina bifida are either to kill them or to do everything possible for each one of them. Basically, he is saying that there is no category of babies with spina bifida who can be "allowed to die."

Lorber and some other pediatricians say that the mortality rate is high for babies they place in the "worst" category of spina bifida, but Zachary maintains that these physicians do not simply withhold treatment. According to Zachary, they "push the infant towards death" by giving:

> eight times the sedative dose of chloral hydrate recommended in the most recent volume of Nelson's Pediatrics and four times the hypnotic dose, and it is being administered four times every day. No wonder these babies are sleepy and demand no feeding, and with this regimen most of them will die within a few weeks, many within the first week.[39]

Prognoses about the intelligence of impaired people seem to be influenced by social views. Down's syndrome is a good example, especially because of the external characteristics associated with it. Let's briefly consider Down's syndrome in more detail.

During the last 50 years, a Copernican revolution has occurred in thinking about Down people.[40] Many earlier studies of IQ on those who were institutionalized were flawed. A sampling bias failed to take into account the higher IQs of Down people who lived with supportive families.

At present, although most Down people will have IQs below 70, less than one-third (some studies say only 10 percent) will have IQs lower than 25 (profoundly retarded and untrainable).[41] Most Down people who receive good early care, maximum stimulation, and support will have IQs between 50 and 70.

What does this imply about quality of life for a Down person? IQ is a measure of intelligence, of course, and academics and physicians often associate intelligence with happiness. However, it is an unwarranted conclusion to infer that people with IQs between about 50 and 70 must be unhappy, unless we simply define unhappiness in those terms.

Given reasonable stimulation, love, and supervision, most Down people will, to use a phrase made important in ethics by philosopher Tom Regan in another context, "have a life."[42] Almost every Down person will have a narrative history, and lives that will go (to use another famous phrase from Regan), "better or worse for them." Under almost any criteria of quality of life, most Down people would not be better off dead.

Note the mention of early care, stimulation, and support; the prognosis for Down's syndrome varies with treatment: early stimulation can raise IQ, whereas merely custodial care will lower it. At birth, we cannot predict whether a Down baby will be at the low or the high end of the IQ range; consequently, the best interest of these babies is maximal treatment. Whether maximal treatment best benefits their families is another question.

Sanctity of Life versus Quality of Life

It is interesting to realize that although the ethical frameworks loosely described as sanctity of life and quality of life are commonly held to be incompatible, these two standards would agree on the early treatment of most Down babies and babies with spina bifida.

It would seem that a neonate with spina bifida has a good chance of "a life"—that is, neither genetics nor probable IQ predetermines a life of misery. Often, it cannot be predicted at birth whether a child with spina bifida will be in the high, normal, or low range of IQ, but most such children will *not* be profoundly retarded. If we cannot assume that low IQ precludes any happiness in life, it can be argued that such children should live—that an IQ described as "borderline," "trainable," or even "imbecile" does not make life so bad that nonexistence would be better.

However, sanctity of life and quality of life diverge when a prognosis predicts a life of total pain: in such a case, considerations of sanctity of life or "the good of the child" support nontreatment. If this outcome could be known in advance, it would be immoral, from a quality of life standpoint, to save the neonate. These cases are the ones that traumatize pediatric neurologists. Because most of these children die, nontreatment is best—but not all of them die, and those who do not die will be worse off.

What about the *family's* quality of life? How does that figure into moral thinking? Into family values? Caring for an impaired child imposes enormous burdens on other children and stressed parents. If the quality of life standard applies to the entire family, rather than just to the baby ("the good of the child"), it implies nontreatment.

This interpretation of quality of life is unusual. When we think of quality of life in, say, cases of PVS or physician-assisted suicide, we are of course thinking of the *patient's* quality of life. Applying this standard to a neonate's family is like arguing that a patient in PVS should be allowed to die, or that a terminally ill patient should be helped to die, not for their own good but for that of the family.

Wrongful Birth versus Wrongful Life

Today, few parents simply accept birth defects as God's will. Standards of health continue to rise, and couples expect healthy babies. Parents often blame physicians for the birth of impaired babies and can sue physicians in civil courts for allegedly causing babies to be impaired.

Both wrongful life and wrongful birth suits fall into the general classification of tort law, and in both kinds of actions compensation for a harm or "tort" is sought.

It is important to distinguish between different meanings of "harm." Like the concept of good, the concept of harm covers a broad range of meanings. For our purposes here, we can distinguish three broad meanings of harm.

In the first way, both a baseline and a temporal (time) component are necessary, so that a change occurs that makes someone worse off. *Baseline harm* requires an adverse change in someone's condition. With baseline harm, someone who doesn't yet exist cannot be harmed, because he or she has no baseline from which change can occur.

The second way of defining harm compares a present deficiency with what normally would have been. In this *abnormal harm,* someone is injured by being brought into existence with some defect that could have been avoided by taking reasonable precautions. Here, the event or omission that causes the defect is the cause of harm.

Third, harm may be defined as a life of total pain and injury, such that no hope exists. Perhaps this is the lot of many pigs raised in industrial factory farms, confined their whole lives and squashed together for maximal profits in tiny metal pens with their tails cut off. Let us call this third way *total harm*. To some of its critics, reproductive cloning would be so bad for the child as to constitute total harm.

Preventing abnormal harm underlies the belief that parents should do everything possible to have healthy, unimpaired babies; that anything less than the maximal effort is blameworthy; and that it is wrong for a woman to take risks with a future person's intelligence or health. In this sense, deaf parents harm their children when they implant only embryos genetically disposed to be deaf.

Total harm in the law is called *wrongful life*. In such cases, lawyers claim that the lives of some babies are so miserable that their existence is a tort. In contrast, *wrongful birth* assumes abnormal harm, and claim not that the child's life is totally miserable, but that the child has been damaged by being born less than normal, and that a physician's action or omission caused the relevant defect. Courts have almost always rejected wrongful life suits because courts have rejected the implication that killing a baby can benefit it.

Several well-publicized wrongful birth suits by parents against physicians have transpired. In New Jersey, parents of a baby with Down's syndrome sued pro-life obstetrician James Delahunty, whom they say discouraged them from pursuing amniocentesis when a sonogram showed a fetus with a thick neck (a possible sign in utero of this condition).[43] The jury awarded the couple nearly $2 million and found Dr. Delahunty guilty of "failing to recognize, appreciate, and discuss the results of the tests, particularly ultrasound" with his patients. The verdict may have stemmed partially from Delahunty's combative behavior in the courtroom.

At least 27 states allow parents to sue for wrongful birth, although Michigan and Georgia recently disallowed them. In a case in 1999, as well as another case in 1990, the Georgia Supreme Court ruled that a couple with a Down child could not sue their physician for failure to perform amniocentesis or other prenatal tests.[44]

In France, an uproar occurred when, after 13 years of litigation, a court ruled in 1995 that parents of a child born with German measles and not offered an abortion were entitled to compensation for wrongful birth. In two subsequent cases, damages were also awarded to parents of children with disabilities where parents argued that had they known prenatally of the disability, they would have aborted. Critics in France assailed these results, saying they had established a "right not to be borne" and restarted Nazi eugenics, and would increase premiums for malpractice. The French legislature in 2002 banned wrongful birth suits.[45]

New Legislation

In 1984, Congress amended its Child Abuse Prevention and Treatment Act of 1974 (not the Rehabilitation Act), to count nontreatment in Baby Doe cases as *child abuse*. The Child Abuse Amendments (CAA) circumvented the injunction against the Baby Doe rules. They made states, not the federal government, responsible for such cases—getting Uncle Sam out of the neonatal nursery. These amendments were never repealed and are technically still in force today.[46]

The only exceptions to the CAA are: (1) when an impaired child is (1) "chronically and irreversibly comatose," (2) when a child is inevitably dying, and (3) when treatment would be "futile and inhumane." These exceptions are often interpreted narrowly, so as to give parents few choices. As one law professor sums it up, "Since passage of the CAA, ethical and legal controversy over parental authority to withhold treatment from handicapped or disabled newborns . . . has largely ceased."[47]

Problems resulting from such narrow interpretation were illustrated dramatically in the Rudy Linares case, which took place in Chicago in 1989. Dan Linares held an NICU staff at gunpoint while he disconnected the respirator of his 16-month-old son Rudy, who had gone into PVS nine months earlier, after swallowing a balloon at a birthday party; Rudy soon died, and Dan Linares was charged with first-degree murder.[48] Because there was no doubt that Dan Linares was a caring parent, a grand jury refused to indict him for homicide; he later received a suspended sentence on a minor charge arising from his use of a gun.

In 1992, the ADA went into effect; this act protects Americans with a wide range of disabilities from discrimination. The application of ADA to newborns with congenital defects—and thus to Baby Doe cases—is so far unresolved.

In 1994, a federal court specifically cited ADA in mandating treatment for a 16-month-old anencephalic infant, Baby K, who had been brought to a hospital emergency room in Virginia in respiratory distress.[49] Baby K had been on a respirator since birth. When the case was heard, her physicians wanted to disconnect it and let her die; but for religious reasons, her mother insisted on continued care. At its heart, Baby K's case was about whether physicians may overrule parents' decisions about continuing futile, expensive treatment without incurring charges of discrimination against the handicapped. For over a year, Baby K continued to receive treatment, but she died in 1995.

After two decades of legal wrangling about Baby Doe cases, the results are equivocal. On the one hand, some impaired babies who would once have died as a consequence of nontreatment now undoubtedly survive to lead meaningful lives. On the other hand, the right of parents to make choices in cases of disabled newborns has declined dramatically. As a result of the amendment to the child abuse act, most NICU physicians usually *overtreat* severely impaired newborns.[50]

The ADA does not make it criminal for physicians to withhold treatment from impaired newborns. Rather, it threatens to withhold federal funding from a state for its programs. Even under this threat, *no state has ever been found to be out of compliance.* Moreover, although thousands of such infants have had life-sustaining treatment withheld or withdrawn, contrary to the guidelines in these regulations, *no legal charges have ever been brought against physicians, hospitals, or states for doing so.*

Nevertheless, while the ADA imposed no criminal charges on physicians who failed to comply with their regulations, most obstetricians perceived it as requiring a presumption in favor of treatment. And subjected to a barrage of lawsuits with every disabled baby, obstetricians these days take few unnecessary risks.

History is repeating itself in bioethics with premature babies, whose numbers have recently soared.[51] The prospects are dire for such babies under 750 grams, yet they do not fall under exceptions to the ADA, so most physicians treat them aggressively. This treatment takes away choice from parents; such lack of choice is being increasingly challenged by parents in court.[52]

The Rise of Disability Advocates

Many pediatricians claim that in the 1950s, it was rare for a baby with Down's syndrome to live long.[53] Even after institutionalization, nontreatment intending death was the norm, not the exception. Babies who survived were sent to be warehoused in custodial institutions, where they were never stimulated or educated. They almost always became severely retarded.

Within pediatric neurology, opinion about treatment in Baby Doe cases changed dramatically over the past decades. In the 1960s and early 1970s, the consensus was that many such cases should not be treated; today, all but the most hopeless cases are treated.[54]

For example, Lorber's criteria concerning spina bifida initially swung the pendulum toward nontreatment in many NICUs; but during the 1980s, right-to-life organizations and disability advocates swung the pendulum back toward treatment. Also, breakthroughs were made in urology, neonatology, neurosurgery, and CAT scan diagnosis, and these not only increased the accuracy of prognoses but also improved quality of life for such children. These changes have led to a new understanding:

> Mild to moderate degrees of microcephaly are compatible with normal or even exceptional intellect. This is particularly true in cases of untreated meningomyelocele in which loss of cerebrospinal fluid through the unrepaired hole in the back may decrease the total mass of the head. . . . Essentially all children with severe meningomyelocele have hydrocephalus. . . . Children with hydrocephalus who are treated reasonably early and who do not develop meningitis have a better than 50 percent chance of being intellectually normal.[55]

The Spina Bifida Association has stated:

> Since we have found it virtually impossible to predict at birth which infants with meningomyelocele will become competitive, ambulatory, and intellectually able, we have not relied on arbitrary guidelines to determine which children should or should not be treated. On the contrary, we believe that all such children should be treated, and we feel that our data show this philosophy to be correct.[56]

The outcome in the Baby Jane Doe case, chosen for discussion because of its fame but otherwise typical of spina bifida, makes this statement seem reasonable. Moreover, the unexpected outcome of the Mueller case and the newer prognoses for Down's syndrome suggest that similar reasoning may be appropriate regarding other defects.

Conceptual Dilemma: Supporting Both Choice and Respect

The parents of spina bifida child Leilani Duff-Fraker, born in 2004, love their daughter, but if their obstetrician had ordered the right tests, they would have aborted her and tried again for a healthy child.[57] Is that inconsistent? Can you love a child who you might have deliberately stopped developing as a fetus?

In some aspects, this question is analogous to the Ayala case, where parents deliberately conceived a child to be a source of bone marrow for her older sister with leukemia. The Ayala parents claimed that they would and could love Marissa, and not just see her as a resource for her sister. Jodi Picoult's *My Sister's Keeper,* a work of fiction, tells a different story.

Public policy reveals a similar dilemma writ large. Is it consistent to do prenatal testing for genetic diseases while at the same time telling adults with the same diseases that they are respected? Is it consistent to test babies at birth for genetic conditions such as phenylketonuria (PKU), and at the same time tell adults with PKU that they are valued? Do funds for prevention of disabilities compete with funds for services for disabled adults?[58]

On another front, is history repeating itself with the half million premature babies born in America each year? Given that the ADA has taken away almost all choices about treatment from physicians and parents, must all extremely premature babies be aggressively treated? Notice that if some are "let die" and do not die as planned, we repeat the scenario of the Baby Jane Doe case.

Finding a consistent, defensible policy on these questions is not easy. Each day, bioethicists and physicians struggle to find it.

FURTHER READING AND RESOURCES

Fred Frohock, *Special Care: Medical Decisions at the Beginning of Life,* Chicago, University of Chicago Press, 1986.

Loretta Kopelman, "Are the 21-Year-Old Baby Doe Rules Misunderstood or Mistaken?" *Pediatrics,* 115: 3, March 2005, pp. 797–802.

John Freeman, "On Learning Humility: A Thirty-Year Journey," *Hastings Center Report,* May–June 2004, 13–16.

John Robertson, "Extreme Prematurity and Parental Rights After Baby Doe," *Hastings Center Report*, July/August 2004, 32–39.
Peggy and Robert Stimson, *The Long Dying of Baby Andrew*, Boston, Little, Brown, 1983.
U.S. Commission on Civil Rights, *Medical Discrimination against Children with Disabilities*, September 1989.

DISCUSSION QUESTIONS

1. Suppose you were expecting a healthy baby and discovered that you were going to have a Down baby or a baby with spina bifida. Would you be able to care for it?
2. Suppose you discovered the above in the first trimester of pregnancy. Would it be selfish of you to abort the baby then and try again for a healthy baby?
3. Is testing of fetuses for genetic conditions, followed by abortions, a new kind of eugenics? Should it worry people with disabilities?
4. Because it harms fetuses/babies so much, should it be illegal to smoke, drink, or use drugs during pregnancy?

CHAPTER 8

Can Medical Research on Animals Be Justified?

The Gennarelli and Taub Cases

The essential question of this chapter concerns whether using animals in medical research can be morally justified. The chapter surveys philosophical opposition to such research and describes the famous cases of Thomas Gennarelli, who injured primates to model head injuries in humans, and Edward Taub, who injured primates to study stroke in humans. Publicity about these cases changed the way animals are used in American research. (Note: In this chapter, although humans are animals, "animals" refers to "nonhuman animals.")

THE GENNARELLI CASE

The Animal Liberation Front and Gennarelli's Research

On Memorial Day, 1984, with labs vacant, members of the Animal Liberation Front (ALF) quietly entered the University of Pennsylvania Medical School in Philadelphia. They broke into a laboratory where they stole 32 audiovisual tapes documenting experiments on primates.

The stolen tapes had been made by neurologist Thomas Gennarelli, who hoped to produce exact brain damage in adult baboons. According to the *New York Times,*

> One sequence showed a monkey strapped to a table pulling against its bonds. The animal's head was encased in a steel cylinder to a pneumatic machine called an accelerator. Suddenly, a piston drove the cylinder upward, thrusting the animal's head sharply through an arc of about 60 degrees.

Doing this for over 15 years, from 1970 to 1985, Gennarelli tried, but failed, to create reproducible head injuries.

The ALF edited the 70 hours of tape to create a 25-minute piece showing the worst abuses and distributing it to television stations. (The Wikipedia article on this film "Unnecessary Fuss," contains free links to it.[1])

Researchers claimed that they sedated the baboons prior to injury and that the baboons felt no pain. Just before the pneumatic hammer smashes their heads, however, the tape shows obviously unsedated baboons struggling to free themselves.

The researchers, all men, sound adolescent and macho on the tape. As the *Times* reporter continues:

> In another sequence, as an animal lay in a coma, a researcher's recorded voice was heard saying, "You'd better have some axonal damage, monkey," and calling him "sucker."[2]

Researchers use profanity, perform unsterile surgery, and execute sloppy techniques. They hold up conscious baboons with broken arms and laugh at them.

In 1984, People for Ethical Treatment of Animals (PETA) gave the edited tape to Congress and ABC News. The public did not like what it saw and demanded suspension of Gennarelli's studies.

The National Institute of Health (NIH) appointed a committee to review the tapes, consisting of a neurosurgeon, a veterinary anesthesiologist, and a veterinary pathologist, all of whom used animals in research. It assumed nothing was intrinsically wrong with injuring baboons to study head injuries in humans: "The research, as proposed," it said, and despite 15 years of failure, "is likely to yield fruitful results for the good of society."[3]

Nevertheless, the committee found Gennarelli guilty of nine of ten charges against him: lack of anesthesia, inadequate supervision, poor training, inferior veterinary care, unnecessary multiple injuries to the same animals, humor, smoking, statements in poor taste around animals, and improper clothing. It concluded: "Taken collectively, these conclusions constitute material failure to comply with the Public Heath Service Animal Welfare Policy." "Material failure" is serious, like "lack of institutional control" over a college's athletic program.

NIH suspended Gennarelli's research, the first time a lab had been closed because of abuse of animals. To Carolyn Compton—a physician, pediatric researcher, and (paid?) spokeswoman for scientists using animals—this was a "tragedy."[4]

To ALF, this meant victory. One member of the original ALF team defended the break-in:

> We may seem like radicals to you, but we are like the Abolitionists, who were regarded as radicals, too. And we hope that 100 years from now, people will look back on the way animals are treated now with the same horror as we do when we look back on the slave trade.[5]

Six weeks after its Memorial Day raid, ALF struck the University of Pennsylvania's veterinary school, taking three cats, two dogs, and eight pigeons. The dean of this school said the raid "would set back research efforts, including a study to determine the cause of sudden infant death syndrome."[6] Another dean said the stolen cats modeled breathing during sleep, a missing dog had a steel plate inserted to study osteoarthritis, another dog had been given ear-canal infections to study cures, and the bones of pigeons had been broken to benefit all birds.[7] He said that the work on dogs would benefit other dogs, adding that such research had to be done and that more dogs would now be needed to use as subjects.

In 1984, ALF struck in California, taking two rabbits injected with oral herpes and numerous dogs with cancer, along with 100 other animals, from the City of Hope National Medical Center in Duarte. Inside the lab was painted: "ALF is watching and there's no place to hide!" Ingrid Newkirk of PETA called City of Hope a "concentration camp" where animals were "being used for painful experiments."[8]

The associate director of City of Hope said the theft of these animals had disrupted $500,000 worth of research on emphysema, cancer, and herpes. ALF had targeted a study testing tobacco carcinogens in dogs. The dogs were forced to breathe air full of tobacco smoke, a model that has never been proven to give lung cancer to dogs.

The associate director refused to comment on whether the abducted animals had been treated cruelly, but did say that 36 cancerous dogs, 12 cats, 12 rabbits, 28 mice, and 18 rats had been stolen and added, "We're concerned that very important research work may not now be completed."[9]

In 1985, the ALF hit the biology and psychology laboratories of the University of California, Riverside, taking 467 animals, including a stump-tailed macaque whose eyes had been sewn shut to study a device to help the blind navigate. PETA said these animals had been used in painful, unnecessary experiments, some involving starvation. NIH investigated the charges but found no evidence of abuse. The university claimed $683,000 in damages.

In 1987, arson gutted the $2.5 million veterinary research animal lab at the University of California, Davis; ALF claimed responsibility. In California in 1988, ALF destroyed a new building for animal research at the medical school in San Diego and burned down a veal-packing plant in Oakland. In televised interviews, masked ALF spokespersons took credit, vowing to continue the attacks "until the killing of the innocent animals stops."

Also in 1988 in Connecticut, Stephanie Trutt planted a bomb outside a company that made surgical staples and used animals to train surgeons in handling them. She was arrested for attempted murder.[10] About this time, the Federal Bureau of Investigation started to monitor and infiltrate the ALF, listing it as a terrorist, violent group.

Several experiments reviewed by NIH in the 1980s fared poorly. The City of Hope Medical Center was fined $25,000, lost $1 million in grants, and lost its Animal Care Assurance, a legal document whereby an institution promises to abide by federal regulations. After ALF released pictures of poor lab conditions and inspectors made an unannounced visit, Columbia University lost grants involving vertebrates.

To prevent further abuses, Congress mandated in 1986 *Institutional Animal Care and Use Committees* (IACUCs) for all institutions receiving federal funds for research on animals. Although IACUCs are composed mostly of researchers themselves, they do force experimenters to justify their projects to fellow scientists, some of whom can be critical. The existence of IACUCs is directly attributable to the exposure of Gennarelli's experiments.

In 2009 at the University of California at Santa Cruz, the ALF took responsibility for starting a fire at the home of animal researcher David A. Feldheim and may have burned a car outside the home of another researcher who lived nearby.[11]

Evaluating the Philadelphia Study

Gennarelli can be described as working at the bottom of a pyramid of basic research on head injury. To him, it seemed obvious that the first step in such research was to produce one head injury precisely and reliably, so others could study it. Similarly, knowing how to produce different kinds of burns in animals is the first step in studying the physiology of burns and the metabolism of healing.

Activists held that Gennarelli had bashed heads for a decade and gotten nowhere. They argued that even if he had succeeded in devising a reproducible model of head injuries, such a model would offer little help in treating such injuries.

A committee of his peers reviewed Gennarelli's grant and said that his research would contribute information about the drug mannitol in reducing brain swelling after trauma and about management of metabolic balance in comatose patients.

Critics said these conclusions papered over a lack of findings. Nedim Buyukmichi, an activist and veterinarian, argued that Gennarelli's studies were too inconsistent to result in a reproducible model of head injuries and too limited in scope to adequately mimic injuries sustained by human victims of accidents: "After 15 years and $11 million to $13 million, essentially nothing has come out of this research that hasn't already been known from studies of human head trauma."[12]

On the tapes workers in Gennarelli's lab appear to treat animals badly. Gennarelli's defenders claim the insensitive comments and behavior of researchers resembled gallows humor among medical residents, but that is no ethical justification, because today such humor is considered unprofessional.

Defenders also ask: even if the animals were mistreated and the researchers were insensitive, does that necessarily affect the scientific value of the research? For activists, Gennarelli's treatment of his animal subjects proved that his project was immoral, but perhaps the two claims should be separated.

PETA AND EDWARD TAUB'S RESEARCH ON MONKEYS

In 1981, Alex Pacheco volunteered in the primate lab of psychologist Edward Taub in Silver Spring, Maryland, a suburb just across the northern boundary of Washington, D.C. Pacheco told Taub that he wanted to become a research scientist, but he really wanted to videotape Taub's research for PETA.[13]

Taub there studied "somatosensory deafferentation" in monkeys by surgically cutting all the nerves in one limb and trying to stimulate regrowth. He hypothesized that, based on the famous idea of psychologist Martin Seligman of learned helplessness, voluntary nonuse caused some damage in stroke. Each year, stroke disables a half-million Americans, who often lose use of a limb.

Pacheco entered the lab late one night and photographed Taub's experiments. As a result, authorities tried Taub in Maryland on charges of cruelty to animals and, after drawn out legal maneuverings where various research organizations backed Taub, convicted Taub of one charge of failing to provide adequate veterinary care.

Pacheco's tactics here raised questions. To obtain evidence for the trial, Pacheco invited activists such as Donald Barnes, John McArdle, and Michael W. Fox to search Taub's lab at night; when warrants were served on Taub, several television stations recorded the event while PETA leaders distributed press releases.

During the trial, PETA's handling of the media was brilliant and it orchestrated each element for maximal impact.

Convicted of failing to provide proper veterinary care, a charge based on the fact that he did not bandage the animals' wounds, Taub testified that it was better to leave the wounds unbandaged. Years of experience had convinced him that the monkeys would only tear the bandages off, making their wounds worse.

Veterinarians disagreed. In response, the American Psychological Association's Ethics Committee, the NIH, and an ad hoc committee of the American Physiological Society exonerated Taub of failure to provide good care. After its own investigation, the psychology department at UAB hired him as a full professor, but to work only on humans, not animals.

The 1991 Story of the Year for ethics in *Discover* magazine concluded that four of Taub's monkeys showed:

> . . . dramatic new evidence of the adult brain's capacity to "rewire" itself, something previously thought to be impossible. And ironically, it was PETA's success at keeping the monkeys away from research for a decade that made the discovery possible.[14]

The 15 surviving monkeys had been transferred in 1986 to the federally funded Tulane Regional Primate Center in Covington, Louisiana. In 1990, in an experiment that PETA opposed, a brain researcher—Timothy Pons—tested Taub's hypothesis by examining the brain of a dying monkey before euthanasia. Pons was "flabbergasted" to discover that "the entire patch of the cortex corresponding to the arm—about half an inch wide—had been rewired to receive input from the face." Pons concluded, "The results offer hope that the brain can be coaxed into rewiring itself after injury." Data from other monkeys in the study supported this finding.

Neural rewiring is the Holy Grail in rehabilitative medicine, offering hope to victims of stroke and spinal cord injury. As such, critics wanted more evidence.

In 2000, Taub achieved a breakthrough, which CNN and ABC News reported extensively.[15] Taub reported that all stroke patients using his *Constraint-Induced Movement Therapy* (CI therapy), had significantly improved in function. For an affected arm, 30 percent of patients gained close to normal use.[16]

So can the brain reorganize after a stroke? Some people think that CI therapy jump-starts self-repair of surviving, healthy cells in the brain or spinal cord. CI therapy tries to "wake up cells that have been stunned," says Taub.[17] "CI therapy appears to produce a re-wiring in the brain that leads to improved motor function of the affected limb."[18]

"Right after a stroke, a limb is paralyzed," he says. "Whenever the person tries to move an arm, it simply doesn't work." But often the cells that represent the arm are still alive. The patient assumes the arm is permanently dead, expects failure from trying to use it, and does not. "We call it learned nonuse," Taub said.

The more the patient relies on the good arm, the less likely recovery becomes in the bad arm. Timing is critical. If movement is induced in the bad limb immediately after a stroke, damage increases to the brain. But in the second or third week, therapy can begin.

Requiring rehabilitation therapists trained in the new techniques, the therapy goes six to seven hours every weekday for ten consecutive weeks. Patients move around with good limbs tightly bandaged. Because of lack of therapists and space, most patients seeking the new treatment cannot be accommodated.

To meet the demand, in 2001 UAB opened the Taub Clinic for CI therapy. Although neither private insurance nor Medicare pays for CI therapy, which runs $6,000 to $13,000, over 5,000 stroke patients now wait for it. Demand for CI therapy has also created ethical problems similar to that of Seattle's God Committee in 1962.

In 2004, the NIH funded the first multicenter national trial to study the benefits of CI therapy.[19] In 2006, a placebo-controlled study proved that CI therapy's benefits last two years after the intervention.[20] Taub claimed a separate result showed benefits five years later. In another study, 21 survivors of stroke underwent the standard CI therapy, while 21 other survivors merely had a general fitness program. Two weeks after CI therapy, patients in the treatment group had a "large to very large" improvement in use of the affected arm, whereas those in the control group had no change.

The Law and Animal Research

In 1992, the Farm and Animal Research Facilities Protection Act made it a federal crime to break into a research facility or the premises of a company that breeds research animals. Violators face prison sentences up to one year for illegal entry and fines up to $5,000. A vice-president at UAB Medical Center, which had originated the bill, said that this legislation would protect scientists against "activists who use terrorist techniques to interfere with potentially life-saving research."[21]

In 1993, animal rights activists won a significant victory for dogs and primates used in laboratory research. Judge Charles Richey ordered the Agriculture Department to enforce the Improved Standards for Laboratory Animals Act of 1985, the act creating IACUCs. The judge concluded that the Agriculture Department had violated the act by giving all power to interpret it to local IACUCs. He implied that IACUC members, including veterinarians and one non-scientist member, protected too much the institutions they were supposed to regulate.

Richey also criticized the government for taking nine years to implement some of its own rules, and he implied that some of the rules increased profitability more than protected animals.

Judge Richey recently rejected the claim by Ingrid Newkirk of PETA that "a rat is a pig is a dog is a boy" and dismissed claims that American researchers had to keep detailed records for their 21 million rats and mice. He said researchers could treat rats and mice differently from dogs and primates. That is significant because medical researchers claim that rats and mice constitute 87 percent of animals they use.[22]

Animal activists see IACUCs as window dressing and claim they do little good. They say that the Department of Agriculture, which must inspect labs, has a too-cozy relationship with animal-abusing agribusiness. They lament that veterinarians on IACUCs are caught in the middle, charged with protecting animals but salaried by researchers.

During the 1980s, faced with what they perceived as devastating losses in public confidence, scientists went on the offensive, establishing the Foundation for Biomedical Research, a lobby for 350 universities, drug companies, manufacturers of medical devices, and commercial animal-supply companies. To counter PETA's lobbyists, it has its own lobbyists in Washington, D.C., and a paid staff member in most states to work with students in high schools and colleges.

Numbers and Kinds of Animals in Research

Animal rights activists made two tests controversial: the LD-50 tests and Draize tests. LD stands for "lethal dosage." LD-50 tests determine what amount of a substance will kill 50 of 100 animals. Done routinely across species for substances ranging from soap to chemotherapies, these tests have been criticized as crude measures (one witness said they tell mice how much of something to take for mass suicide). Because of criticisms, since the early 1970s, use of LD-50s declined 96 percent, replaced by LD-10s.[23]

The Draize test estimates whether products irritate human eyes; samples are dripped into rabbits' eyes, which are particularly sensitive. Activists seek alternative tests using cell cultures and computer models.

Over the last decades, activists and researchers agreed on the 3Rs, made famous by researcher/activist Barbara Orlans, of replacement, refinement, and reduction. "Replacement" means use tissue culture instead of animal skin or a mouse instead of a dog. "Refinement" means improving the quality of life of research animals, as well as the methodology. "Reduction" means reducing the number of animals used, e.g., LD-10s rather than LD-50s.

As of 2010, the European Union banned use of animals to test cosmetics, so the Draize test is no longer done there. Instead, blush or eyeliner made by L'Oréal is tested on artificial human skin called Episkin and EpiDerm (the same skin grown for burn victims from a sample of their own skin).[24]

How many animals and what kinds of animals do American researchers use each year? The answers are controversial. The Foundation for Biomedical Research claims that, "Many people think that abandoned or stolen pets are used in research. This is completely untrue and is banned in this country."[25] However, a May 2009 report by the National Academies of Science implies that, even though demand has declined and that the system should be phased out, some "Class B" dealers have previously been selling "random source" dogs and cats to researchers.[26]

Activists have claimed that researchers use a vast number of animals in research, with estimates in the past from 14 to 71 million.[27] The Foundation for Biomedical Research claims that the number has fallen from a peak in the 1970s of 5.5 million to the present level of around 2.5 million. They attribute this reduction to the 3Rs, to refining techniques, to finding alternatives, and by substituting mice for higher mammals.

Whatever answers are correct, basic research uses far more animals than most people realize. For every practical success in human medicine, such as cyclosporin or knee replacements, dozens of failures occur in studies with human subjects and dozens of failures occur in animal studies. To arrive at each success, the sad truth is that researchers use millions of animals each year.

Descartes on Animal Pain

Since prehistoric times, humans have used animals for many purposes, but experimentation on animals did not arise as a specific issue until the beginning of modern science. Rene Descartes in the seventeenth century set the premises for the modern debate.

Not only a mathematician and philosopher, Descartes also studied physiology and the circulation of blood by dissecting live animals without anesthesia (which was not discovered until 1846). To understand why he considered that permissible, it is necessary to understand his basic philosophical approach, which is known as *Cartesianism* and which deeply influenced Western science and philosophy.

Descartes is known for his famous argument "Cogito ergo sum": "I think, therefore I am." According to him, what distinguishes human beings from other animals is *res cogitans,* or "thinking stuff," a substantial mind or soul. For Descartes, this mental substance held together transient mental states such as perceptions, feelings, thoughts, and dreams and served as a ground for free will, reason, and moral values. Nonhuman animals, Descartes believed, lack *res cogitans,* mind or soul, and are therefore ultimately only *res extensa,* or "extended, physical stuff." Thus in Cartesian philosophy, animals were merely fleshy machines; their eyes reflected no soul and no pain lay behind their external "pain behavior."

Descartes's idea that animals lack a soul was not unique as this was also Christian doctrine. Descartes accepted Christian teaching that humans have souls created by God, whereas animals do not. Descartes assumed further that *soul* is identical to *mind,* so if animals have no soul, neither do they have a mind; and if animals have no mind, they are not conscious and if they are not conscious, they cannot feel pain.

For Descartes, in order to feel pain, a mind is needed, and—to repeat—only human beings have minds. In Descartes's view, no middle ground exists between a human being, who has a soul and a capacity to experience pain, and an animal that has no soul and no capacity to experience pain.

Cartesianism represents an attempt to deal with the tension between science and religion by demarcating proper areas for each: the province of science is the study of matter, mathematics, animals, and the human body; that of religion and the humanities is mind, art, and ethics. Obviously, however, it has not come to represent a consensus, or even a widely accepted solution—even for Christians, who are still struggling with the concept of how mind and soul are related and whether animals count in the grand scheme of things.

Among Descartes's followers during his own century were an infamous group of early physiologists and *vivisectionists* (researchers operating on live animals without anesthesia) at the Jansenist seminary of Port Royal. Here is how eighteenth-century writer Nicholas Fontaine describes them:

> They administered beatings to dogs with perfect indifference, and made fun of those who pitied the creatures as if they felt pain. They said the animals were clocks; that the cries they emitted when struck were only the noise of a little spring that had been touched, but that the whole body was without feeling. They nailed poor animals up on boards by their four paws to vivisect them and see the circulation of the blood that was a great subject of conversation.[28]

To some extent, the Cartesian concept of animals has persisted into modern times. Some behavioral psychologists argued against assuming rats were conscious and drew a distinction between "pain behavior" and the experience of pain. Rats and chickens, they said, exhibited "pain behavior," but whether they had mental states and thus had an experience of pain like humans was another matter.

C. S. Lewis on Animal Pain

The twentieth-century Christian writer C. S. Lewis tried to find a middle ground between the Cartesian view and a view equating animal and human pain. Lewis rejected the view that animals feel nothing and argued that animals indeed do feel. But in what sense? Lewis distinguished between *sentience* (the ability to feel pain) and *consciousness* (awareness of feeling pain). All mammals are sentient, he argued, but only humans are self-conscious.[29]

According to Lewis, animals feel pain, but not as humans do. A rat receiving three electric shocks feels the pain of each shock—the rat is sentient—but it does not think, "I have had three shocks." The thought, "I have had three shocks," requires what Lewis calls "consciousness or soul" (he runs these together).

Lewis agreed with the eighteenth-century philosopher David Hume, who argued that self-identity requires a permanent self or mental substance which unites all of a person's thoughts as "his" or "hers" (Hume famously thought that, even for humans, this deep self was a myth).[30] For Lewis, a baboon would have a "succession of perceptions," but not the human experience of pain as "my pain."

Lewis identified consciousness with self-consciousness or soul (for which he also used the term "deep self"). Some critics have disagreed with this idea, particularly since Lewis assumed that memory depends on self-consciousness. These critics observe that if self-consciousness were needed for memory, animals would never remember anything, and studies of learning in animals would be senseless. But everyone knows that animals remember—a dog who has been given a treat by a human remembers that human.

Philosophy of Mind and Ethics

Today, philosophy of mind and animal ethics agonize over answers to the following questions: how much pain do animals feel? To what extent is their pain like our pain? On the ladder of evolution from an amoeba to baboons, at what point does an organism become sentient? When can an animal remember pain as "my pain"?

These are not simple questions. They raise some of the deepest problems in philosophy of mind and lie behind many controversies about animal research.

As we consider various answers to such questions, do we have, as a species, a conflict of interest? Do we have any bias toward accepting some answers and rejecting others? Remember that for centuries, societies considered people of color and women to be "obviously" and "naturally" inferior to white men.

Finally, even if animals are not aware of pain, or do not remember pain as humans do, that does not mean they suffer less in medical experiments. When humans consent to be subjects of medical experimentations, we explain to them the purposes and risks of the study so they understand the experiment. This does not occur with animals, who have no idea why they are being used. Having no way to understand the research, they may suffer more.

In discussing abortion and end-of-life care, we explored the gradient theory of personhood. To extend that theory to animals, we should note that on a cross-species gradient of characteristics of persons, adult baboons will possess more characteristics than newborn humans or profoundly brain-injured humans. Therefore, adult baboons will be more persons than human embryos or end-stage vegetative humans.

Peter Singer on Speciesism

Before 1975, groups promoting animal welfare focused on humane treatment of research animals. In that year, the Australian philosopher Peter Singer published *Animal Liberation,* where he argued that animals should count for something.[31] To say animals do not count because they are inferior by nature, Singer held, is like saying slaves or women do not count because they are inferior by nature. Just as racism and sexism are evil, Singer said, so is *speciesism.*

According to him, the argument that supports equal rights for minorities and women also supports animal rights. If our moral concern for children, women, and minorities stems from their sensitivity to pain, family ties, and ability to reason, why wouldn't these factors also be a basis for concern for animals?

Note that we treat humans with *equal* human rights despite the obvious fact that they are *unequal* in their ability to suffer, in their intelligence, strength, and character. Inequality of ability does not dictate inequality of treatment. Such arguments put speciesists on the defensive: if the principle of equality applies to all people, despite their obvious differences in ability and intelligence, why should it not apply to animals?

Singer also argued that a medical experiment using animal subjects must be speciesist unless humans would be willing to substitute irreversibly comatose human subjects. This is an interesting approach. Most people who accept the idea of using, say, a chimpanzee in medical research would cringe at the idea of using an anencephalic baby (an infant born lacking a normal brain). But if the chimpanzee is active, gregarious, sensitive, and responsive whereas the anencephalic baby is hopelessly mute, comatose, and dying, why should the chimp be the victim? If the answer is simply that the baby is human and the chimp nonhuman, that answer is mistaken because it assumes what it must prove; in other words, it's speciesist.

Let us put the point differently. Suppose an institution exists with hundreds of profoundly retarded human children and adults who have been abandoned by their families to the State. They are so profoundly retarded as to have virtually no recognizably human interactions with each other or the staff. Even so, most people would be horrified to learn that a drug company was using them as subjects to test promising drugs for toxicity in humans.

Now move to a large center for primates, such as one near San Antonio, Texas, that holds hundreds of chimpanzees and baboons. Only these primates are *more* social, *more* interactive, and *more* intelligent than the humans described above. Yet these are precisely the beings drug companies use to test new drugs for toxicity. Why do we tolerate such testing on them and not on the retarded humans?

In addition to his argument about speciesism, Singer also used *utilitarian reasoning*. According to utilitarian ethical theory, right acts produce the greatest good for the greatest number; for instance, research on presently sick patients is right if it helps a greater number of future sick patients.

Singer maintains that stipulating that the "greatest number" must refer only to humans begs the key question. Once animals count for something, however small, in utilitarian reasoning, then radical conclusions follow. Experiments that inflict horrible pain on many animals cannot be justified on the ground that they save a few human lives because the number of animals suffering outweighs the small good to humans.

Yale philosopher Shelly Kagan, in an interview in 2000 about Singer's brilliance, pointed out that Singer often argued "a utilitarian view without limiting itself to utilitarianism."[32] That accurately sums up *Animal Liberation,* where Singer graphically described the many ways that animals suffer in vast, industrialized hog factories to become tasty flesh for humans.

Singer and other activists emphasized how pigs are more intelligent than horses, dogs, and cats, which we revere as pets. Pigs suffer the sad quirk of fate that humans like the taste of their smoked, cooked flesh, a fact less true of deer, buffalo, and bison. Singer also explained how farmer-businessmen raise pigs, veal calves, and chickens in small, confining cages in industrial-type farms.

So Singer argued that current factory farming is evil. Billions of animals suffer and die each year so humans can enjoy their flesh. Arguably, vegetarian eating is healthier for humans today than a meat-centered diet, and in addition, saves animals much pain.

Tom Regan on Animal Rights

Tom Regan, an American philosopher and animal rights activist, argues that all research on animals is wrong:

> I argue that the whole system of animal experimentation [and] the whole system of commercial and sport trapping and hunting are morally bankrupt institutions. The only way you change these things fundamentally is by eliminating them—in much the same way as with slavery and child labor.[33]

Regan argues that human beings have rights because they *have a life*. That is, humans have lives that can go better or worse for them, and this is true for each human being independently of whether or not others value him or her. In other words, people have inherent, not instrumental, value. Where Singer loosely applied utilitarianism to animals, Regan loosely applied a Kantian ethics to animals, asserting the rights-based idea that each animal's life should be treated as an "end in itself."

So Regan condemns research on animals because it treats them as a means to the good of helping humans. For Regan, animals have rights not to suffer at the hands of humans, rights to be respected in their own habitat, and rights to enjoy a natural lifespan. So eating them is also immoral. In other words, each animal's life has *inherent value.*

Once the premise is accepted that each animal's life has inherent value, it follows that medical research to benefit humans is unjustified. For if a life has inherent value, no competing value trumps it.

For Regan, animals have lives that can go better or worse for them: "They too have a distinctive kind of value in their own right, if we do; therefore, they too have a right not to be treated in ways that fail to respect this value."[34] If humans count in the moral calculus because they possess X, and if animals possess X, then it is inconsistent not to count animals equally. Those who claim that animals differ about X must prove why.

Regan's critics say that his argument runs several unjustified inferences together. First, they ask, if any being (human or nonhuman) has a life that can go better or worse, does that fact give every life a distinctive value? Second, and more important, just because an animal "has a life" doesn't mean it is equal in value to that of humans.

Note, however, that Regan includes a qualification: he says that animals (like humans) have lives which can go better or worse *for them*. By qualifying his claim this way, no comparison is possible between human and animal lives. If fish in an aquarium "have a life" that can go better or worse *for them,* from that standpoint, we do not have a right to destroy them.

Consider the Lifeboat Test: only a dog or a man can remain in a lifeboat. Which should survive? Regan implies that because "animals aren't there to be used as our resources," it is wrong to kill the dog to save the man, and scientist Charles McArdle concurs—"I would seriously have to question whether I would allow an animal to die just to protect me."[35] On the other hand, the pediatric researcher Carolyn Compton disagrees: "I love animals, but there's no question in my mind that if I were able to sacrifice an animal life to save a human being, I would do it."[36]

The philosopher Carl Cohen states, "Rights arise, and can be intelligently defended, only among beings who do, or can, make moral claims against one another."[37] For Cohen, because animals cannot make claims, they lack rights.

But this seems to assume that claims can be made only with vocal cords. When a dog pesters his owner to be taken for a walk, isn't he claiming a right to a walk?

Cohen rejects the analogy among racism, sexism, and speciesism: although racism and sexism are bad, speciesism is not. "Speciesism is not merely plausible; it is essential for right conduct, because those who will not make the morally relevant distinctions among species are almost certain, in consequence, to misapprehend their true obligations." That is, they will take the dog from the burning building, not the child; give money in their wills to ensure that their pets are taken care of but ignore their nephews and nieces; and support the Humane Society but not famine relief.

Why We Need Animals in Research: The Official View

According to the Official View, which federal law expresses, drugs must first be tested on animals to screen for toxicity and to indicate possible benefit to humans. Sometimes this view approaches religious fervor: "Every major medical advance of the century has depended on animal research," says a neuroscientist from Rutgers University.[38]

For example, scientists use mice to test extract of grapes to prevent cancer and also give mice cancer in order to test such drugs.

In Phase I of testing drugs on humans, scientists strive to see how much of the drug can be given without producing toxic effects. Phase I is done only after extensive testing of the drug in animals. Without such testing, the Official View claims, many more toxic reactions would occur in humans.

The Official View argues similarly for how scientists test new heart pumps, artificial pumps, salves for burns, antibiotics, and new kinds of surgery. If they did not test these first on animals, making their mistakes and gaining skill, more humans would be injured or harmed.

If no animals were available, such tests would need to be done on humans. It is inconceivable that humans would be given cancer to have subjects to test anti-cancer drugs, so progress against cancer would slow.

As evolution teaches, humans evolved through primates from even lesser animals. As such, we share nervous systems, receptors for pain, and fight-or-flight reactions with our predecessors. Moreover, it is precisely because of sharing so much with primates and mammals that the latter make such good subjects for medial research: they predict well how drugs and surgeries will work in humans.

Finally, the Official View emphasizes Taub's research. Condemned originally as cruel, Taub's studies led to his breakthrough and stroke victims now benefit.

In sum, on the Official View, if we want medical research to continue, using animals in research is indispensable and also reduces harm to humans from medical research.

Critiquing the Official View

For too long, the Official View has not been challenged in medicine or science, but perhaps it is time to do so. Three different critiques of it are commonly made.

1. *Inherently Wrong*. The most basic criticism of the Official View is that the infliction of pain on animals is inherently wrong, that just as we should not experiment on some humans to help the majority, as Mengele did with Jewish subjects, so we should not harm animals to benefit humans. This argument assumes *equivalence,* that animal and human suffering are equivalent and that one should not be accepted to advance the other.

Many people reject equivalence, believing that animals, compared to humans, are either of no moral value or of inconsequential moral value. Others may believe that, although animals count for something, human welfare counts for so much more that animal suffering in research can be allowed.

2. *Bad Science.* Some scientists think that the Official View is based on bad science. This objection has two parts: first, testing drugs, devices, and techniques on animals does not in fact predict harm to humans; second, some drugs, devices, and techniques that harm animals may help humans, but are screened out, thus potentially beneficial tools are lost due to testing on animals. So testing these things on animals is both too broad and too narrow: it allows too many bad things to go through and wrongly screens out too many good things.

Philosopher of science Niall Shanks and anesthesiologist Ray Greek studied whether testing of drugs on animals predicts their toxicity or benefits to humans and concluded that most extrapolations rest on shaky grounds:

> Drugs such as Practolol, Opren, Fialuridine, Clioquinol, Zelmid, Troglitazone, and others (such as Avandia), came to market, in part, because they tested safe in some animal species. They went on to prove dangerous in humans. It is still difficult to induce lung cancer in animals from cigarette smoke. Animals that were fed a high fat, high cholesterol diet failed to develop coronary artery disease, and so this diet was thought safe for humans. Asbestos, benzine, glass fibers, and other environmental poisons were all proved "safe" in animals and consequently kept on the market long after epidemiological data proved them carcinogenic or otherwise dangerous.
>
> From 1976 to 1985, 209 new drugs were approved for use in the United States after extensive animal testing. . . . Of these, 198 were followed . . . by the FDA and 102, or 52 percent, were either withdrawn or relabeled as having secondary to severe unpredicted side effects such as lethal dysrhythmias, heart attacks, kidney failure, and stroke.[39]

Such recalls make one wonder how well responses in animals of drugs predict responses of the same drugs in humans. Testing drugs on embryonic cells might be preferable and save both suffering in animals and prevent harm to adult humans.

What about Taub's study? Well, notice that Taub made his advance with humans only *after* he was banned from experimenting on primates (a condition of his hiring at UAB). What if he had directly tried to help humans overcome stroke? Were the animal studies necessary? One could argue that, if he had been blocked from using animals, he could have gone directly to using humans and more quickly have discovered his breakthrough.

What about evolution? Doesn't our common genetic history mean that drugs tested on nonhuman mammals will be likely to predict their effects on humans? Yes and no. Although we share 98 percent of our genes with apes and baboons, we also have many variations in the human genome, such that some drugs that work well in Caucasians do not work well in African Americans. Similarly, the variations between nonhuman primates and human primates mean there are many slips between the cup and the lip in predictive drug testing.

Also, if we are 98 percent the same genetically as apes, shouldn't we regard apes as 98 percent persons? Shouldn't they have rights not to be kept in cages or used against their wills to provide organs for humans, as in the Baby Fae case?

Another problem is that many labs use mice or rats or primates bred to be a uniform type. In that way, the results are more easily reproducible by other scientists. But using only one genetic strain of mouse also limits testing of a new drug to that strain, whereas using many kinds of mice and animals would better mimic the variation in humans.

3. *Cost/Benefit.* Most people do not understand how many animals scientists use in research or how much such animals suffer. Once a year in medical school, students pause in a ceremony to remember those who dedicated their bodies to be cadavers for students to learn on in gross anatomy. We need the same kind of ceremony to commemorate what animals have given us.

However, if the benefits of using animals to screen drugs and devices are questionable, and if good arguments can be made that we should go directly to testing on human embryos or human volunteers, then the use of vast numbers of animals in research becomes morally unjustifiable. For example, it would seem that studies of vaccines for HIV on chimpanzees and monkeys offer little guidance for how the same will work on humans.

The Medical Retort

Let's assume that some pharmacological results on animals generalize poorly to humans. That does not prove that research on animals itself is unjustified. Rather, like implementing the 3Rs, it suggests that refined planning of experiments would benefit animals, humans, and scientists.

But assume humans get some benefit by having a drug or surgical technique first tested on animals and that, without animals, humans would need to be used. Is that justifiable?

Brain-dead cadavers and anencephalic newborns could be used to substitute for many mammals, but some would fear a slippery slope of degrading humans to the kind of degradation now faced by research animals.

Moreover, what about democratic voting? If Americans were polled, wouldn't most want new drugs and devices tested first on animals before humans? Are most Americans wrong about the usefulness of such research? Most Americans have pets or livestock, so they may be more knowledgeable than activists admit. Is it OK for a whole society to be democratically speciesist?

CONCLUSION

The question of using animals in medical research inflames passions. The Gennarelli and Taub experiments lead us in different directions, for the former's research went nowhere and abused animals, but the latter's had unexpected good results for humans.

Perhaps the final thought should be no on whether any animal research is justified but on whether the current *scale* of such research is justified. Perhaps we should make use of animals—especially primates, pigs, dogs, and cats—a rare event in medicine, like experimenting on live-born fetuses or separating conjoined twins. In that way, we might get the most out of the pain we inflict on such unwilling, uncomprehending subjects.

FURTHER READING AND RESEARCH

Deborah Blum, *The Monkey Wars,* New York, Oxford University Press, 1994.

Peter Carruthers, *The Animals Issue: Moral Theory in Practice,* New York, Cambridge University Press, 1992.

Gary Francione, *Introduction to Animal Rights: Your Child or the Dog?,* Philadelphia, PA, Temple University Press, 2000.

R. G. Frey, *Rights, Killing, and Suffering,* Oxford, England, Basil Blackwell, 1983.

Jean Swingle Greek and Ray Greek, *What Will We Do If We Don't Experiment on Animals?* Bloomington, IN, Trafford Publishing, 2004.

Gil Langley, *Animal Experimentation: The Consensus Changes,* New York, Routledge, 1989.

Tibor Machan, *Putting Humans First,* Lanham, MD, Rowman & Littlefield, 2004.

Jim Mason and Peter Singer, *Animal Factories,* New York, Crown Publishers, 1980.
F. Barbara Orlans, *In The Name of Science: Issues in Responsible Animal Experimentation,* New York: Oxford University Press, 1993.
James Rachels, *Created from Animals,* New York, Oxford University Press, 1990.
Denise Radner and Michael Radner, *Animal Consciousness,* Buffalo, NY, Prometheus Books, 1989.
Richard Ryder, *Victims of Science: The Use of Animals in Research,* London, Davis-Poynter, 1975.
Tom Regan, *The Case for Animal Rights,* Berkeley, University of California Press, 1983.
Peter Singer, *Animal Liberation,* New York, Random House, 1975.
Susan Sperling, *Animal Liberators,* Berkeley, University of California Press, 1988.

DISCUSSION QUESTIONS

1. If someone is against all use of animals in medical research, should he or she refrain from using medicines or products tested for safety on animals? The White House was built by slaves. Should American presidents therefore refuse to live in it? Are the arguments properly analogous?
2. "I agree that animals suffer in being raised for my food, but I don't care. I enjoy eating bacon, barbecue, and ham, and I will never change." Does this person commit any mistake of reasoning in admitting that he doesn't care enough about suffering of animals raised for his food to become a vegetarian?
3. "I'd rather be your pet than your fetus." Do people concerned with animal rights too often discount the suffering of fetuses in abortion? Shouldn't pro-life people be against both kinds of suffering?
4. What about the dog and the man in the lifeboat? If only one can stay, should we draw straws to see who goes overboard? (and don't keep the dog to eat him!)
5. Would it be acceptable for humans to volunteer to spare animals? Could we imagine a scenario where, if enough humans volunteered to test, say, new vitamins, no animals at all would need to be used in testing?

CHAPTER 9

Research on Human Subjects

This chapter describes the Tuskegee Study of untreated syphilis in Alabama, experimentation by Nazi physicians, secret American medical research, two controversial experiments in Africa, Jesse Gelsinger's death and financial conflicts of modern researchers.

Its essential question for discussion is: Were the experiments on African women to prevent infection with HIV of their babies like the Tuskegee Syphilis Study?

INFAMOUS MEDICAL EXPERIMENTS

William Beaumont

In 1822, physician William Beaumont, the father of gastric physiology, treated patient St. Martin for a bullet wound in the stomach; St. Martin survived, but the wound healed strangely, leaving a hole. To observe the hole, Beaumont employed St. Martin as a servant, and proved the previously unknown fact that stomach juices digest food. St. Martin ran away and Beaumont had him caught to continue to exhibit him. Hospitals today in Texas and Michigan bear Beaumont's name.

Nazi Medical Research

Besides participating in the Holocaust, physicians during the Nazi regime conducted heinous experiments on humans. They reasoned that if victims in concentration camps were going to die anyway, why not use them to benefit medical science?

Across the globe during the same war, Japanese physicians carried out deadly experiments on Chinese prisoners at unit 731 in Harbin, killing 3,000. To study the natural course of diseases, physicians injected prisoners with anthrax, syphilis, plague, and cholera.[1]

From 1943 to 1945, gay men, convicted criminals, Russian officers, Polish dissidents, Jews, and Gypsies on Ward 46 at Buchenwald in Germany got experimental vaccines against typhus. Physicians injected blood infected with typhus into 40 involuntary subjects, who served as a treatment group. Overall, they infected 1,000 prisoners, 158 of whom died. They established no thresholds of infection.[2]

In experiments at Buchenwald, physicians tried to cure gay men with hormone shots, had inmates shot to study gunshot wounds, starved inmates to study the physiology of nutrition, and amputated women's bones and limbs to study regeneration. To study malaria, physicians used anopheles mosquitoes to infect subjects. Physician Ernst Grawitz infected legs of women with staphylococci, gas, and tetanus bacilli. In testing sulfa drugs, he rubbed into wounds particles of glass and stone.

In experiments at Ravensbrück, physician Sigmund Rascher devised his "sky ride wagon" to simulate rapid changes in altitude. Victims were locked inside an enclosed box on wheels with monitoring equipment inside.[3] Rascher froze 100 nude Jewish and Russian prisoners in icy waters to study techniques to revive downed pilots in similar waters. He also forced nude Jewish women to revive the subjects sexually. Since such women would be unavailable to revive pilots downed in icy seas, this exercise simply degraded the subjects for the amusement of the guards.

Josef Mengele

The most infamous Nazi physician, Josef Mengele, known as the Angel of Death, participated in the death of 400,000 victims in concentration camps. Ambitious, the young Mengele sought fame. To get it, he studied medicine and anthropological genetics between 1930 and 1936 in Munich, when eugenics movements swept Germany and America. Munich then headquartered the Nazi Party and its ideology of racial purity.

Contrary to some accounts, German medical schools did not resist Nazi eugenics and killing undesirables, but led these movements. To advance, Mengele joined the Brownshirts, a fanatical Nazi movement.

Mengele needed groundbreaking research to reach his goal of appointment as a professor. In 1943 at the Auschwitz concentration camp, he experimented to overcome the effects of genetics by modifying environments. He wanted to produce blue eyes, blonde hair, and healthy bodies free of genetic disease.

As subjects, he needed identical twins, natural controls for environmental differences. So Mengele examined incoming trains of boxcars filled with Jews destined for execution, looking for twins and other usable subjects, signaling his choices with a flick of his wrist.

Describing Mengele's experiments is painful. He injected blue dye into children's eyes to see if he could create blue eyes. To see if twins could be produced, he forced female twins to engage in coitus with male twins. He interchanged blood of identical twins to observe results; he interchanged blood between pairs of twins.

One pair of fraternal twins consisted of a hunchback and a normal child; Mengele surgically grafted the hunchback to the normal child's back, creating the effect of conjoined twins; he accentuated this effect by sewing their wrists back to back. A witness reported that when these conjoined children returned to the barracks: "There was a terrible smell of gangrene. The cuts were dirty and the children cried every night."[4]

Mengele obtained between 150 and 200 twins, most of who died. He also tested endurance by subjecting 75 prisoners to electric shock; 25 of them died immediately. To study sterility, he severely burned Polish nuns by giving them high dosages of radiation.

Mengele once found a hunchback and the hunchback's son; he had both of them killed, their bodies boiled, their flesh stripped, and their skeletons dipped in gasoline for preservation for his anthropological studies of body types. When he came upon seven dwarfs from a Rumanian circus family, he kept them alive to exhibit them to visiting physicians.

When 300 Jewish children escaped a gas chamber and fled to a nearby field, Mengele cool, impersonal, and detached, had them recaptured, lit a gasoline fire set in a large pit, and had the children thrown in. On fire and screaming for their lives, some children clawed their way over dead bodies to the top, where Mengele and his men kicked them back in.

When the Russian army approached Auschwitz in 1945, Mengele escaped to Paraguay. He lived there for 40 years, eluding Israelis who tried to capture him as a war criminal. In later conversations with his grown son Rolf, he expressed no regret for his actions: it was not his fault that Jews had to die at Auschwitz, he said, so why not use them to advance medical knowledge and his own chances for a professorship? Never captured or tried as a war criminal, Mengele died in Brazil in the summer of 1985.[5]

American Military Research during World War II

In 1941, American researchers experimented on orphans at the Ohio Soldiers and Sailors Orphanage, on retarded inmates at New Jersey State Colony for the Feeble-Minded, and on patients at a mental institution in Dixon, Illinois.[6] To develop a vaccine against shigella, they injected deadened forms into subjects. None died, but many got sick.

Some questionable research used military personnel as subjects. Cornelius Rhoads, Director of Memorial Sloan-Kettering Cancer Hospital in New York City, became head of the military's secret chemical warfare service. Rhoads:

> supervised the long secret and now infamous tests where thousands of American troops were intentionally exposed to mustard and other poisonous gases. Rhoads discovered that the mustard gas killed white blood cells and other cells that divided rapidly. After the war he and others began to experiment with mustard gas as a cancer treatment and also to search for other systemic poisons that kill dividing cells.[7]

In research conducted by the armed forces on poisonous agents, 60,000 subjects did not know what they were undergoing.[8] About 4,000 to 5,000 subjects inhaled mustard gas in gas chambers.

During the war, Franklin Roosevelt established the Committee on Medical Research, which approached its work with a wartime mentality that carried over into researchers' attitudes after the war: disease was the enemy, researchers were the soldiers, and victory could be won—with enough resources and enough will. During the war, ethical concerns about experiments carried little weight:

> A wartime environment also undercut the protection of human subjects, because of the power of the example of the draft. Every day thousands of men were compelled to risk death, however limited their understanding of the aims of the war or the immediate campaign might be. By extension, researchers doing laboratory

> work were also engaged in a military activity, and they did not need to seek the permission of their subjects any more than the selective service or field commanders did of draftees. . . . In a society mobilized for war, these arguments carried great weight. Some people were ordered to face bullets and storm a hill; others were told to take an injection and test a vaccine. In philosophical terms, wartime inevitably promoted utilitarian over absolutistic positions.

When subjects of secret chemical research later applied for treatment at veterans' hospitals, the Veterans Administration (VA) denied that they had been exposed to these agents. This scenario recurred after the war in Vietnam and after Operation Desert Storm.

World War II institutionalized some doubtful attitudes in medical experimentation. When war came to an end, the fight against diseases did not: "The prospect of winning the war against contagious and degenerative illness gave researchers in the 1950s and 1960s a sense of both mission and urgency that kept the spirit of the wartime laboratories alive."[9]

The Nuremberg Code

After World War II at the Nuremberg trials in 1946, German physicians defended themselves against charges of war crimes by saying that they had merely been following orders, that their experiments had been properly related to solving medical problems of war, and that what they had done did not differ from similar research done on captives by American physicians.

The judges at Nuremberg lacked a code of ethics for experimentation on captive populations, so they created ten principles for ethical experimentation, known as the *Nuremberg Code*. Its most important principle was that people should freely consent to participation in any experiment.

Postwar Criticisms

By the 1970s, faith waned in scientific and medical progress. Rachel Carson's *Silent Spring* described the ravages of pesticides; the Cuban missile crisis brought America close to nuclear war; and scientists discovered that drugs such as thalidomide (an antinausea drug during pregnancy), once hailed as miraculous, caused children to be born lacking arms and legs.

In 1966, Harvard medical professor Henry Beecher criticized 22 specific medical experiments published in medical journals that had not obtained consent from subjects, asserting that this was the norm.[10] About the same time, physician Henry Pappworth similarly criticized 500 medical experiments.[11] That year, the United States Public Health Service began to require informed consent of subjects.

THE TUSKEGEE STUDY

Nature and History of Syphilis

In the past, victims who suffered from untreated syphilis included Cleopatra, King Herod of Judea, Charlemagne, Henry VIII, Napoleon Bonaparte, Frederick the Great, Pope Sixtus IV, Pope Alexander VI, Pope Julius II, Catherine the Great,

Christopher Columbus, Paul Gauguin, Franz Schubert, Albrecht Dürer, Johnann Wofgang von Goethe, Friedrich Nietzsche, John Keats, and James Joyce.[12]

Between 1900 and 1948, and especially during the two world wars, American reformers mounted the *Syphilophobia Campaign*. Reformers emphasized that prostitutes spread syphilis, and that syphilis rapidly killed. As an alternative to visiting prostitutes, they advocated clean, active sports, or "Muscular Christianity."

Antisyphilis crusaders split twice over methods to prevent spread of syphilis: once during World War I over giving out condoms, and again during World War II over giving out penicillin. In each conflict, reformers who wanted to reduce the harm of syphilis battled those who wanted to reduce illicit behavior.[13]

This conflict repeated over the next century in battles about venereal diseases, prostitution, alcoholism, drug addiction, gambling, and sex education. The *Harm Reduction Movement (HRM)* focuses on reducing the associated harms of these behaviors, not on moral censure or eliminating the behaviors. Popular in public health, moralists who oppose HRM attack the illicit behavior and view HRM as enabling it, for example, by teaching men how to use condoms.

The armed services during the world wars adopted pragmatism. Commanders who needed healthy troops overruled moralists and ordered the release of condoms in the first war and penicillin in the second. After the wars, returning troops continued to use condoms and got penicillin, normalizing these practices among Americans.

Schaudinn discovered in 1906 the spirochete that causes syphilis. It is a chronic, contagious bacterial disease, often venereal and sometimes congenital.

Syphilis has three stages. In the first, *primary syphilis,* spirochetes mass and produce a primary lesion, a chancre (pronounced "SHANK-er"). During this stage, syphilis is highly infectious. After the chancre subsides, the disease spreads silently for a time, but then produces an outbreak of secondary symptoms such as fever, rash, and swollen lymph glands.

In the second stage of *latent syphilis,* spirochetes disseminate from the primary lesion throughout the body, producing systemic and widespread lesions, usually in internal organs. Syphilis then spreads silently from 1 to 30 years. During this stage, symptoms vary so widely that syphilis was once known as the Great Pretender.

In its last stage of *tertiary syphilis,* chronic destructive lesions damage the cardiac and neurological systems. Syphilis then may produce paresis (slight or incomplete paralysis), gummas (gummy or rubbery tumors), altered gait, blindness, or lethal narrowing of the aorta.

Today penicillin treats syphilis. Such treatment has been possible only since 1948, when penicillin became available to everyone.

Beginning in the sixteenth century, to treat syphilis, physicians applied the heavy metal mercury as a paste on the back. During the nineteenth century, they similarly administered another heavy metal, bismuth. Neither mercury nor bismuth killed the spirochetes, though they ameliorated symptoms.

In 1909, after the spirochete of syphilis had been identified, two researchers—a German, Paul Erlich; and a Japanese, S. Hata—tried 605 forms of arsenic and discovered a "magic bullet" against it in combination 606 of heavy metals (which included arsenic). Erlich humbly called this Salvarsan (implying salvation from syphilis) and patented it; its generic name is arsphenamine.[14] After finding that it cured syphilis in rabbits, Erlich injected it intramuscularly into men with syphilis.

At first, Salvarsan seemed to work wonders, and during 1910, physicians greeted Erlich with standing ovations. Later, syphilis recurred in some patients treated with Salvarsan, and some of them died, from syphilis and worse, from Salvarsan. Erlich maintained that the drug had not been given correctly, but he also developed a less toxic form, Neosalvarsan.

Physicians injected Neosalvarsan intramuscularly in 20 to 40 dosages over a year, charging patients a dollar a visit. To get full treatment, patients needed both the time and money for these visits. As most did not have time and money, it was no one-shot, magic bullet for syphilis, like penicillin later was.

Between 1890 and 1910, Norwegian Caesar Boeck studied the natural course of untreated syphilis in 1,978 subjects. He believed that heavy metals removed only the symptoms of syphilis. Because heavy metals killed some syphilitics, he studied whether they might fare better untreated.

In 1929, Boeck's successor, J. E. Bruusgaard, selected 473 of Boeck's subjects for further evaluation.[15] Bruusgaard learned that of subjects who had had syphilis for more than 20 years, 73 percent were asymptomatic. Because this discovery dramatically contradicted the Syphilophobia Campaign, the leaders of this movement resisted the fact that syphilis did not universally kill, much less did not do so rapidly (foreshadowing similar battles later about AIDS). Even more disturbing to the Syphilophobia Campaign, Bruusgaard confirmed that some latent syphilitics might never develop symptoms at all.

So when the Tuskegee Study began in 1932, Boeck's and Bruusgaard's studies had caused physicians to question the received views about the natural course and treatment of syphilis.

The Racial Environment

In the 1930s, American medicine was racist. Most physicians condescended to African-American patients and held stereotypes about them, as in this example from a 1914 *Journal of the American Medical Association:*

> The negro springs from a southern race, and as such his sexual appetite is strong; all of his environments stimulate this appetite, and as a general rule his emotional type of religion certainly does not decrease it.[16]

Physicians saw African Americans as dirty, shiftless, promiscuous, and incapable of personal hygiene. In 1900, a Georgia physician wrote, "Virtue in the negro race is like 'angels' visits'—few and far between. In a practice of 16 years in the South, I have never examined a virgin over 14 years of age."[17] In 1919, a medical professor in Chicago wrote that African-American men were like bulls in *furor sexualis,* unable to resist copulation around females.[18]

Given such racism, white physicians around 1929 saw syphilis as a natural consequence of low character in African Americans, described by one white physician as a "notoriously syphilis-soaked race."[19] Such physicians also assumed that African-American men would not seek treatment for venereal disease.

Historian Alan Brandt argues that in the early 1900s, many white American physicians were racially biased and most remained so throughout the decades of the Tuskegee Study. Brandt writes, "There can be little doubt that the Tuskegee researchers regarded their subjects as less than human."[20]

DEVELOPMENT OF THE TUSKEGEE STUDY

A Study in Nature Begins

Physiologist Claude Bernard in 1865 distinguished *studies in nature* from normal *experiments* by saying that in normal experiments, some factor is manipulated, whereas in studies in nature, someone merely observes what would have happened anyway. In centuries before the Tuskegee Study, physicians sought to understand the natural history of diseases and in doing so, they relied on studies in nature.

The great physician William Osler once said, "Know syphilis in all its manifestations and relations, and all other things clinical will be added unto you."[21] Yet as late as 1932, syphilis's natural history had not been documented, and because of Boeck's and Brussgaard's results, physicians doubted the inexorability of its course.

This explains why the United States Public Health Service (USPHS) believed it needed a study in nature, and then it discovered an opportunity. Around 1929, six counties in America had high rates of syphilis—above 20 percent—and a charity, the Julius Rosenwald Foundation of Philadelphia—tried to treat with Neosalvarsan all syphilitics in those counties. In 1930, this foundation surveyed African-American men in Macon County, Alabama, where Tuskegee is the chief town. It citizens were 82 percent black, and its rate of syphilis was then the highest in the nation, 36 percent. The foundation treated or partially treated some of these 3,694 syphilitics with Neosalvarsan.

Then something unforeseen happened: in 1929 the Great Depression began. As its years ground on, funds for charity plummeted, and the Rosenwald Foundation left, hoping that USPHS would continue its program. But funds for public health also plummeted and by 1935, the USPHS budget had fallen from $1 million to less than $60,000.

In 1931, USPHS repeated the Rosenwald foundation's survey of syphilis in Macon County, testing 4,400 African-American residents, and found that 22 percent of men had syphilis, as well as a dangerous 62 percent rate of congenital syphilis. Of great importance for the Tuskegee Study, this survey identified 399 African-American men who had had syphilis of several years' duration, but who had never been treated.

Identification of these 399 untreated men created the opportunity for a study in nature of syphilis. The Surgeon General himself, Raymond Vonderlehr, wrote in 1936 in the *Journal of the American Medical Association* that the Tuskegee Study was "an unusual opportunity to study the untreated syphilitic patient from the beginning of the disease to the death of the infected person."[22] His decision began the Tuskegee Study.

Three points deserve emphasis. First, the 399 subjects had *latent* syphilis, not infectious syphilis. During this stage, syphilis is largely noninfectious during sexual intercourse. Second, researchers did not divide the 399 subjects into the typical experimental and control groups: they were all simply observed. There was, however, another group of natural controls, 200 age-matched African-American men living in Macon County who had never had syphilis.

Third, the 399 men with syphilis and the 200 men without it were perfect for a study in nature because they were *so vulnerable:* they were poor, illiterate, and tied to the land as tenant farmers. As such, unlike other people with syphilis over the next four decades, *they were unlikely to ever leave Macon County*. Partly because of this vulnerability, Vonderlehr implied, they presented an "unusual opportunity."

Vonderlehr had no sense that it might be wrong to use such vulnerable subjects in a lifelong experiment. Like many of his time, he may have assumed that people with syphilis got what they deserved, and that these poor black men would never have had the means, will, or opportunity to get any treatment, even though the Public Health Service itself might have one day provided treatment to them.

The Middle Phase: Poor Design

No single physician oversaw this study. It lacked written protocols, and later investigators often mixed up the subjects in the no-treatment group of 399 syphilitics with the 200 controls without syphilis. Nurse Eunice Rivers, an African-American nurse permanently assigned to stay in Tuskegee to keep track of the study, kept poor records, lost them, and because many of the men had the same last names, often confused a "Johnson" in the no-treatment group with one in the control group.

Researchers assumed that controls would remain uninfected, but in a county where one in three people had syphilis, many controls eventually contracted the disease. Unfortunately, when this happened, some were switched to the no-treatment group of syphilitics.

There were gaps in the study. Federal doctors visited in 1939 and then not again until 1948; seven years passed between visits in 1963 and 1970. Only Nurse Rivers held the shaky study together.

During the course of the research, many of the 399 syphilitic subjects, who were supposed to remain untreated, obtained Neosalvarsan or penicillin outside Macon County. James Lucas, a Centers for Disease Control (CDC) physician, said, "effective and undocumented treatment had been given to the vast majority of patients in the syphilitic group."[23] As a result, researchers could not know whether a subject observed really represented the consequences of untreated syphilis or when a particular subject had gotten it.

So the study proved nothing. Before it began, physicians knew that syphilitics had greater morbidity and mortality than nonsyphilitics, and from Bruusgaard's discovery, that not all men in the latent phase died of syphilis. But the Tuskegee Study added nothing to that knowledge.

Spinal Taps

When physicians returned, they wanted to know, first, if they had a subject in the study group; and second, if so, how far his syphilis had progressed. To determine progression, they did spinal punctures on 271 of the 399 syphilitic subjects.

In doing spinal taps, they inserted a ten-inch needle between two vertebrae into the cerebrospinal fluid to withdraw a small amount of fluid. Because this is a delicate and uncomfortable process, physicians warned subjects to stay still, lest the needle swerve and puncture their fluid sac, causing infection and possible paralysis.

Some physicians then and now regard spinal taps as insignificant, justified by the need to prove a diagnosis. On the other hand, professionals who describe a spinal tap this way may be thinking about administering one rather than receiving one.

A spinal tap is not a minor procedure, like taking blood. Some patients experience side effects, such as being unable to stand for a week without a severe headache. One person in a million will become paralyzed or permanently comatose.[24]

Tapping someone involuntarily, without obtaining informed consent, is legally a battery. Researchers who need healthy volunteers for spinal taps offer as much as $1,000 for them. Even then, some people will not undergo a nontherapeutic tap for $5,000 or for any amount. That should tell us something.

Deception

To induce subjects to travel to town and undergo these painful taps, physicians offered a series of freebies: transportation, hot lunches, medicine for any disease other than syphilis, and burials—all free. In return for these benefits, physicians did spinal taps and later, autopsies, to inspect for damage from syphilis.

But these freebies and the persuasion of Nurse Rivers failed to get all the men to come to town for the "round-ups," so researchers resorted to deception. *Infamously, they told the black men that they had "bad blood" and that the spinal taps were treatment for their bad blood.* Researchers sent the subjects the following letter, under the imposing letterhead "Macon County Health Department," with the subheading "Alabama State Board of Health and U.S. Public Health Service Cooperating with Tuskegee Institute":

> Dear Sir:
>
> Some time ago you were given a thorough examination and since that time we hope you have gotten a great deal of treatment for bad blood. You will now be given your last chance to get a second examination. This examination is a very special one and after it is finished you will be given a special treatment if it is believed you are in a condition to stand it.[25]

The "special treatment" mentioned was the spinal tap to culture for neurosyphilis. The subjects were instructed to meet Nurse Rivers for transportation to "Tuskegee Institute Hospital for this free treatment." The letter closed, in capitals:

> REMEMBER THIS IS YOUR LAST CHANCE FOR SPECIAL FREE TREATMENT. BE SURE TO MEET THE NURSE.

To repeat, the researchers never treated the subjects for syphilis. *Although penicillin was developed around 1941–1943 and was widely available by 1948, the subjects in the Tuskegee Study never received it, even during the 1960s or up to 1972.* In fact, during World War II, the researchers contacted the local draft board, which prevented eligible subjects from being drafted, and hence from being treated for syphilis with penicillin by the armed services.

The First Investigations

In 1966, USPHS venereal disease investigator Peter Buxtun learned about the study. By this time, supervision of the study (and Buxtun) had moved to the newly created CDC in Atlanta. When Buxtun asked about the study, the CDC threatened to fire him.

By 1969, Buxtun's protests led to a meeting of a small group of physicians at CDC to consider stopping the Tuskegee Study or revealing it. At the end, they voted to continue the study and to keep it secret.

In 1970, American Public Health Association published a monograph on syphilis. It stated that treatment for late benign syphilis should consist of "6.0 to 9.0 million units of benzathine penicillin G given 3.0 million units at sessions seven days apart."[26] The first author was William J. Brown, head of CDC's Tuskegee section from 1957 to 1971. Brown had been on the CDC committee in 1969 and had argued for continuing the study, where subjects with late benign syphilis received no penicillin.

The Story Breaks

Buxtun eventually contacted Jean Heller, who worked for the Associated Press. On July 26, 1972, her story appeared on front pages of newspapers nationwide.[27] She described a study run by the federal government in Tuskegee, Alabama, where poor, uneducated African-American men had been used as guinea pigs. After noting the terrible effects of tertiary syphilis, she noted that in 1969 a CDC study of 276 of the untreated subjects had proved that at least seven subjects died "as a direct result of syphilis."

Heller's story study stunned Congressmen. Senator William Proxmire called it a "moral and ethical nightmare." In reply, J. D. Millar, chief of Venereal Disease Control at CDC, said that the study "was never clandestine," correctly pointing to 15 published articles in medical journals over 30 years.

The Aftermath

After Heller's story appeared, the Secretary of Health, Education, and Welfare terminated the study. CDC estimated that 28 syphilitics had died of syphilis during the study; it then gave penicillin to the remaining subjects.

In 1973, on behalf of the Tuskegee subjects, lawyer Fred Gray filed a class-action suit against the federal government. In 1974, the U.S. government settled out of court. According to the settlement, living syphilitics received $37,500 each; heirs of deceased syphilitics, $15,000 (since children might have had congenital syphilis); heirs of living controls, $16,000; heirs of deceased controls, $5,000. Controls and their descendants received compensation because they and their families had been deprived of antibiotics during the decades of the study. The government also provided free lifetime medical care for Tuskegee subjects, their wives, and their children.

In 1972, and as a direct revelation of the study, the federal government required all institutions that conduct human medical experimentation and receive federal funds to have Institutional Review Boards (IRBs). Today, IRBs must scrutinize written proposals and defend against abuses in medical research.

In 1988, 21 of the original 399 syphilitic subjects were still alive, each of whom had had syphilis for at least 62 years.[28] In addition, 41 wives and 19 children had evidence of syphilis and had received free medical care.

In 1997, President Clinton met four of the eight living survivors to apologize for the Tuskegee Study, saying, "What the United States did was shameful, and I am sorry."[29] The youngest survivor then was 87, the oldest between 100 and 109.[30] By then, the government had paid $10 million to the study's original 600 members or to their families or heirs, who by then numbered more than 6,000. Because of lack of treatment for syphilis of men in the study, any of these other people might have contracted syphilis.[31]

Perhaps the worst effect of revelation of the study was distrust by African Americans of medical experiments, a legacy that researchers still struggle to overcome.

ETHICAL ISSUES

Informed Consent and Deception

In the Tuskegee Study, the subjects did not know they were part of a government study lasting throughout their lives, did not even know what syphilis was, and did not know that they weren't being treated with available drugs. In other words, they had no informed consent, which many critics considered to be ethically outrageous.

R. H. Kampmeier, an emeritus professor of medicine at Vanderbilt Medical School, worked as a syphilologist during the decades of the study.[32] He argued that a study undertaken in the 1930s could not be faulted for lack of informed consent, which began only after 1966. Would it make sense, he argued, to judge Pasteur unethical because he, too, did not get consent?

Kampmeier cited another landmark study by USPHS in 1943 that studied giving penicillin to 35,000 syphilitics; it did not get consent from subjects. He claimed that during the 1930s and 1940s, physicians often walked into a patient's room and simply announced they were taking out the patient's gallbladder. Medical historian and physician Thomas Benedek dismisses informed consent in the Tuskegee Study as "anachronistic," emphasizing that USPHS did not require informed consent until 1966.[33]

While it is true that informed consent in medical experiments was not mandated by court decisions until 1966, the presumption had always been that physicians would "First, do no harm" to their patients. Not obtaining consent for procedures that might benefit subjects differs from procedures that might *harm* subjects.

Finally, and granted that telling patients the truth was not *legally* required before 1966, was it *ethical* for the Tuskegee researchers to lie to their subjects for all those decades? Isn't the truth what one person owes another, especially as doctor and patient?

Racism

The Tuskegee Study took place in Alabama in the Deep South and all its subjects were African American. Under such circumstances, was it only a coincidence that no subjects were white? Would white subjects have been deceived and left untreated the same way?

In his classic work *Bad Blood,* medical historian James Jones saw the Tuskegee Study as a result of pervasive racism in American medicine during the 1930s. How bad was that? To take one example, black students at Tuskegee Institute in the 1930s lived in fear of rural white toughs just outside their campus.

Although studies in nature occurred in medicine during the early 1930s, why did the study in nature of syphilis use only African-American subjects? Some physicians believed then that syphilis ran a different course in different races, and this implied the need for a parallel study of untreated white syphilitics. That the USPHS did no parallel study of white subjects shows that it saw black subjects as expendable.

Media Coverage

In defending the Tuskegee Study, Kampmeier objected to the "great hue and cry" in the media in 1972, and to journalists' claims that "treatment was purposefully withheld to evaluate the course of untreated disease." He said about *Time* and *American Medical News:* "In complete disregard of their abysmal ignorance, members of the fourth estate bang out anything on their typewriters that will make headlines."[34]

With regard to the first objection, Kampmeier exaggerated the "hue and cry" of the media. Indeed, the media botched the story. Coverage shrank within days, and the story moved to the back pages, where only short paragraphs followed it.

In terms of Kampmeier's second objection, he attacked the media for reporting the damaging aspects of the study, such as the withholding of treatment. In defense of the media, researchers *did* intend to withhold treatment. That was precisely the intention of the study.

The Tuskegee Study deserved far more attention than it got. True, it had complex issues that involved racism at a time when racial turmoil upset Americans, but today such a story would receive weeks of nationwide scrutiny, and probably get a Congressional hearing on television.

The relation then between medicine and the media can also be questioned. Before Heller's story broke, the Tuskegee Study had been reported repeatedly in medical journals in at least 17 articles between 1936 and 1972. Researchers did not conceal the study within medicine. Despite this, no professional publication, physician, or editor alerted the nation to the story.

Between 1966 and 1971, one African-American professional at CDC did mail boxes of documents about the study to several national newspapers and magazines.[35] Nothing happened. Why is that?

The answer is important to understanding many issues in medical ethics and to whistle-blowing about corruption. Print and television reporters need an expert to help them understand such complex stories and, equally important, to take responsibility for claims about wrongdoing. Virtually no reporters then or now have the medical background to understand such complicated stories and, without that, cannot risk charging physicians with possible crimes.

A natural tendency also exists to want *someone* else to be the whistle-blower and to bear the brunt of retaliation. As a result, merely mailing information or passing it along conversationally is not enough for reporters to publicize wrongdoing.

Harm to Subjects

Kampmeier argued that if the Tuskegee Study had never occurred, its subjects would have received no treatment and would have been no worse off. Such a claim can never be proved. If the Tuskegee Study had not occurred, many things might have happened. Another charity might have provided Neosalvarsan. A writer like John Steinbeck might have soon written a novel about syphilis in Macon County, arousing national concern and getting penicillin to people there infected with syphilis.

So what harm, if any, resulted to subjects with syphilis from nontreatment? This question might seem even absurd: if subjects were left untreated, of course they must have been harmed! However, the issue is not that simple.

In 1931, penicillin was unavailable, so physicians withheld Neosalvarsan from subjects. Because Neosalvarsan was expensive and cumbersome to administer, even if this study had not occurred, subjects might not have received it. Boeck and Bruusgaard had also undermined claims about the benefits of heavy metals, so harm is difficult to prove. In a review of medical evidence available in 1940, medical historian Benedek concluded that in 1937, untreated syphilitics actually lived longer and better than those partially treated with heavy metals.[36]

Not everyone agrees. UAB Professor of Internal Medicine Benjamin Friedman, whose career spanned the decades of this study, countered that:

> In the 1940s it was known that patients receiving as few as 20 injections of arsenicals rarely developed symptomatic aortic disease. Since we could not determine in advance which of the latent syphilitics would, after 20 or 30 years, develop symptomatic aortic disease, it was necessary to treat all of them. One cannot maintain that some small number of syphilitics deprived of treatment did not therefore suffer injury.[37]

By 1934 the major professional organization of physicians treating syphilis, the Cooperating Clinical Group, proved that use of heavy metals improved Bruusgaard's statistics and recommended that all syphilitics get Neosalvarsan, mercury, and bismuth.[38] Even if many patients could not afford such therapy, they should have been told about it.

Later during the study, penicillin became available. Although Alexander Fleming discovered penicillin in 1929, the world did not appreciate his discovery until 1941, and only around 1946, as a result of wartime production to treat soldiers, did penicillin become available to most Americans. By 1948, anyone could get it.[39]

Kampmeier argued that withholding penicillin in 1946 did not harm subjects with latent syphilis, which he said, was a "chronic, granulomatous, self-limiting disease" and not fatal. He argued next that proof of penicillin's effectiveness did not come until 1948 and then only for primary syphilis. So the study's subjects by 1948 could no longer have been helped by penicillin; the damage to them had already been done.[40]

Benedek disagreed. He concluded that giving penicillin to latent syphilitics in 1948 "might have exerted a definitely beneficial effect on the prognosis of only 12.5 percent of the subjects."[41] Still, that penicillin would have helped 50 subjects.

Effects on Subjects' Families

Recall that Macon County had a rate of congenital syphilis of 62 percent. "Virtually all subjects were or had been married" and had an average of 5.2 children.[42]

When we consider the subjects' families, wouldn't the men in the study want to know they had syphilis? Even in latency, wouldn't they want to know they could become infectious again? Did the researchers withhold the truth because they thought these men couldn't refrain from sex?

These researchers subjected women and children in Macon County to harm. Either the researchers discounted this harm, or thought it didn't matter.

Kant and Motives of Researchers

When physicians at CDC and USPHS debated the Tuskegee Study in 1969, many assumed that if no harm could be proved, nothing unethical had been done. This is also Kampmeier's unstated assumption.

Focusing on consequences, however, is only one way to judge morality. We can also adopt, not a consequentialism or utilitarianism, but a Kantian ethics focused on motives or a virtue ethics focused on the character of researchers.

Although we cannot prove that being left untreated harmed the study's subjects, it may have been only good luck that the study caused no more harm than it did. Why is that?

Historical evidence cuts both ways. We cannot use differing historical standards at differing times to excuse lack of informed consent but not pay attention to what else researchers believed at the time. Let us put ourselves in the minds of researchers in the late 1940s. *The crucial fact is, that when penicillin became available, most physicians believed it would help latent syphilitics.*

So they believed that subjects would be harmed by not getting penicillin. For all anyone knew in 1948, penicillin could have helped patients with aortic heart disease or would have prevented or ameliorated it.

For Kantian ethics, researchers deliberately willed harm on these subjects. They used them as "mere means," as guinea pigs, and could not universalize such behavior as a universal maxim for all physicians to act on. Not only did they lack what Kant calls a "good will," they also had an *ill will* toward vulnerable subjects.

It is no good appealing to sophisticated knowledge that came later about how the damage from syphilis had already occurred. Researchers then believed they were depriving syphilitics of something likely to help them, or depriving them of a way that could help them not pass syphilis on to their female partners. But out of a desire by researchers to prove the final ravages of syphilis, or lack thereof, researchers deceived subjects and believed they were allowing subjects to be harmed.

HIV PREVENTION IN AFRICA: ANOTHER TUSKEGEE STUDY?

Researchers proved in 1994 that giving AZT (zidovudine) during pregnancy cut by two-thirds transmission of HIV from mother to child in North America.[43] CDC, NIH, and WHO then set out to study whether doing a quicker version in Africa would prevent HIV in the 800 infected babies born there every day by doing a randomized control study on infected mothers.

One might well ask, "As the ability of AZT to block vertical HIV transmission had already been proven, why do such a study at all in Africa?" One answer is that the strain of HIV in Africa differs from that common in North America. So the study commenced. The second answer is that researchers felt that in Africa they needed a speedier course of AZT.

In 1997, Marcia Angell, executive editor of the *New England Journal of Medicine,* claimed that such research resembled the Tuskegee Study because researchers gave half of pregnant, HIV-infected black women placebos, and thus babies were born with preventable HIV infections.[44]

So this study had subjects who were: (1) black, (2) female, (3) poor, (4) illiterate, (5) victims of sexually transmitted diseases, and (6) without other available treatment. Like the Tuskegee Study, magisterial but distant governmental agencies conducted the research. Like the Tuskegee Study, vulnerability and powerlessness characterized the subjects. Columnist Ellen Goodman noted that the Tuskegee Study had not ended; it had been merely exported.[45]

Researchers passionately retorted that, had their research not been done, infected mothers would not have gotten AZT and their babies would have been infected anyway.

Angell replied that it had long been established that placebo-controlled studies could not be done on American women. Giving AZT to pregnant women to prevent transmission of HIV to their babies became *the standard of care* for all pregnant, HIV+ women. Angell argued, "If it is unethical to do placebo-controlled trials in America, it should also be unethical to do them in third-world countries."[46]

African officials replied that Angell and Goodman were ethical imperials imposing American ethical standards on African countries.[47] Such officials were also black and had lost children to HIV, unlike the white USPHS physicians of the Tuskegee Study.[48]

They also replied that if they could prove—via a placebo-controlled trial—that a shorter regimen of AZT could reduce HIV transmission by half—they could save 150,000 thousand children a year. If skeptics such as Angell caused delays of proof, more children would die.

Officials also claimed that a placebo-controlled trial of HIV transmission could be done faster and with fewer subjects than a AZT-controlled study, and that once they had good results, African governments would give all pregnant, HIV+ women the new, smaller dosage of AZT.

Researchers also argued procedurally that review committees in both countries had approved the studies and that, unlike the Alabama men, the women themselves had consented. Subsequent interviews by the *New York Times* cast doubt on how much the women understood.

Angell argued that researchers didn't need placebo-controlled studies, that comparing dosages of AZT to other anti-HIV drugs could prove the same thing. Given the poverty of such countries, she denied that a proven, reduced dosage would later be given to all pregnant women because—even at $80—AZT cost 11 times more per year than that normally spent on such African women.

Both sides invoked justice.[49] Philosophically, one side invoked Jeremy Bentham, utilitarianism, and public health ethics. The other side hailed Immanuel Kant, his axiom that people can never be used as a "mere means," and his belief that ethical principles are not local but universal.

For researchers, the risk-benefit ratio had to be different for poor, illiterate women in backward countries who otherwise would not have gotten treatment. For critics, the same reasoning had led to the Tuskegee Study and to Nazi experiments: "they're going to die anyway, so we might as well study them to learn something."[50] As Angell retorted, "People can't be used as a means to a noble end."[51]

In 1998, CDC proved that $80 worth of AZT in the last four weeks of pregnancy cut transmission in half and suspended the study.[52] At this early cessation, both sides claimed victory.

Meanwhile many thousands of subjects in third-world countries continued to be subjects of HIV-vaccination studies, many of them placebo controlled. One occurred in 1996 by Pfizer in Kano, Nigeria, during an epidemic in children there of deadly meningitis. Pfizer researchers flew to Kano and gave half of 200 infected children either a low dosage of the standard antibiotic ceftriazone or Pfizer's experimental drug Trovan. Pfizer had never tested this drug in oral form in children.[53] Researchers commonly create conditions most favorable to proving efficacy of their own drugs, such as giving low dosages of standard drugs or "washing out" all traces of previous drugs in subjects, making them worse off.[54] In this study, five children died who took Trovan, six died who took the lower dose of ceftriaxone, and "many others [were] blind, deaf, paralyzed, or brain-damaged." Parts of this study resemble the trial of a TB vaccine for HIV-infected Africans portrayed in the 2005 movie *The Constant Gardener.*

Secret American Governmental Medical Experiments

During the 1940s, radiation enthralled some physicians. Joseph Hamilton of the University of California at Berkeley injected plutonium into 18 unsuspecting patients diagnosed with cancer. According to Kenneth Scott, a scientist who later investigated these abuses, two patients were mistakenly diagnosed with cancer but nevertheless given "many times the lethal dose of plutonium."[55]

Physicians also studied radioactive isotopes used in diagnosis and research. In the late 1940s at Vanderbilt University, physicians injected 819 pregnant women with radioactive iron in a nutritional study. A study in 1960 found that three of their children died of rare forms of cancer.[56] In 1945, Eda Charlton entered Strong Memorial Hospital in Rochester, New York, with a mild case of hepatitis and was secretly injected with plutonium-239 to study how her body eliminated radiation. Physicians there covertly followed her for years to observe the effects (she died of a heart attack in 1983).

From World War II to the mid-1970s, physician-researchers subjected over 16,000 American patients to radiation experiments.[57] The Department of Energy or its predecessors conducted at least 435 experiments in 21 states. From the 1940s to the 1960s, physicians exposed 1,500 military aviators and submarine crewmen to encapsulated radium on the end of wires inserted high into their nostrils for several minutes.[58] In another experiment, they paid 130 male prisoners $200 to undergo X-ray radiation of their testicles; afterward, these men got vasectomies. In another trial, physicians injected plutonium into an indigent 36-year-old Texan's injured leg, which surgeons then amputated.

In 1995, the President's Committee on Human Radiation Experiments investigated these experiments and concluded that the government should apologize to involuntary subjects and should compensate people who had been injured.[59]

In 1991 in Operation Desert Storm, officers forced soldiers to take experimental vaccines against biological agents. Federal law stated that, under operational conditions, soldiers could not refuse such vaccinations. Many soldiers subsequently became sick. For years afterward, the Pentagon and Department of Defense denied that their sickness was service related. Yet the military's own records showed many causes of such sickness, especially acting in combination, such as sandstorms, biological weapons, oil fires, contaminated water, rare microorganisms, the above vaccines, chemical vapors from bombed Iraqi storage areas, unspent rocket fuel, and high levels of stress.[60]

The Krieger Lead Paint Study

In 2001, after Ellen Roche died in a study of a drug to prevent asthma, the federal Office of Protection from Research Risks (OPRR) halted all federally funded research at Johns Hopkins Medical School. When she volunteered for the study, Ellen was healthy; soon, she was dead.

After its research stopped, a physician from Hopkins on television denounced suspension of Hopkins' research monies, claiming Hopkins had killed only one person in many decades of medical research and that lives would be lost from such a suspension because of delayed cures.

Normally, when a hospital kills someone, its spokesperson should say it's sorry, not complain about being disciplined. Such lack of remorse motivated reporters to dig further, and they uncovered interesting details about the workings of Hopkins' IRB and its Krieger Institute.

The Krieger case was conducted by a branch of Johns Hopkins Medical School that studied retardation in children from lead paint, and which six of seven judges on Maryland's highest court likened to the Tuskegee Study.[61] The study, conducted in the mid-1990s by Hopkins's Kennedy Krieger Institute, recruited 108 poor, black families to live in East Baltimore in houses with lead paint.

Ingesting lead-based paint is a known cause of mental retardation in small children. According to the Krieger Institute, the study sought cheaper ways to reduce lead contamination in houses, so landlords in East Baltimore would not abandon them.

Did the parents understand the nature of the study? Did they understand the risk to their children by living in these houses? "It can be argued that the researchers intended that the children be the canaries in the mines but never clearly told the parents," one critic said.[62] Moreover,

> Maryland Court of Appeals Judge Dale R. Cathell, who wrote last week's scathing opinion, said the board [had] instructed Kennedy Krieger researchers to write consent forms for study participants that skirted federal regulations requiring disclosure about risks.

> The Court of Appeals ruling ordered trials to be held in lawsuits filed against Kennedy Krieger by two women, Viola Hughes and Catina Higgins, whose children were involved in the study. Hughes's daughter now suffers from learning disabilities and cognitive impairments, both of which are often associated with lead poisoning. . . . Higgins says researchers withheld test results that showed high levels of lead contamination from her. . . .
>
> Kennedy Krieger is a major institution in the study of lead paint abatement. Marc Farfel, who conducted the study, said today that it identified more effective ways to remove lead hazards and prompted legislation forcing landlords to remove those hazards.[63]

Amazingly, an investigation by Office for Protection from Research Risks (OPRR) revealed that the IRB at Johns Hopkins, which supposedly had reviewed and discussed the ethics of the Krieger study and all other research at the medical school, had rarely met face to face.

The Krieger Study resembled the Tuskegee Study in that poor black people were deliberately recruited to a study where physicians foresaw harm to subjects. Researchers rationalized the harm by saying that if the study had not occurred; the subjects would have lived in such housing anyway. Revelation of the Krieger Study further damaged already bad relations between Baltimore African Americans and Hopkins.

The Death of Jesse Gelsinger

In 1999, the death of teenager Jesse Gelsinger from gene therapy, like revelations of the Tuskegee Study or Gennarelli's head injuries on baboons, changed regulation of American medical research.

In 1999 in Tucson, Arizona, 17-year-old Jesse Gelsinger worked as a clerk and rode a motorcycle on weekends. He heard about experimental gene therapy at the University of Pennsylvania for his inherited disorder, ornithine transcarbamylase deficiency (OTC).

In the genetic disease OTC, the liver doesn't properly cleanse blood of ammonia produced in normal metabolism, resulting in toxic levels. Many OTC newborns die around birth; half don't live to age five. A new regimen of drugs and diet enabled Jesse to live to be a teenager, but without a cure, he would eventually die.

Jesse entered the study as a healthy research volunteer. A friend said he "wanted to prove he was a man."[63] Penn researchers claim they Jesse that the experiment wouldn't help him, but that it might help OTC babies. Jesse wanted "to help save lives," his father said.

But why weren't studies done on dying OTC patients? Answer: Because OTC babies are born dying, their parents will consent to anything, no matter how dangerous the experiment.

So Penn researcher James Wilson sought adults with OTC whose livers still functioned. He wanted to inject an adenovirus into them that contained copies of the gene lacking in OTC patients. Quite common, adenoviruses can transmit genes to patients with genetic diseases.

What actually happened when Dr. Wilson injected his adenovirus into Jesse was quite grim:

> Four days after scientists infused trillions of genetically engineered viruses into Jesse Gelsinger's liver . . . the 18-year old lay dying in a hospital bed at the University of Pennsylvania. His liver had failed, and the teenager's blood was thickening like jelly and clogging key vessels while his kidneys, brain, and other organs shut down.[64]

The wrongful death lawsuit claimed that Wilson knew the virus had injured other OTC adults and that he failed to use simple, direct language to explain this to the Gelsingers. As Penn bioethicist Arthur Caplan said,

> Not only is it sad that Jesse Gelsinger died, there was never a chance that anybody would benefit from these treatments. They are safety studies. They are not therapeutic in goal. If I gave it to you, we would try to see if you died, too, and if you did, OK.
>
> If you cured anybody, you'd publish it in a religious journal. It would be a miracle. All you're doing is you're saying, "I've got this vector." I want to see if it can deliver the gene where I want it to go without killing or hurting or having any side effects.[65]

Doctor Wilson had a financial conflict of interest from his biotech company, Genovo, which owned patents on the adenovirus, should it prove therapeutic. Biogen, Inc. had paid Genovo $37 million for rights to genetic therapies.

Wilson denies that money influenced his decisions, but that he wanted to be the first to cure a genetic disease.[66]

Wilson reported to the FDA only 39 of 700 problems about the virus, although the law required reporting all of them. In 2000, researchers concluded that adenoviruses should be used only as a last-resort, not on healthy volunteers. Until it could be proved safe, they curtailed gene therapy.

After an investigation of Wilson's research, the NIH in 2000 suspended medical research at Penn. After a Congressional hearing into Jesse's death, the NIH vowed to better monitor medical research. As a result, it suspended medical research at the University of Colorado Medical Center, the University of North Carolina, Johns Hopkins hospitals, and at the University of Alabama at Birmingham. The Gelsinger family settled out of court with Penn for undisclosed monies. After improving their regulation of medical research and conflicts of interest, these medical centers regained their grants, although Wilson's protocols were stopped.

Financial Conflicts and Twenty-first Century Research

The Bayh-Dole Act of 1980 erased an ethical bright line between academic and corporate medicine and allowed universities and their researchers to patent and reap royalties together. Since then, scandals about money keep recurring in medical research.

Twenty-five years later, pharmaceutical companies fund most research into drugs and devices at universities; they do not fund independent peer review of their new drugs and do not publicize bad results. By indirectly paying physicians to test new drugs and by financially encouraging physicians to recruit patients for experiments, drug companies cause physicians to choose *their* drug and not the best drug for their patients.

In 1998, a study by the Department of Health and Human Services concluded that IRBs could no longer handle the job of protecting subjects from abuses in medical experimentation.[67] It found that IRBs were underfunded, overworked, and that the volume of work expected of volunteers could not be accurately and conscientiously performed. Another study in 2002 by the Institute of Medicine reached similar conclusions.[68] Since then, several medical research centers improved their structures for reviewing research, although financial conflicts continue.

In 1991, the federal government adopted *The Common Rule,* under which universities' IRB must review all protocols the same way, regardless of funding. This rule in effect subjects all protocols to the same standards as those required by NIH and the FDA.

Several scandals erupted in the 1990s wherein a few physicians appeared to have taken millions of dollars from drug companies for dubious research.[69] Some doctors in Georgia allegedly made $4 million over seven years from aggressively soliciting people with schizophrenia for drug trials; they made another $6 million over the same period from testing other drugs.[70] Some physicians who worked for drug companies made an extra $100,000 a year flying around the country to give talks to physicians to promote a drug for a pharmaceutical company.

Today, all medical journals continue to take expensive ads from drug companies and almost all medical practices allow drug representatives to buy them and their staffs expensive daily lunches or dinners. Drug companies give these gifts because they work. Learning to take free stuff from drug companies begins in medical school, when students learn to expect free lunches paid for by drug companies. Everyone ignores the corrupting influence of taking these gifts on their later decisions about prescribing drugs to patients.

The Olivieri Case

In 1996, Apotex, Inc. tried to suppress adverse findings by Nancy Olivieri, a Canadian hematologist.[71] When using its experimental iron-chelating drug (deferiprone) on patients with thalassemia, a hereditable blood disorder, in a clinical trial paid for by Apotex, she discovered serious risks and attempted to publish them, but Apotex threatened to sue her for doing so. Olivieri claimed that because of its financial ties to Apotex, her employer, the University of Toronto, failed to support her against the drug company. In a scenario that invokes *The Constant Gardener,* she published her findings anyway in 1998 and was terminated from her position at the university. The case became famous in Canadian medicine for its suppression of academic freedom and for its exposure of ties between medical universities and drug companies. An investigation by the Canadian Association of University Teachers vindicated Olivieri in 2001.[72]

FURTHER READING AND RESOURCES

Thomas Benedek, "The 'Tuskegee Study' of Untreated Syphilis: Analysis of Moral Aspects versus Methodological Aspects," *Journal of Chronic Diseases* 31, 1978.

Alexee Deep, "Placebo-Controlled Zidovine Trials in the Developing World," *Princeton Journal of Bioethics* 1, no. 2, Fall 1998, pp. 21–39.

James Jones, *Bad Blood,* New York, Free Press, 1981.

DISCUSSION QUESTIONS

1. Even if subjects can't be proven to have been harmed by not getting penicillin in the 1940s, explain how Kant would say the research was still wrong.
2. Were the studies to prevent vertical transmission of HIV in Africa really like the Tuskegee Study? What was the same and what differed?
3. Why did the controls without syphilis also get compensation?
4. Knowledge of the Tuskegee Study has prevented many black patients from participating in medical research. Is it time now to get over that? If blacks don't participate in medical research, will studies be done to help them?
5. Wasn't Mengele a sadist? Can you do such things just because of ambition?
6. Was the Krieger Lead-Based Paint Study like the Tuskegee Study?
7. Given his conflicts of interest, should Wilson have been allowed to experiment on Jesse Gelsinger?
8. Does the Olivieri case show that medical research is too closely tied to private industry?

CHAPTER 10

Surgeons' Desire for Fame: The Ethics of the First Heart, Hand, and Face Transplants

Many people desire to be famous, but do we wrongly honor those in medicine who were first? This chapter's key question concerns whether surgeons harm too many patients in trying to be first.

This chapter begins with the race to be the first to transplant a human heart, then the implantation of the artificial heart, and finally, the first hand and face transplants. Along the way, the chapter discusses the dismal history of organ transplants, before cyclosporin the sad history of artificial hearts, and low quality of life and high costs of these exploits for patients.

THE FIRST HEART TRANSPLANT

In 1966, two American surgeons had been patiently developing programs to transplant the first human heart: Richard Lower of Virginia and Norman Shumway of Stanford University. Both had tried for years to overcome the problem that the immune system rejected another person's heart, and both had made progress.

Yet in a race to achieve surgical immortality, South African surgeon Christiaan Barnard beat both of them and on December 3, 1967, transplanted a human heart in Cape Town. Controversially, Barnard used the careful results of these two men and jumped the gun, transplanting a heart before he knew how to control rejection but getting the world's fame for being first.

Barnard grew up poor in South Africa and attended medical school there. Between 1955 and 1957, he trained under surgeon Owen Wangansteen in Minneapolis-St. Paul. When Barnard returned to South Africa in 1967, Wangansteen gave him a heart-lung machine, expecting him to transplant kidneys, not hearts.[1] Until surgeons overcame the problem of immune rejection of a foreign heart, no one expected a heart to be transplanted.

After spending a decade transplanting hearts in dogs, Stanford University's Norman Shumway announced on November 20, 1967 that he was now ready to transplant the first human heart and actively sought a suitable candidate and donor.[2] Two weeks later, Christiaan Barnard, an unknown surgeon in a faraway country, would surprise him.

Yearning for international fame back in Africa, Barnard had secretly decided to try to transplant a human heart. With his physician-brother Marius, he quietly assembled a team at Groote Schuur Hospital in Cape Town.

In 1967, Louis Washkansky, aka "Washy," suffered from end-stage cardiac disease. He had diabetes, coronary artery disease, and congestive heart failure; his flabby heart extended across the inside of his large chest, from wall to wall.

As a young man, Washy had been a weightlifter and amateur boxer. A big, intelligent man with a ferocious desire to live, he had an exuberant, macho personality and liked to flirt with nurses.

Knowing that he would die soon and that his last two years had been hellish, when approached about the transplant, he did not hesitate. Barnard told his patient, "We can put a healthy heart into you, after taking out your heart that's no longer good, and there's a chance you can get back to normal life." To that, Washy replied, "So they told me. So I'm ready to go ahead."

After obtaining Washy's permission, Barnard waited three weeks for a donor. Meanwhile, Washy developed fulminant pulmonary edema—a sign of imminent death—and Barnard feared his chance would pass.

In California, Shumway also waited for the right patients and had to be especially careful that any donor was dead because brain death had not yet been legally defined. In Richmond the next year, and when VIrginia lacked any brain-death statute, Richard Lower narrowly missed criminal conviction for taking the heart for transplant of a black man.

On December 2, 1967, as she walked with her mother to a bakery a half mile below Groote Schuur, a speeding car smashed into 25-year-old Denise Ann Darvall. The accident crushed her head, and a few minutes later, an ambulance took her up to Groote Schuur's emergency room. While driving up the mountain to visit her husband, Washy's wife passed the accident.

Shortly after Denise's arrival, Barnard spoke to Edward Darvall, who had just learned of his daughter's death. "We have a man in the hospital here, and we can save his life if you give us permission to use your daughter's heart. . . ." Edward replied, "If you can't save my daughter, try and save this man."

Barnard summoned his team. As the story is told, the car of one physician broke down, but he ran up the mountain to the hospital, arriving breathlessly in pajamas. The operation took place during the early hours of December 3, 1967.

After her heart had stopped beating, the Barnards declared Denise dead.; surgeons then opened her body, preparing it for Barnard's excision. In an adjacent room, surgeons gave Washkansky drugs to produce paralysis and to prevent spontaneous breathing. They then placed him on the heart-lung machine that had come from Minnesota.

At this point, everything almost failed. Washkansky's femoral artery, where Barnard had attached a tube, had been narrowed by buildup of cholesterol and the machine couldn't force blood into his heart. The pressure on the tube climbed to 290, just below the point where the lines would blow, spilling liters of blood over the room. Barnard and other surgeons frantically reattached the line directly to Washkansky's aorta. Gradually, the pressure dropped.

Barnard then walked to the next room and excised Denise Darvall's heart, leaving part of the wall attached to it like the lid of a jack-o-lantern. He put her heart into a basin of chilled fluid and walked 31 steps back to Washkansky's operating room, where he gave the basin to a nurse to hold. Barnard then cut out Washkansky's flabby heart. Peering down into Washkansky's empty chest cavity, he said, "This really is the point of no return."[3]

He next sewed Denise Darvall's heart with its attached wall into Washkansky's chest, where it looked small. After some false starts, the new heart started to beat. After working all night, the surgeons finished the operation at 7 A.M. on December 3. An hour later, Washy regained consciousness and tried to talk. Thirty-six hours later, he ate a soft-boiled egg.

He then had five rough days, when his urine output, enzymes, and heart rate seemed problematic. Also worried about immunological rejection of the heart, Barnard flooded Washy with gamma ray radiation and administered prednisone (steroids) and azathioprine, but Washy didn't tolerate them well. By day five, he said, the constant tests were "killing me. I can't sleep. I can't do anything. They're at me all the time with pins and needles. It's driving me crazy."[4]

On the sixth day, Washy received more steroids to prevent rejection, and this began five good days when he laughed, visited with his family, and wanted to go home. At this time, Barnard told a press conference that if his patient's progress held, he would "have him home in three weeks."[5]

In retrospect, these five days were the eye of the hurricane; soon Washkansky's body would start to reject the new heart. As this rejection started, Washy began to feel terrible and he suffered from constant pain in the shoulders; dark circles formed under his eyes; his heart and breathing rates climbed; on the 13th day, a shadow of unknown origin appeared on his lung X-ray. Moreover, his personality changed. This vibrant, forceful man became sullen and irritable.

In addition to the threat of rejection, dangers of infection loomed. At the time, most posttransplant symptoms could indicate either rejection or infection, and treatment of one problem could exacerbate the other. So Barnard waited for a definitive diagnosis, even if waiting risked Washy's death.

By the 14th day, Washkansky felt he was dying. He couldn't eat. He lost bowel control. He had such severe pain in his chest that he preferred to lay in his own feces than try to move. Barnard said that he was "constrained" to insert a nasogastric tube to feed his patient, but Washkansky didn't want it. To him, it didn't look as though he would ever be normal again; he had lost his dignity and hence his will to live.

On day 15, mottled patches appeared on Washkansky's legs, indicating circulatory failure. He breathed with difficulty, and X-rays showed ominous patches on his lungs. As he gasped for breath, Barnard decided to place him on a respirator. Washkansky resisted. He had been on the respirator when he first woke up after the operation, and he knew that reconnecting it meant giving up speech. He also felt death to be near.

Barnard disagreed; on December 18, he told Washkansky that there was "a chance" he'd be home by Christmas. Washkansky replied, "No, not now." Living in a sterile tent, and despite his extreme weakness, he grabbed its sides to prevent Barnard from entering to reopen his tracheotomy hole.

As Barnard entered, Washkansky persisted, saying, "No, Doc."

Barnard replied, "Yes, Louis," and put him on the respirator."[6] Washkansky never spoke again. Such is the way of surgeons who, when they want to achieve a breakthrough, push patients.

On December 19, new X-rays showed that bilateral pneumonia—Klebsiella and Pseudomonas—had infiltrated Washkansky's lungs. Earlier treatment with penicillin had killed one organism but allowed others to grow. Barnard had guessed wrong: the immune suppressants had allowed all these organisms to flourish.

On December 20, 17 days after the operation, Washy received 40 percent oxygen; then, as his breathing worsened, 100 percent. By day 18, infection overran his lungs and he began to suffocate.

After two hours of Washkansky's dying gasps, the transplanted heart went into wild fibrillation from lack of oxygen and stopped beating. Even then, Barnard would not give up; he rushed a team together to put Washy on a heart-lung machine. At this point, his brother Marius argued passionately that it was "madness" to continue because Washkansky was "clinically lost." Reluctantly, Barnard agreed. On December 21, after having lived 18 days with a transplanted heart, Louis Washkansky died.

Meanwhile, another patient, dentist Phillip Blaiberg, wanted a heart transplant and was going downhill fast. Nevertheless, and repeating a pattern he would continue the rest of his career, Barnard jumped at the chance for fame and abandoned both Blaiberg and the chance to build a cardiac unit of international quality.

So Barnard flew to the United States, skipping Washy's funeral, where he appeared on television, met the president, and stayed in the States for ten days. Back home later, he transplanted a black heart into Blaiberg, who walked out of the hospital on his own, and thus became a real success.

Fame Cometh

Perhaps no physician before or after would get the kind of saturation coverage by television, magazines, and newspapers that now came to Christiaan Barnard. Long before people talked of "superstars," Barnard became one. A few months later and after 20 years of marriage, he divorced his first wife, Loki, who told reporters, "He was more famous than the Beatles and he loved it."[7]

In 1968, Christiaan Barnard may have been the most famous person in the world. His handsome face smiled from the cover of *Time* magazine, he appeared on television in England, and American president Lyndon Johnson entertained him.

He looked younger than his age, was tall, in good physical shape, witty, worldly, ambitious, and lusty. In his two autobiographies, he admits that fame went to his head and brags about bedding beautiful women, including the actress Gina Lollobrigida. He admits that fame ruined his first marriage to Loki, his second in 1970 to a 19-year-old model, and his third at age 60 to a 19-year-old waitress who bore him two children before leaving him.

Even in 1967, he had the beginnings of crippling arthritis and soon, could no longer operate. In 1984, he took $4 million for saying that a facial cream named "Glygel" reverses aging in skin (it doesn't), for which he was expelled from the American College of Surgeons and a cardiology society. In 2001 he died of an asthma attack, alone at age 78 at a swimming pool in Cyprus, lured there in hopes of signing a contract for an olive oil bearing his name and picture.

Barnard's fame influenced surgeons far more than his surgery. As journalist Donald McRae writes, "Which red-blooded cut-master among [surgeons] would not wish to bed Gina Lollobrigida, lunch with Sophia Loren, and then have Gregory Peck suggested as the perfect actor to play him on the big screen?"[8]

In Plato's *Republic*, Socrates relates the story of the Ring of Gyges, a ring that made its wearer invisible (like the film *Hollow Man*). When Gyges found it, he killed the king, married his beautiful wife, and became king himself. The moral of Socrates's story is that when luck gives a person the opportunity to do anything he wants, that person's true character emerges. In Gyges's case and in Barnard's case, that character failed to measure up.

The Posttransplant Era: "Surgery Went Nuts"

Following Barnard's success with Blaiberg, surgeons around the world went wild trying to transplant hearts. Magazines called 1968 the "Year of the Transplant." During that year, 105 hearts were transplanted. After one year, of the 105 heart-transplant patients, 19 had died on the operating table, 24 had lived for three months, two had lived for 6 to 11 months, and only one had lived for almost a year. Of 55 liver transplants in 1968 and early 1969 (the 15 months after Barnard's landmark operation), 50 of the 55 patients failed to live even six months. Almost all these early transplants failed because the immune system rejected the organs.

Most reporters also missed the fact in 1968 that 25 percent of transplant recipients became not just depressed or irritable but also temporarily psychotic. Massive dosages of immunosuppressive drugs produced initial euphoria, followed by catatonia, severe depression, hysterical crying, and even permanent psychosis. Few deaths could be more distasteful than as a psychotic patient in a postoperative bed in a hospital.

One of the great figures of medicine, Francis Moore, says that the year 1968 saw "epidemics" of chauvinism and of surgeons' egos: "It was the only example I know in the history of transplant medicine where everyone went nuts."[9] Nobel Prize winner (1954) Andre Courmand of Columbia University called Barnard's operation a stunt: "Merely demonstrating that it is technically feasible" to transplant a human heart, he said, was unethical.[10] Physician Norman Staub said Barnard's operation was "grandstanding," a blatant grab for fame.[11]

Many cardiac surgeons criticized heart transplantation with reason. In animals or humans, heart transplants rarely lasted more than a month, let alone years, and the death rate in early heart transplants appalled knowledgeable observers. While 1968 may have been the "year of the transplant," the following two years were the years of the high-tech last gasp.

Because of poor results, the Montreal Heart Institute in 1969 suspended heart transplants, followed by suspensions at Harvard and Pittsburgh. Surgeon John Kirklin at UAB refused to start in the first place, despite pressure to do so. Threatened with Congressional investigation and oversight, by 1970 almost all surgeons had stopped transplanting.

BARNEY CLARK'S ARTIFICIAL HEART

Barney Clark practiced dentistry in Utah for decades. He was A Latter-Day Saint and for 30 years he smoked cigarettes. In 1970 at age 49, he felt unwell. Eight years later, he was diagnosed with emphysema, an incurable, obstructive lung disease, and cardiomyopathy, a disease where the muscles of the heart weaken and quit pumping blood. Too late, he quit smoking.

Over the next four years, powerful drugs dilated his blood vessels and kept him alive, but by November 1982, he was dying. Although he initially scoffed at an artificial heart, approaching death gave him a new perspective and he decided to go for it.

At the University of Utah in Salt Lake City, physician Willem Kolff had been working on an artificial heart for two decades. In many ways, Kolff symbolizes the pros and cons of the desire to achieve a medical breakthrough.

In 1943, Kolff invented the first hemodialysis machine in the Netherlands. He converted a fuel pump from an automobile to force blood through a semipermeable membrane to clean it before it returned to the body. His first patient, a woman who had belonged to the Nazi Party during World War II, lived a few days. Unlike modern dialysis machines, his machine could not sustain patients indefinitely because each time it was used, physicians had to make new connections between arteries and veins for its cannulas. Only in 1960, when Belding Scribner of Washington invented a permanent indwelling shunt, could dialysis sustain patients for years (see Chapter 11).

Despite the simplicity of his machine, Kolff was lauded for decades as a genius, as a brave man of vision, and as one who pushed back the frontiers of medicine. Even though his breakthrough had been crude and showed little elegant scientific understanding, it had brought him fame, honorary doctorates, and the Lasker Award for medical research. Some dubbed him the "Father of Artificial Organs." At Utah, he got his own research lab and didn't need to see patients to make a living. No wonder physicians emulated him.

In 1985, 40 years after inventing the dialysis machine, Kolff paired with Robert Jarvik, an ambitious young student whom Kolff had helped get into Utah's medical school. After medical graduation, Jarvik directly went to work in Kolff's lab, never did an internship or residency, and never directly cared for patients. Jarvik modestly named the first artificial heart after himself.

The surgeon who implanted the Jarvik-7 was 36-year-old William DeVries, a tall, blonde-haired Nordic man with a lean, tanned face. Because of his rugged good looks and macho daring in surgery, some American reporters lionized him as a surgical John Wayne.

Like Christiaan Barnard, DeVries wanted to make surgical history and to place Utah on the world's medical map. Jarvik, Kolff, and DeVries worked hard to push back the frontier of surgical-biomedical engineering, all motivated by the desire to be first in something.

The Implant

In a heart, the ventricles—its two, powerful, lower parts—pump the blood. The Jarvik-7 consisted of molded polyurethane with two chambers of plastic and aluminum holding an inner diaphragm. A wall of thin membrane separated these chambers, through which the diaphragm's contraction forced blood. An air compressor moved the diaphragm, brought by 6-foot tubes inserted through the upper abdomen. The compressor weighed 375 pounds and rolled around on wheels on a large metal cart.

The Jarvik-7 contained the same commercial valves used by heart surgeons and, as in a natural heart, there were four of them (analogous to mitral, tricuspid, etc.). Someone pressing his ear to Barney Clark's chest could hear their clicking sounds as the valves opened and closed against the walls of the Jarvik-7.

DeVries operated on Barney Clark on December 1, 1982, almost 15 years to the day after Washkansky's transplant. On his way to the operating room, Clark joked, "There would be a lot of long faces around here if I backed out now."[12]

Upon opening the chest, DeVries found a flabby, enlarged heart: Twice the size of a normal heart, it merely quivered and didn't contract: one physician there described it as looking like "a soft, overripe zucchini squash." DeVries first cut away the lower part of the heart, the two ventricles; then he stitched two Dacron cuffs to the intact upper part, the atria. He then connected these Dacron cuffs with Velcro fasteners to the plastic ventricles of the Jarvik-7. However, when DeVries snapped the Velcro fasteners, the pressure ripped out the stitches from the paper-thin, atrial walls, so the cuffs had to be restitched into a new section of heart wall and the fasteners gently snapped into place.

The cuffs then held, but when DeVries turned on the Jarvik-7, its left ventricle didn't pump blood. Frustrated, DeVries tried for an hour to get it to work. Three times he opened the ventricle by hand, each time risking introduction of air into the blood and a stroke. At one point, DeVries reportedly exclaimed, "Please, please, please work this time!"[13]

DeVries finally replaced the faulty Jarvik-7 with parts from another one and got the rebuilt machine working, two hours later, all during which Barney Clark was being maintained on a heart-lung machine, subjecting him to risks of mental damage and stroke-causing clots from being under anesthesia so long.

The implant took all night and concluded about 7 A.M. on December 2. A few hours later, the anesthesia wore off and DeVries watched anxiously to see how Clark had fared. If he had a stroke, he wouldn't be able to move his hands. Clark could move them and everyone felt relieved.

Later that day at a press conference, university physicians falsely described the operation as a "dazzling technical achievement," something "as exciting and thrilling as has ever been accomplished in medicine." Hospital administrators also hyped it as "one of the most dramatic stories in medical history."

Back in the recovery room, like most post-op cardiac bypass or transplant patients, Clark's condition shocked visitors, and this held for Una Loy Clark. She saw a man pierced by five tubes: a breathing tube ran through a hole in her husband's throat, a feeding tube went into his stomach, a catheter emptied his bladder, and two hoses connected the Jarvik-7 thumping through his upper abdomen to the 375-pound air compressor at his bedside.

Like Louis Washkansky after his operation, Clark felt horrible. Though he had not suffered a massive stroke, he had experienced intensive care psychosis and felt confused, delirious, amnesiac; at times, he was unconscious.

On December 4, DeVries operated to repair ruptured air sacs in Clark's lungs. On December 6, Clark felt better and asked DeVries how he was doing. DeVries replied, "Just fine." Seconds later, Clark had seizures—involuntary shuddering from head to toe—perhaps caused by the dramatic increase in blood flow from the Jarvik-7.

DeVries injected muscle tranquilizers and anticonvulsants. Clark lost consciousness for the next several hours and his seizures continued, though gradually the quivering became confined to his left leg and left arm. At this point, he probably had some small strokes.

During the following days, Clark wanted to die and once asked DeVries directly, "Why don't you just let me die?"[14] Such a reaction is not uncommon after traumatic surgery and often passes. His lack of energy, difficulty in breathing, and stupor depressed Clark; he told a psychiatrist several times, "My mind is shot."

One of the $800 welded commercial valves broke inside the Jarvik-7 on December 14. Clark's blood pressure dropped dramatically, threatening his life, and DeVries had to operate yet again to replace the valve. Each of these many operations and anesthesias subjected Clark to more risk, more injuries.

Nineteen days after the operation, Clark improved, and DeVries hinted he might one day go home, but soon massive complications began. Devries gave Clark a blood thinner to prevent clots, but it caused severe bleeding. On January 18, DeVries surgically sealed a severe nosebleed. Clark's underlying emphysema created pneumothorax, escape of air from lungs into the chest cavity, and that required DeVries to operate yet again to relieve pressure on his weak lungs.

From January to March, Clark complained of conditions caused by his emphysema. He was suffocating and could never get a good breath. On February 14, he left the surgical ICU for a private room, but because he needed a respirator, he returned on February 15.

On February 24, he moved to a private room and had a good week. On March 1, DeVries filmed several interviews with Clark. On March 2, Humana Hospital released a short, highly edited clip to the public. According to cardiologist Thomas Preston, this clip "came from an extensive interview in which, encouraged by Dr. DeVries, Clark issued a semblance of a positive statement."[15]

Although the clip showed his best moment, even then Barney Clark, tethered to a huge machine, in pain and not fully alert, looked miserable. Prompted by DeVries, he claimed to be glad to be alive and not sorry to have undergone the operation.

The next day he developed severe nausea, aspirated vomit, got pneumonia, and ran a high fever. By March 21, his kidneys failed. On March 23, 1983, having lived 112 days with an artificial heart, Barney Clark died. Inside his body, after someone "called" the death, the Jarvik-7 continued to pump. Asked if she wanted to be present when DeVries turned off the Jarvik-7, Una Loy Clark said, "He's already dead," and left the room.[16]

Following Clark's death, public opinion varied. Some people called the operation "one of the boldest human experiments ever attempted"; others concluded that it had failed to prove its worth, and that even if it had returned Clark to normal, it cost too much, both in money and suffering.

Until the experiment could be studied, Utah's IRB and the FDA postponed any further implants. Kolff defended the project: "A number of doctors were opposed to the artificial kidney and wrote articles against it. I decided not to respond at all. . . . I still have the same policy now for people [who] tell us that the artificial heart has no future."

DeVries surprisingly commented: "After the first two days, 95 percent of the issues we were dealing with concerned ethics, moral value judgments, communications with the press—problems I had never thought about."[17]

A few weeks after Barney Clark died, the hospital revealed that it had not previously disclosed that a valve had broken and killed Ted D. Baer, a 220-pound ram who had lived 297 days with a Jarvik-7. Heart surgeons understood the import of this revelation: even if Clark had lived a few more months, breaking valves later would have killed him.

This is an important point for bioengineering students. Unlike hemodialysis, in which the machine can fail and the patient lives on by getting another machine, if patients leave the hospital and their Jarvik-7 fails, they immediately die. The challenge of creating a totally implantable artificial heart, such that patients could pass the "walk-out-of-the-hospital-on-their-own" test, is that the mechanical heart needs to be flawless, subject to no breakdowns, interruptions, or failures. Otherwise, patients with them inside immediately die.

Post–Barney Clark—Not Fame but Infamy

After Barney Clark died, the FDA allowed DeVries three more such operations. On November 25, 1984, nearly two years after Barney Clark's operation, DeVries implanted a second Jarvik-7 into William Schroeder at Humana.

"Bionic Bill," age 51, younger and healthier than Clark, had no emphysema. Not surprisingly, he lived much longer, 21 months. But his quality of life suffered. Only 19 days after his operation, he suffered a stroke from a clot formed by the Jarvik-7. Schroeder then had a cascade of strokes, repeated bouts of endocarditis, and eventually underwent a tracheotomy. On August 6, 1986, he suffocated to death, a horrible way to die.

On February 17, 1985, Murray Haydon received the third Jarvik-7. On the 17th day after the implant, he started to suffocate and had a tracheotomy. He then experienced various infections, but lived for ten months. After his death, an autopsy revealed that a hole from a catheter in part of his natural heart wall had not healed, so blood had poured into his lungs.

The fourth recipient, Jack Burcham, had an awful death. Going into surgery on April 16, 1985, Jack thought he had nothing to lose by going for the implant, but he was wrong. During the operation, DeVries made the amazing discovery *that the Jarvik-7 wouldn't fit inside Jack's chest*. When Jack Burcham left the operating room, "his chest, draped with sterile dressing . . . [was] only partly closed around the device."[18]

It is almost unbelievable that a surgeon would take out a man's heart and not measure in advance whether a replacement, mechanical heart would fit inside the new cavity. This is in the same territory as amputating the wrong leg.

An autopsy showed that large blood clots had clogged the valve openings in his artificial heart. Afterward, DeVries admitted that the surgery had shortened Burcham's life.[19]

Three years later in 1988, after a long dispute, William DeVries left Humana Heart Institute, claiming that he was unhappy with its red tape. Divorcing his wife of 24 years, he then moved to Humana Hospital in Louisville, Kentucky, a for-profit center where he hoped for a freer hand and three times his former salary.

Over the next four years, he left three different surgery practices around Louisville before starting a risky solo practice in 1992. But because they saw only miserable outcomes, grandstanding, and obliviousness to clinical realities, physicians didn't refer patients to him. For some time, he continued to claim that the Jarvik-7 could be successful, but his was a voice in the wilderness. Lacking referrals, he had no patients into which to implant artificial hearts.

After Barney Clark's death, Robert Jarvik sought and enjoyed fame. He modeled Hathaway shirts in ads and gave interviews to *Playboy*, with whom he discussed his sex life. In 1988, he divorced his wife of many years and, after having known her for only five days, married the columnist who calls herself Marilyn Vos Savant ("Marilyn the wise" in French). Billing themselves sometimes as "the world's smartest couple," Jarvik and Vos Savant claimed that their children from previous marriages were their children "only in the biological sense." Marilyn once added, "I don't consider either of us to have children."[20] She writes a weekly column for *Parade* magazine.

In 2006, Jarvik reappeared in television ads for Lipitor, rowing across the screen. Pfizer eventually cancelled the ads, as they used a body double for Jarvik, who apparently doesn't row. In the intervening years, he founded Jarvik Heart, a small company developing not an artificial heart but a cardiac pump.[21]

William DeVries struggled as a cardiac surgeon between 1992 and 1999, and then retired. After the bombing of the World Trade Center in 2001, he joined the Army Reserve and entered the Army Medical Department Basic Officer course, graduating in 2002 at age 58, as one of the oldest officers to do so.[22] He now operates on hearts with the 324th Combat Support Unit in Florida.

ETHICAL ISSUES

The Desire to Be First and Be Famous

In 1967, surgeon Norman Shumway at Stanford University Hospital in California had trained the longest and most rigorously in hopes of performing the first safe, successful heart transplant. After Barnard jumped the gun, a few months later Shumway transplanted the first heart in America. But both Shumway and Richard Lower felt bitterly disappointed that Barnard had grabbed their results, transplanted a heart, and gotten the world's fame.[23]

A dozen heart surgeons around the world could have done what Barnard did. Isn't it arbitrary to glorify the surgeon who did the first heart transplant, but to ignore the great heart surgeons who laid the foundation and who could have done the transplant but were held back by ethics?

Soon after Barnard's operation, Brooklyn surgeon Adrian Kantrowitz transplanted a heart into a newborn. Kantrowitz needed an anencephalic infant as a source of a heart and found one the day after Barnard's operation. If he had found it sooner, Kantrowitz would be known today.

Reporters describe breakthrough surgeons as "brave," "brilliant,"and "dedicated," but rarely do they report on those who were second or third or those who built the foundation for the breakthrough. Nor do reporters explain how many patients suffered before surgeons obtained good results, or how hard the surgeon pushed these patients.

One factor in being first is the media, which feeds public hunger for medical breakthroughs. On the journalistic side, this hunger leads to inaccuracy and sensationalism. On the medical side, this hunger leads to haste and imprudence. In Brazil, a surgeon so raced to do the first heart transplant there that his patient only learned of the event when he woke up with another heart inside him.

Barnard wanted fame and seemed to relish it. He loved talking to reporters and held daily briefings. When leaving the hospital, he paused for photographers and shook the hands of waiting South Africans. For access to himself and Washkansky, he took money from American journalists, justifying doing so to supposedly raise money to benefit future patients.

Although Barnard wouldn't allow Washkansky's wife to touch him after the operation, citing dangers of infection, such dangers mysteriously vanished when Barnard allowed a film crew to tape the first conversation between Washkansky and his son inside the hospital room.

Reporters understandably focused on the symbolism of the operation: a heart that once lived inside one human now pumped inside another. But this symbolism and Barnard's resulting fame blinded them to clinical realities. Most reporters lacked medical background and the public wanted medical miracles, not messy clinical details.

DeVries criticized the "media circus." The media had changed since Barnard's operation 15 years before; now they were more skeptical. At one point, when told there would be no further briefings, reporters exploded. The hospital later relented, but reporters became angry as weeks passed and the hospital kept spinning the facts. *New York Times* physician-reporter Lawrence K. Altman especially held DeVries's feet to the fire.

What was going on? DeVries and the University of Utah had encouraged hundreds of television and print reporters to follow the operation, but when it didn't turn out well, they tried to stonewall them. The desire to manage the news conflicted with their desire for fame.

Medically, is it ethical to try to achieve a "first" when the essential, underlying problem remains unsolved? The artificial heart presented medical problems similar to that of heart transplants before cyclosporin in that poor trade-offs for the patient existed in both cases. Preventively treating one kind of problem worsened another.

With transplants, surgeons fought infections with antibiotics, and by holding off immunosuppressive drugs, thereby increased chances of rejection of the foreign heart. If they gave immunosuppressive drugs, infections flourished. With artificial hearts, blood clots (thrombi) formed on joints and surfaces of mechanical surfaces. When such clots break free (embolism), they travel in the blood to the small vessels in the brain, lodge there, and cause brain damage (strokes). Blood-thinning medications such as Heparin reduced or prevented clots, but when given to postoperation patients such as Barney Clark, the patients bled out of their sutures.

In 1988, three heart experts reviewed DeVries's surgeries and concluded that his implants created clots and the longer patients' implants were in place, the more clots patients had.[24] So they wrote the epitaph of the artificial heart, a verdict that 20 years of subsequent work has not reversed.

Concerns about Donors: Criteria of Death

In 1968 and after Barnard's operation, cardiac surgeon Werner Forssmann publicly criticized Barnard for taking a beating heart out of one patient to transplant it into another.[25] For Forssmann, before it became a candidate for transplantation, a heart should stop. Because of similar concerns, Japan banned heart transplants for many decades.

Although Barnard did not discuss this with Edward Darvall, he must have been concerned about whether Denise Darvall's death would be accepted. Critics would scrutinize him for any sign of Dr. Frankensteinian overeagerness.

Barnard turned off Denise's respirator and waited for her heart to stop. The longer he waited, the more her heart would be damaged. Washkansky needed a heart in the best possible condition, and Barnard's brother Marius, who was also a surgeon, wanted to remove Denise's heart before it stopped beating.

But Denise Darvall had a healthy heart, so why did her heart stop at all? First there was a problem. Because brain death had not yet been defined, death only came by *whole-body standards* when the heart and lungs stopped. As surgeon Thomas Starzl explained much later, "The steps to donation began with disconnection of the ventilator. . . . During the 5 to 10 minutes before the heart stopped and death was pronounced, the organs to be transplanted were variably damaged by oxygen starvation and the gradually failing and ultimately absent circulation"[26]

So recipients like Louis Washkansky received damaged hearts that could have been supplied in better condition. On the other hand, most transplant surgeons at the time realized that they had little choice in this matter. Transplant surgery depended entirely on altruistic, voluntary donations, and any suspicion of doubtful procedures would sabotage donations.

However, Marius kept secret a detail for nearly 40 years: rather than wait for her heart to stop beating, at Marius's urging, Christiaan had injected potassium into Denise's heart to paralyze it and thus, to render her technically dead (by the whole-body standard).[27]

Responding the next year to this emergency, Harvard appointed a committee to decide when beating hearts could be ethically removed from head-damaged patients. This committee gave birth to the famous Harvard Criteria of Brain Death (discussed in Chapter 2 on comas), which requires the entire brain to be nonfunctioning before organs can be removed.

After Barnard's operation, in trying to be first in their area, surgeons hoarded possible donors and did not share them with other surgeons, even if they better tissue-matched a patient at another hospital. Everyone in the 1970s needed a system that matched donor organs and patients, but the United Network for Organ Sharing (UNOS) would not begin for another decade.

Even as late as 1985, a Gallup poll showed that 44 percent of Americans hadn't signed organ cards because they feared being declared dead prematurely. In the

United States today, by law in all states, physicians who declare a potential organ donor brain dead may not belong to the surgical transplant team.

Quality of Life

An important ethical issue concerned the resulting quality of life for the recipients. In both cases, it was poor.

Barnard and DeVries emphasized that for the first case, the question was not how long the patient could live, but whether. But then reflection set in. Did Washy have 17 days worth of living? Did Clark have 112? Or was it merely, as the *New York Times* said, "112 days of dying"?[28] The same *Times* dubbed research on the artificial heart, "The Dracula of Medical Technology," a phrase that stuck.[29]

In the early 1980s, Sandoz pharmaceutical discovered cyclosporin, a drug that selectively blocks immune rejection of foreign tissue and that revolutionized organ transplants. Thereafter, the number of organs transplanted soared dramatically.

Today, 75 percent of heart transplant patients survive for at least three years and more than 61,000 heart transplants have been performed in America. By 2009, American surgeons had performed 46,000 heart transplants.[30]

Dirk van Zyl, Barnard's sixth heart transplant patient, died in 1996 of diabetes unrelated to his transplant, the longest-living heart transplant recipient at 23 years. Sara Remington, the first infant in the world to receive a heart transplant in 1984, survived to reach her 13th birthday.

Still, life after a heart transplant does not live up to the wonderful life reported in the popular media. Taking cyclosporin for life often causes cancer, and many recipients are in and out of hospitals frequently for repeated operations and complications.

In 2001, Abiomed implanted AbioCor, a titanium artificial heart, in patients at Jewish Hospital in Louisville (DeVries was not involved), the Texas Heart Institute in Houston, UCLA Medical Center, and Hahneman University Hospital in Philadelphia. Abiomed aimed to extend lives of dying patients from an expected 30 to an actual 60 days of life.

Robert Tools received the first AbioCor in 2001 and lived 151 days. Three other patients lived for 92, 78, and 32 days, but another died on the operating table. The biggest success was Tom Christerson, who lived 17 months.

By 2005, Abiomed had tested 14 patients, two of whom died immediately, the rest of whom lived for an average of five months. The widow of one, James Quinn, sued because her husband went through two months of hellish dying, constantly worried about who would pay for his round-the-clock nursing care.[31] Abiomed asked a panel of physicians advising the Food and Drug Administration to let it implant one more heart at a cost of $250,000, but the panel balked.[32]

In October 2004, a rival company, SynCardia of Tucson, Arizona, won approval for a trial of its CardioWest mechanical heart, a direct descendant of the Jarvik-7.[33] Approval was not as a substitute for heart transplants, but as a temporary bridge to transplant for patients on waiting lists.

In 2001, Norman Shumway doubted whether artificial hearts would ever be successful. "An artificial heart is a tremendously difficult problem because the human body is living tissue. . . . [The body] always is going to be opposed to plastic materials."[34]

Expensive Rescue versus Cheap Prevention

In 2002, a heart transplant cost about $210,000, and bills for immunosuppressants for the rest of the patient's life were $15,000 a year.[35] Eighty percent of commercial insurers and 97 percent of Blue Cross Blue Shield plans covered heart transplants. Medicaid in most states also covered them.

In 1999, about 2,200 hearts were transplanted in America, plus 4,700 livers and over 12,000 kidneys. Remarkably, about 900 lung transplants were also done that year.

What about costs? Was the program cost effective? How much is one more year of longer life worth? Is every life worth the same amount? What's the opportunity cost of spending so much money this way?

Artificial hearts could cost society dearly. NIH invested over $8 million in research leading up to the Utah project and over $200 million nationally in similar projects between 1964 and 1982. Was this the best way to spend limited funds? Should such expenditures be continued? If artificial hearts were successful, could society afford to pay for them? The now-defunct Office of Technology Assessment estimated in 1990 that 60,000 Americans might use artificial hearts, at a cost to Medicare of $5.5 billion a year.[36]

All of which is a lot of money and effort to rescue a damaged heart. Glamorous, high-tech operations are dramatic, but might not the money spent do more good for more people if spent to prevent smoking, promote exercise, and create healthier hearts?

The *Progressive* magazine complained that a "medical establishment grown fat on chemicals and technological wizardry is not willing to empower people so they can prevent illness."[37] *Progressive* argued that artificial hearts would benefit only the small number of cardiac patients who could afford them and hence were "qualitatively different from the basic advances in immunology which have saved million of lives, even among populations not directly treated."

Saving bad hearts illustrates again the rule of rescue. Our society cares more about saving an identifiable life than about preventing future deaths from heart failure.

One way to prevent such deaths is to tax cigarettes out of existence. Around 2002, New York and Washington put high state sales taxes on tobacco. In these two states a pack of cigarettes from a vending machine—often used by teenagers to get cigarettes—costs over $8. Such taxes discourage smoking in people when they are young—just when cigarette companies want them to become addicted as happened to Barney Clark.

Real Informed Consent?

How much does a candidate for a new kind of transplantation understand about its experimental nature? How much can such candidates understand, given that they are seriously ill and desperate? In their situation, how is *informed* consent obtained?

The media paint a sunny picture of organ transplants, typically equating success with surviving one year. Within surgery, transplants have grown from being merely *experimental* to being *therapeutic*.

Nevertheless, laypeople believe that healthy transplanted organs will function for a lifetime. The reality is different. If the recipient lives long enough, almost all recipients will reject their organs. One-third to one-half of recipients reject their heart transplants after five years. Kidney transplants began in 1951 and today are closest to being truly therapeutic rather than experimental; but even so, over 50 percent of patients reject transplanted kidneys after ten years.

To prevent rejection, surgeons prescribe continuous cyclosporin, which over years often causes malignant lymphoma and which often destroys kidneys, the liver, or the brain. Cyclosporin also makes women grow facial hair. After several years, its efficacy fades.

Some scholars believe that reclassification of organ transplants in the 1990s as "therapeutic" stemmed not from medical progress, but to make transplants eligible for reimbursement and to obtain publicity and increase donors. So organ donation was framed as a "gift of life" and "making a miracle happen, ignoring the darker emotional and existential implications of what it involved."[38]

After miserable results from heart surgery, one wonders about the relationships between surgeon and patient. One surgeon confesses: "It is sometimes hard to meet the eyes of patients who have improved enough to have been moved to the regular post-op floor and finally become alert enough to communicate their despair and disappointment. . . . Often, after entering the experience with great hope, patients for whom transplantation has been a series of setbacks clearly articulate their feelings of betrayal: 'No one ever told me it could be like this.'"[39]

Growth of Left Ventricle Assist Devices: More Rescues?

In 1998, the FDA allowed cardiac surgeons to insert left ventricle assist devices (LVADs) into patients as bridges to heart transplants. Being on the pump gave patients 408 days of life compared to 150 days on drugs. In 2001, average first-year costs were $222,000.[40]

By 2005, "the workhorse of mechanical support for patients with heart failure today is the left ventricle assist device, which piggybacks onto the native heart, pumping blood directly out of the left ventricle into the aorta."[41] Between 1,000 and 2,000 patients a year get LVADs now.[42]

One wonders about LVADs as a final destination. Is this a good way to live? In any given years, five million Americans live with heart failure, with a half a million new cases diagnosed each year. Can each get an LVAD at $200,000?

Overall, patients on LVADs fare poorly. About half return to the hospital within six months, and a year after surgery, only 30 percent are alive. Worse, many complained of pain and poor quality of life, creating ethical dilemmas. Some turned off their power, committing suicide, or requested physicians or ethics committees to let them die.[43]

HAND TRANSPLANTS AND THE DESIRE TO BE FIRST

In 1998, surgeon Jean-Michel Dubernard performed the first hand transplant in France. A 41-year-old man who had died in a motorcycle accident was the source and the recipient was 48-year-old New Zealander Clint Hallam. A year later, Louisville's Jewish Hospital did the first hand transplant in America on 38-year-old Matthew Scott, who lost his hand to a firecracker.

Before these hand transplants, doctors debated the ethics of transplanting a nonvital organ. Unlike heart and liver transplants, humans did not need a hand transplant to survive, and the recipient had to take antirejection drugs for life, increasing his risks of later getting cancer.

In 2001, Clint Hallam demanded that his transplanted hand be amputated. He felt pain and had no normal feeling in the new hand. Because his antirejection drugs gave him diarrhea and influenza, Hallam had not taken them. He also did not undergo physical therapy.

In contrast, Mathew Scott began to feel cold and heat in his palm and within a few months, nerve growth reached his wrist. He could write his name, tie his shoelaces, and wears a new wedding ring on the new hand. In January 2009, Scott reached a historical ten-year milestone, celebrated at a press conference. In an amazing video (posted on YouTube) Scott can later be seen throwing out a pitch at a baseball game. Another video shows a successful patient threading a needle after a double hand transplant

In another case, which should have been front-page news in ethics, surgeons in South Africa considered but declined to try to be first in transplanting fingers in children.[44] Citing the significant dangers of taking immunosuppressive drugs over many decades, which include cancer, hypertension, opportunistic infections, and diabetes, the surgeons decided that the children might be able to adapt easier and live better without the transplanted digits.

By 2006, surgeons around the world had completed 30 hand-forearm transplants, including three in Lyon, France.[45] Double amputees reported the best psychological results. All patients survived and after two years, none had rejected their new limbs. All had to endure immunosuppressant therapy, including steroids. Despite taking these medications, 12 had acute rejection episodes.[46] In 2001, John Irving explored some of these issues in his novel *The Fourth Hand*.

FACE TRANSPLANTS AND THE DESIRE TO BE FIRST

In the early 2000s, history repeated itself when an unknown surgical team in France beat experienced surgeons around the world to do the world's first full, real face transplant. American surgeon Maria Seimionow of the Cleveland Clinic had been preparing for 20 years to do a face transplant and in April 2005, had been given permission by the IRB of her hospital to go ahead.[47] A year before, John Barker in Louisville had been given similar permission by his IRB, as had surgeon Peter Butler in London in 2005.

Meanwhile in France, Jean-Michael Dubernard, the surgeon who performed the first successful double hand transplant, yearned to make more medical history before his upcoming mandatory retirement. In 2005, Isabelle Dinoire, an unemployed, divorced mother of two teenage daughters living in government housing, attempted suicide by taking sleeping pills.[48] These pills caused her to pass out, and as she was losing consciousness, her head hit a piece of furniture.

While Dinoire was unconscious, her newly acquired black Labrador retriever bit off her nose, chin, mouth, and supporting facial muscles and tissue, allegedly trying to wake her up (the dog later was inadvertently destroyed).

After the mauling, and according to her transplant surgeon, Dinoire's wounds were so severe that she struggled to speak and had to eat through a tube

Questions surround selection of her for the transplant. Was this case like Barney Clark's? In other words, "She's got nothing to lose, so why not try it?" A surgeon in Paris, who had been carefully preparing and playing by the rules, accused Dubernard of bypassing established ethical and legal guidelines for doing transplants.[49]

At the university hospital in Amiens and at Dubernard's urging, Dr. Devauchelle, the head of maxillofacial surgery, decided to transplant onto Dinoire a triangular flap of a brain-dead cadaver's chin, nose, and mouth.[50]

When asked about the face transplant, Ms. Dinoire consented. A French national ethics committee dismissed it: the very notion of informed consent [in this case] is an illusion.[51]

Dr. Devauchelle had already identified a potential candidate in a hospital in Lille, Maryline St. Aubert, who had committed suicide by hanging and who was brain dead. The hanging might have damaged her facial veins, but Devauchelle claimed not to know about this. He cut a triangle of facial tissue from St. Aubert, put it on ice, then sewed it onto Dinoire.

Following the surgery, Devauchelle turned over Dinoire's care to Dubernard. Thomas Starzl, who performed the world's first liver transplant, said of Dubernard, "There's a big brain behind him and steely will to confront massive criticism."[52]

Dubernard, a former deputy mayor of Lyon, also served as an elected deputy in the French National Assembly. A self-described workaholic and chain-smoker, Dubernard commuted from Lyon two days a week to Parliament and on other days doctored in Lyon. Under French law, he faced mandatory retirement in 2008. Like Christiaan Barnard, he confessed to love international publicity and to want a huge "first."

As we know from 30 years of transplants, the real key to success is not the surgery but preventing rejection of the transplanted tissue. Through a steady treatment of immunosuppressants, as well as use of hematopoietic stem cells from Dinoire's face and bone marrow, Dubernard tried to prevent her immune system from rejecting the new tissue. After a week, she could speak and drink.

After several months, Ms. Dinoire returned home. When outside, she wore a surgical mask. Without the mask, as she tried to talk, people could see her jawbone move.

Ethical criticisms focused first on the fact that Dinoire had to take immunosuppresant drugs for life. Already in late 2005, surgeons had to give her increased dosages to prevent rejection of her new face. As we know, such drugs increased Dinoire's risk later of cancer, diabetes, and other medical problems. Estimates predict that 10 percent of such grafts will fail the first year and 30 to 50 percent within three to five years, so candidates must be prepared for failure. Because transplanted skin triggers more fierce rejection than any other organ, facial transplantation carries great risk of rejection and more risk of cancer from taking immunosuppressants drugs at higher levels.

Second, ethical criticism focused on selection of Dinoire, a mentally unstable smoker. Would she adhere to rigorous posttransplant regimens? If her face sloughed off in the worst case, did she possess the mental health to continue?

Third, French physicians seemed to have rushed Dinoire into surgery merely to be first. Admittedly, they feared the female American surgeon getting there first.

In contrast, at the Cleveland Clinic in America, Maria Seimionow, the woman who by rights should have been first, emphasized, "First, do no harm." She said, "The thing I'm worried about is, if it fails, what I'm going to be left with." London surgeon Butler said, "My main concern is not to harm the patient." Seimionow's protocol required good health, good personality, and good family support, none of which Dinoire had.

In 2006, Dinoire resumed smoking, which jeopardized the healing and stability of her transplant by constricting blood vessels and increasing chances of infection. The same year, surgeons disclosed that the donor's face lacked a key nerve that controlled the lower portion of her face. That same year in a visit to UAB, Dubernard revealed to this author that in the first weeks after the operation, he feared each phone call might tell him that the transplant had fallen off Dinoire's face.[53]

In 2007, Dubernard revealed pictures and video of Dinoire, who reportedly consented to this release, who looked much better than expected, and who was said to be "satisfied" with the results. Dubernard pronounced the surgery "perfect" and said her new face looks like, and moves like, her old face.[54]

More Face Transplants

In 2006, Chinese surgeons in Xian attempted a copycat operation, transplanting two-thirds of the face of a man mauled by a bear in a 14-hour operation.[55] Before the operation, the patient had been living as a recluse for two years. Two years later, he died. Though the surgery was not directly related to his death, it is possible that his refusal to take immunosuppressant drugs, instead taking herbal treatments, could have caused his death.

Another face transplant in France was performed in 2007 on Pascal Coler, who suffered from neurofibromatosis, which disfigured his face with large tumors. He suffered a life that was reminiscent of Quasimodo and claimed that strangers had fainted when they saw him. By March 2008, his new faced approached the outer boundaries of normality.

Maria Seimionow of the Cleveland Clinic performed the first American face transplant in December 2008. Connie Culp had been shot in the face in 2004 by her husband and over the next four years, underwent 23 reconstructive surgeries without positive results. The 46-year-old mother of two consented to a 23-hour surgical transplant of 80 percent of a face from a female cadaver by Dr. Seimionow, assisted by seven other surgeons at the Cleveland Clinic. In 2009, Culp went on television, her face swollen but her speech and mental adjustment remarkably good (over time, her swelling would go down).

In 2009, surgeons at Brigham and Women's Hospital in Boston performed a second face transplant. Though they did not disclose the patient's name, his "nose, upper lip, palate, muscles, nerves and some skin" had to be replaced.[56]

Beyond the race to be first and be famous, face transplants raise at least four kinds of ethical issues: consent, selection, identity, and motivation of recipient for undergoing the operation.

As for consent, one hopes any possible patient understands the risk of cancer from taking drugs for life to suppress rejection. There is also risk of the entire face sloughing off and ending up with a gigantic hole where nose, mouth, and chin should be.

Second, when someone awakes to a different face, it is natural to ask, "Who am I?" Although personality is not physical appearance, many people could find themselves with an altered personality.

Third, with better surgical techniques, will some patients seek face transplants for merely cosmetic reasons? What exactly is "cosmetic"? Neurofibromatosis?

Right now, the consensus is that face transplants should be done only in cases of lack of physical function, such as not being able to eat or speak. The risk associated with the surgery and drugs is too high for it to become a cosmetic procedure anytime soon.

CONCLUSION

Norman Shumway, regarded inside surgery as the true "father of heart transplant surgery," died at age 83 in 2006, but his passing attracted little notice. Doctors called him "one of the 20th century's true pioneers in cardiac surgery." Philip Pizzo, M.D., dean of Stanford School of Medicine, said of Shumway that "he developed one of the world's most distinguished departments of cardiothoracic surgery at Stanford, trained leaders who now guide this field throughout the world, and created a record of accomplishment that few will ever rival. His impact will be long-lived and his name long-remembered."[57]

Though Maria Seimionow will not be remembered for doing the first face transplant, she should be remembered for doing the first *ethical* face transplant. And when it comes to heart transplants, the name we really should remember is "Shumway."

FURTHER READING AND RESEARCH

Philip Blaiberg, *Looking at My Heart*, New York, Stein and Day, 1968.

Christiaan Barnard and Curtiss Bill Pepper, *One Life*, New York, Macmillan, 1969.

Donald McRae, *Every Second Counts: The Race to Transplant the First Human Heart*, New York, Putnam, 2006.

Renée Fox and Judith Swazey, *The Courage to Fail: A Social View of Organ Transplants and Dialysis*, 2nd ed. rev., Chicago, University of Chicago Press, 1978.

Thomas Starzl, *The Puzzle People: Memoirs of a Transplant Surgeon*, Pittsburgh, PA, University of Pittsburgh Press.

DISCUSSION QUESTIONS

1. Was surgeon Barnard correct to force Washy to go back on a ventilator the last time? In terms of Margaret Battin's ideas, did Washy get a "least worst death"?
2. How did the first heart transplant lead to the first definition of brain death at Harvard? Why was this definition so conservative?
3. What were the medical trade-offs in the first heart transplant and first artificial heart between treating two different things? Do such trade-offs suggest that each operation was premature?
4. Is it wrong for people to want to be famous? For surgeons? Isn't that how great things are accomplished, by people pushing themselves? What's wrong with fame that is deserved?
5. Is the fact that so many famous surgeons got divorced after becoming famous relevant to judging their accomplishments?
6. Why is it so hard to put money into preventing heart disease rather than expensively trying to cure it after it develops?
7. If one is dying and hope is offered, is it possible to get real informed consent? Won't a dying man grasp at any offered hand?
8. The Baby Doe chapter and this one suggest that many reporters may not have the medical background to inform readers of the true issues of a breakthrough. Has this situation gotten better or worse with the demise of some famous newspapers?

CHAPTER 11

Allocation of Artificial and Transplantable Organs

The God Committee and Live Donors

Every day in American medicine, someone decides who gets expensive medical resources and who does not. But are such decisions governed by principles of justice? The chapter discusses the famous God Committee in Seattle in the 1960s that decided which patients in renal failure would receive dialysis and hence, live. Its essential question asks who *deserves* a scarce resource, and specifically, whether bad decisions about personal health justify denial of that resource. Should smokers with emphysema be eligible for lung transplants? Alcoholics for liver transplants? Chapter 14 also discusses such questions in connection with genes for diabetes, breast cancer, and dementia.

BACKGROUND

An Artificial Kidney: Hemodialysis

The kidneys remove toxins accumulated by normal cellular metabolism in the blood. When both kidneys fail, toxins accumulate to lethal levels.

Hemodialysis (literally "tearing blood apart") substitutes for the kidneys: It removes blood from the body and sends it through cannulas (tubes), where a surrounding solution absorbs toxins by osmosis through a semipermeable membrane; then the cleansed blood is returned to the body. Patients in renal failure must undergo hemodialysis (more simply, "dialysis") for several hours, two or three times a week.

The process doesn't cure kidney (renal) failure, and leaves patients tired and cranky, with lives revolving around appointments. To get off dialysis, most patients want to get a kidney transplant.

Dutch physician Willem Kolff invented the hemodialysis machine in the Netherlands in 1943 and later worked on artificial hearts with Robert Jarvik. Kolff converted an automobile's fuel pump to force blood to and from the body for cleansing. Each session of dialysis required surgeons to connect cannulas to arteries and veins. Because an artery or vein can be used only once, surgeons soon exhausted all sites.

In 1960, physician Belding Scribner in Seattle invented the permanent indwelling shunt, a piece of tubing permanently attached to one vein and one artery, which allowed blood to flow continuously. The shunt could be shut off between dialyses, like a spigot.

At first, Scribner did not realize that the combination of a workable dialysis machine and a permanent shunt meant that he and Kolff had created an artificial kidney, a machine that could sustain life indefinitely.

This breakthrough led to something wonderful: thousands of dying patients would now live. It also led to a new ethical issue: if no way could be found to dialyze them, many others would die. Given the scarcity of machines, physicians needed to employ a criteria of distributive justice to select who would live and who would die.

Supply and Demand of Donated Organs

Problems of distributive justice arise in allocating solid organs. Over the past decades, the number of organs available for donation has never matched demand: the number from cadavers hovers around 4,000 a year. Second, the need for transplantable organs has steadily increased, especially as more Americans on dialysis desire kidney transplants. The new source of organs has been live donations from friends and relatives. In 2003, more transplantable kidneys came from such donors than from cadavers, a milestone.

Less than 20 percent of American adults agree to be organ donors. Young adults notoriously do not think about death and resist signing donor cards. Some people reject the idea of desecrating a corpse by removing organs.

Some African Americans refuse to sign donor cards because they consider themselves more likely to be declared dead prematurely. In 1968, surgeon Richard Lower transplanted the heart of African-American Bruce Tucker using the new Harvard criteria of brain death. When Tucker's heart was removed, he was not legally dead by the old, whole-body criteria, but it took a tense trial for a judge and jury in Richmond, Virginia, to decide that the new criteria excused a transplant surgeon from charges of murder.[1]

Of course, without a signed donor card, a family may still donate organs of a brain-dead relative. And even if the brain-dead patient has a signed card, if the family refuses, surgeons do not take organs because they fear lawsuits and bad publicity.

Confusion over the definition of brain death decreases organ donation. For this reason, America has not moved beyond the conservative Harvard criteria of brain death to broader criteria.

For successful transplants, physicians must keep the cadaver's organs in good condition. For their own well-being, victims of head trauma should be kept as dry (internally) as possible, whereas transplant surgeons need well-hydrated organs. As discussed later in this chapter about non-heart-beating donor protocols, what's best for the organs may not be what's best for trauma patients.

Young, healthy adults constitute the best sources of good organs; in practice, this means people killed in motor vehicle crashes. In his first efforts, Dr. Kevorkian worked to allow prisoners on death row to donate organs before execution, but most of them would have had unsuitable organs due to age, abuse of alcohol or other drugs, cancer, or hepatitis B or C.

Preventing car accidents reduces the number of donatable organs: restraints and seats for infants and children, helmets for motorcyclists, a legal drinking age of 21, lower speed limits, and laws and social pressure against drunk driving all reduced deaths among Americans under 40—the age group most likely to have donatable organs. When one state recently allowed motorcyclists not to wear helmets, the number of deaths, and subsequent organs from them, soared.

At least 14 European countries follow France and *presume consent*: a dead person is presumed to be a donor unless he specifically declines in writing to a national agency. Presumed consent has not been tried in America, where mistrust of doctors already prevents donation and where physicians fear lawsuits.

Mandated choice requires adults, in obtaining a driver's license, to indicate whether they want to be organ donors. Most American states require this choice. *Required request* mandates that someone at a hospital must ask a relative of brain-dead patients about organ donation.

THE GOD COMMITTEE

When Belding Scribner developed his shunt in 1962, inpatient dialysis cost $20,000 a year. Because it was an experimental treatment, insurance companies refused to pay for it. To hold down costs, such companies do not cover any experimental treatments until scientists prove them therapeutic. So Scribner's Swedish Hospital dialyzed its first patients without charging them.

Swedish Hospital soon told Scribner he could admit no more patients for dialysis. By then, Scribner had a year's experience with dialysis and decided that patients could undergo it outside the hospital in clinics staffed by nurses. In 1963, Swedish Hospital started an outpatient dialysis center. That center could serve 17 patients, but many more patients were eligible. From its beginning, the ethical problem flared of *who shall live when not all can*?[2]

Instead of leaving this problem of distributive justice to physicians, Swedish Hospital, Scribner, and King's County Medical Society took the unusual step of creating an Admissions and Policy committee to decide who would get a dialysis machine. Scribner wrote in 1972, "As I recall that period, all of us who were involved felt that we had found a fairly reasonable and simple solution to an impossibly difficult problem by letting a committee of responsible members of the community choose which patients [would receive treatment]."[3]

The intent of creating this committee was to take the burden of moral decision off physicians, since a physician would naturally want her patients to be accepted.[4] The committee of seven members represented the community: a minister, a lawyer, a housewife, a labor leader, a state government official, a banker, and a surgeon. Two physicians familiar with dialysis served as advisers and screened applicants for medical unsuitability. The committee worked anonymously and never met candidates.

The committee first limited candidates to residents of the state of Washington who were under age 45; candidates had to be able to afford dialysis or have insurance that covered it. Almost immediately too many patients applied and additional criteria became necessary. The committee then considered a candidate's employment, children, education, motivation, achievements, and promise of helping others—criteria somewhat like those used by admissions committees to medical school.

The committee eventually asked for analyses of a candidate's ability to tolerate anxiety and ability to manage his medical care independently; it considered whether a candidate had previously used symptoms to get attention. In its deliberations, it evaluated the personality and personal merit of the candidate and the family's support for a patient on chronic dialysis. Elderly curmudgeons without siblings or children fared badly.

Shana Alexander Publicizes the God Committee and Starts Bioethics

This committee struggled with distributive justice long before bioethics became a field. In 1962, no philosophers had written about ethical issues of allocating organs; indeed, no one had written about bioethics at all.[5] At least, they had not in the modern sense in which cases are analyzed to find a just public policy. The major previous writings were in Catholic medical ethics.

In May 1962, Dr. Scribner took a patient to Atlantic City for a newspaper convention to lobby publicly for more dialysis machines. In the process, he described the God Committee to reporters, and it was his account of that committee, rather than his appeal for more machines, that made the front page of the *New York Times* the next day.[6]

Life magazine assigned its first woman reporter, Shana Alexander, to write the story of this committee, and she spent three months in Seattle doing so. Her article appeared in November 1962 and carried the phrase "God Committee"—a phrase that stuck.[7] Alexander described the committee as playing a godlike role in deciding who would live and who would die. She described in detail the committee's criteria, which came to be called *social worth criteria*, or criteria about a person's worth to society.

In the spring of 1963, the *Seattle Times* ran on its front page a picture of nine of the center's dialysis patients, with the heading, "Will These People Have to Die?"[8] As a result, the Boeing Corporation and the U. S. Public Health Service offered temporary financial support.

In 1965, television reporter Edwin Newman narrated an NBC documentary on the God Committee, *Who Shall Live?* That year, Congress had added to Social Security two national medical programs—Medicare for the elderly and Medicaid for the indigent, but dialysis was not yet covered by either of them. In the documentary, a congressman asked why, if the United States could have a space program, it couldn't have a dialysis program to save lives. National interest grew about the story, and indirectly, about bioethics.

The media mattered greatly in this case. Shana Alexander said that when Scribner went to Atlantic City, he had been "angling" to get the story into the magazine with the largest circulation. Medical sociologist Judith Swazey agrees that Scribner set out to get publicity.[9]

Thirty years later, Scribner said that he had been "totally naive" about the national publicity, that a 1968 article in *UCLA Law Review* gave him "a lot of flak,"[10] that he had had nothing to do with the committee—which had been created and supervised by the King's County Medical Association—and that when he had a dying patient who wasn't selected, he tried to circumvent the committee.

The story about his work in the *Seattle Times* could not have been written without the initiation and cooperation of Scribner and other physicians at Seattle hospitals. These physicians manipulated *The Seattle Times*, *Life*, and NBC News to obtain funds for their patients. Their success began a pattern of using the media when patients needed organ transplants, a pattern that came to be called the *rule of rescue*.

The End-Stage Renal Disease Act (ESRD)

The God Committee continued to select and reject candidates for dialysis for nearly a decade. By 1971, many stories had dramatized the plight of patients in renal failure, and that year Shep Glazer, the president of the American Association of Kidney Patients, testified before Congress. As the story goes (it may be exaggerated), Glazer dialyzed himself before the House Ways and Means Committee, disconnected a tube from the machine, let his blood flow onto the floor, and said, "If you don't fund more machines, you'll have this blood on your hands."

In 1972, Congress legislated for Americans a one-organ right to medical care. The *End-Stage Renal Disease Act (ESRD)* mandated the federal government to pay for a dialysis machine for any American who needed one. Faced with the problem of distributive justice, of deciding which patients should be funded and how to select them, Congress took the easy way out and funded all patients. It decided not to decide.

Congress passed ESRD in a session lasting only 30 minutes. The impetus came from a coalition of kidney patients, lobbyists for some physicians, concerns over high rates of kidney failure in people of color, and concerns that too much money was being spent on space and the war in Vietnam but too little on dying people who might be saved.

By making dialysis available to all patients, ESRD ended the problem of allocating machines and thus ended the need for the God Committee.

In retrospect, ESRD was hastily conceived, and it set an unfortunate precedent. Other groups, such as hemophiliacs, pressed for similar coverage. No one accurately predicted the long-term costs to society.

Advocates of funding for dialysis predicted that, as more machines were produced, costs would drop. Their prediction is a textbook lesson in how classic supply and demand fails to work in medical finance. Senator Vance Hartke of Indiana predicted that although ESRD would cost $100 million the first year, its cost would drop sharply because of increased efficiencies in production. Willem Kolff said that his machines could be mass-produced for $200 each.

But under *cost-plus reimbursement*, in effect for hospitals during the 1970s and 1980s, hospitals could buy as many dialysis machines as they wanted and pass the cost "plus" a percentage of profit on to Medicare. So they had no incentive to buy $200 machines but were movitated to buy $20,000 machines. The larger the cost, the greater the profits they made.

In 1983 and in efforts to rein in out-of-control costs, reimbursement by *Diagnostically Related Groups (DRGs)* units replaced cost-plus funding. Hospitals still found a way around DRGs and costs continued to soar. As yet another way to control costs, managed care started in the 1990s.

By 2006, instead of costing a few hundred million dollars, the 330,000 Americans on dialysis in ESRD cost Medicare $16 billion a year. This yearly figure was 160 times higher than Senator Hartke's prediction, possibly 1,000 times higher, and Hartke had predicted costs to fall dramatically. When people started talking about funding Kolff's artificial hearts in the mid-1980s, few of them remembered these incorrect estimates.

Under ESRD, Congress also reimbursed kidney transplants. After the development of cyclosporin, the number of successful renal transplants jumped from 3,730 in 1975 to 9,000 in 1986 and to 15,000 in 2003.[11] In addition to the question whether every dying kidney patient should undergo dialysis, this development raised a new question: should every dialysis kidney patient have a kidney transplant? If so, where would the organs come from?

One thing is certain: what drove the expansion of people on dialysis and people getting kidney transplants was the fact that federal funds paid for all treatments for the kidney, a situation that existed for no other organ or disease. In contrast, during the last decades, over 40 million Americans lacked basic medical coverage. At the same time, any American suffering kidney failure had all medical expenses covered and, frequently, could go on disability.

The Birth of Bioethics

For complex reasons, Belding Scribner did something that went against a medical practice that went back centuries: he made public a moral dilemma that hitherto had been discussed only privately among physicians. Bringing this issue to the public's attention created controversy within medicine. As in Karen Quinlan's case, physicians felt that such ethical issues should be handled quietly within the profession.

By making this move, Scribner began a new process—the education of the American public about ethical problems in medicine. Scholars now began to publicly discuss problems such as brain death, assisted reproduction, and just allocation. With these articles and new courses, the new interdisciplinary field of bioethics began.

ETHICAL ISSUES

Social Worth

As we have seen, the God Committee took "social worth" into account (although the committee itself did not use this phrase). Medical sociologists Renée Fox and Judith Swazey, who spent 40 years studying artificial kidneys and transplantation, reviewed the minutes of the committee's meetings and criticized its criteria:

> Within these very general criteria, the specific, often unarticulated indicators that were used reflected the middle-class American value system shared by the selection panel. A person "worthy" of having his life saved by a scarce, expensive treatment like chronic dialysis was one judged to have qualities such as decency

> and responsibility. Any history of social deviance, such as a prison record, any suggestion that a person's married life was not intact and scandal-free, was a strong contraindication to selection. The preferred candidate was a person who had demonstrated achievement through hard work and success at his job, who went to church, joined groups, and was actively involved in community affairs.[12]

Any standard of social worth implies that some people are worth more than others. Is it therefore unjust? Immanuel Kant argued that every human should be treated as an "end in himself" with absolute moral worth. To judge that one human deserves to live more than another is to treat some wrongly as a "mere means."

How then would Kant treat everyone the same? The key question is what rule or maxim could be universalized. For Kant, that would be impartial, random selection by lot, say, by drawing straws.

Two critics of the God Committee, a psychiatrist and a lawyer, raked social worth over the coals:

> ... [*Life*] magazine paints a disturbing picture of the bourgeoisie sparing the bourgeoisie, of the Seattle committee measuring persons in accordance with its own middle-class suburban value system: scouts, Sunday school, Red Cross. This rules out creative conformists, who rub the bourgeoisie the wrong way but who historically have contributed so much to the making of America. The Pacific Northwest is no place for a Henry David Thoreau with bad kidneys. . . .[13]

Law professor George Annas criticized the committee for preferring housewives over prostitutes, working men over "playboys," and scientists over poets.[14] Annas argued that some criteria of social worth can be just at some stage of the selection process, but these criteria must be made public. If the rule is going to be "always prefer housewives to prostitutes," this should be explicit. Secret rules allow discrimination based on race, sex, class, wealth, or other arbitrary qualities.

In fairness to the God Committee, today nephrologists prefer that patients dialyze as out-patients because six patients can be supported outside the hospital for the cost of one inside. For out-patient dialysis to work requires support by the patient's family and a positive attitude by the patient.

Self-Inflicted Injuries

Kant's ethics may also be contradictory because Kant stresses personal responsibility for health. Should someone who behaves irresponsibly get a scarce medical resource?

Take the famous case of the half-Sioux Ernie Crowfeather. A small-time criminal and a charmer, he received dialysis for 30 months but refused to follow the regimen, hated his quality of life, drank, imposed his childlike needs on the staff, and finally turned down further therapy and died.[15] Crowfeather was a patient for whom Scribner went around the committee to get dialysis.[16]

Liver transplants also raise the issue of self-inflicted injuries. By far the most expensive organ to transplant, relocating a liver calls for a highly skilled team and takes a long time. The most common cause of liver destruction, or end-stage liver disease (ESLD), is alcoholism. When alcohol is a factor, the condition is actually called *alcohol-related end-stage liver disease (ARESLD).*

In the 1990s, physicians debated whether patients with ARESLD should be equally eligible for liver transplants. This is partly a medical issue, since it can be analyzed in terms of which patients will benefit most from such a transplant, but it also concerns social worth. Is a nondrinker more deserving of a donor liver? Can someone with ARESLD be blamed for the loss of his liver? Would a drinker keep on drinking, thereby destroying the new liver, or would drinkers be transformed by receiving the gift of life?

With ARESLD, this question is complicated by disagreement over whether alcoholism is a disease or a chosen behavior. The disease model of alcoholism has prevailed for some time, but it has recently been attacked by philosopher Herbert Fingarette, who in turn draws on themes in Kant's ethics.[17]

In 1992, two teams of clinical medical ethicists debated this point. In Chicago, physicians Alvin Moss and Mark Seigler argued that as ARESLD principally causes liver failure, as not enough livers are available for transplant, and as recidivism is likely among alcoholics, patients who develop liver failure "through no fault of their own" should have a higher priority for donor livers than patients with ARESLD, whose condition "results from failure to obtain treatment for alcoholism."[18]

Two medical ethicists at the University of Michigan, Carl Cohen and Martin Benjamin, disagreed. They maintained that alcoholics are not morally blameworthy and, after liver transplants, survive as long as nonalcoholics, so should not be penalized.[19]

Kant and Rescher

Kantian ethics pulls in two directions on the question of penalizing alcoholics for liver transplants. On the one hand, Kant believes that people choose to drink and should be held responsible. For him to claim that, "The alcoholic's actions are caused by a disease" is to treat the person as a "mere means,"as if he were the passive vehicle of causal forces over which he has no control. Herbert Fingarette's research shows that most so-called alcoholics drink voluntarily, given proper incentives and contexts, and can moderate their behavior. Fingarette also emphasizes that Alcoholics Anonymous assumes that drinkers can choose not to drink.

As said, all other things being equal, Kantian ethics also pulls for a lottery in distributing a scarce liver, to treat each person equally and as having equal moral worth. Can these two strains of Kantian ethics be reconciled?

Perhaps. In 1969, philosopher Nicholas Rescher argued that the God Committee had been correct to use criteria that included social worth.[20] Rescher favored considering life expectancy, number of dependents, potential for future contributions to society, and past achievements. Less controversially, he supported screening candidates for medical problems that were likely to make them do poorly on dialysis and waste machines. He suggested that such a system might be based on points, with ties broken by a lottery.

Kant would be sympathetic to Rescher's two-tiered approach. Those who had injured themselves through voluntary behavior do not deserve the same chance as those who lost kidneys through a genetic disease. Once such people are screened out, however, everyone should be considered equally by lottery.

Distribution Systems and Waiting Lists

In the 1970s, no system existed for distributing donated organs, and surgeons with organs in one medical center did not always share them with surgeons elsewhere. This was wasteful. Some hoarded organs soon were lost.

The National Transplantation Act (1984) and the federal Task Force on Organ Transplantation (1986) were combined in 1987 to create the United Network for Organ Sharing (UNOS). UNOS alleviated some regional competition and established national standards about which patient would get the next available organ. UNOS continually grapples with the ethical question: *what is the most fair, just way to allocate organs*?

UNOS deals only with candidates who are already in the system. Thus how and when applicants get onto waiting lists for donor organs remains a pressing issue. Specifically, if you don't have medical insurance or a hospital willing to take you as a charity case, you won't get on the UNOS list.

An especially vexing problem is the practice of *multiple listing*.[21] Some patients get appointments with surgeons at more than one transplant center and have themselves worked up at each; but only people who can take time off from work, can afford to travel, and have generous medical plans can arrange for multiple listings.

In 2009, Apple cofounder Steve Jobs illustrated the advantages of multiple listing when he traveled from California to Memphis to get a liver transplant. Without having the money to get himself worked up in Tennessee, he would not have become the sickest patient on the hospital's list.

For a patient who needs a kidney, being on several lists may not be necessary to get one, but for a patient who needs a heart or a liver, a multiple listing may be a matter of life and death. One criterion for receiving a heart or liver is locality: a candidate must be within the area of the transplant center or have the money to get there fast. A patient who registers at half a dozen such centers could significantly increase his chances of being selected.

Imagine that you are going to die in Memphis of liver failure, but you know that 100 other patients want a liver for the same reason. Then you learn that Californian Steve Jobs received a liver because he gamed the system to get on the right list. It's one thing to feel unlucky because you're in a life-threatening condition, but another to feel that you are going to die because someone else managed to get into line in front of you.

When former baseball star Mickey Mantle came to Baylor University Medical Center in Dallas on May 28, 1995, decades of alcoholism, as well as Hepatitis C, had destroyed his liver. Physicians also diagnosed him with end-stage liver disease.[22] A CT scan found a large tumor on the center of his liver compressing his common bile duct.[23]

Mantle went on the UNOS waiting list for a liver transplant and was classified as a Stage 2, the second most urgent.[24] Two days later, he received a liver.[25]

Many felt that Mantle's celebrity had vaulted him to the top. The transplant team was also criticized for giving a transplant to a person with first, liver cancer and second, lifelong alcoholism. Many felt that Mantle had destroyed his liver on his own and that someone more deserving should have received the transplant.

Three months after his transplant, Mantle died from cancer.[26] His case rocked the public's trust in UNOS and its methods of selecting candidates.

Similarly in 1993, the governor of Pennsylvania from 1987 to 1995, Robert Casey, was diagnosed with Appalachian familiar amyloidosis, a rare genetic disease. Seemingly within ten hours of entering the waiting list, Casey got a combined liver-heart transplant, even though many other candidates were ahead of him.

It was later claimed he had been on the list for a year but did not want his disease known for political reasons. Pittsburgh's famous transplant program in Pennsylvania also defended Casey's selection, saying he was the only person on a list of people needing both a liver and a heart. After the outcry, UNOS revised its criteria to say that a successful candidate must be at the top of one of the lists for single organs (which Casey had not been) in addition to his place on any list for two transplants.

In 1990, New York State banned multiple listing. In 1992, some patients who were multiple listed argued in a hearing before UNOS that forbidding the practice denied their "liberty right" to contract for medical care.[27]

There are two powerful arguments against multiple listing. First, a primary attribute of a just medical system is equality of access, and the use of wealth to jump the line violates this norm. Second, multiple listing compromises the entire UNOS system because some people are getting listed above others arbitrarily. UNOS should be impartial not only in dealing with candidates who are already listed, but also in the actual process of deciding who gets listed.

A similar problem surfaced in the early 1990s, when it was revealed that candidates for neonatal heart transplants were being identified prenatally and then being placed on waiting lists immediately, while they were still fetuses.[28] Because time accumulated on a waiting list gives a candidate extra points, such a practice would offer a significant advantage. In this case, prenatal listing was made possible by the ability to diagnose hypoplastic left heart syndrome (HLHS) in utero, but such early diagnosis is not uniformly distributed in the United States, and early listing of babies diagnosed in utero seemed unfair to babies who were not diagnosed until birth. Moreover, fetuses with HLHS remain relatively safe while they are in the womb, whereas at birth HLHS babies are almost always at great risk and are in NICUs. For these reasons, UNOS changed its policy in June 1992 and put fetuses on a separate list from babies. UNOS also decided to allocate a heart to a fetus only when no baby could use it.

Retransplants

Retransplantation of the same patient raises other issues about justice. Since patients often reject transplanted organs, a second or third transplant can be done. But is it fair to give a particular patient a second heart or kidney when thousands of others never get one? Shouldn't patients get a second organ only when everyone has had a chance at one?

UNOS treats those waiting for retransplants as first-time patients. This does not lead to the best outcomes. Nearly 82 percent of first-time transplants survive one year, but only 57 percent of retransplants do. Retransplanted patients fare worse than first-transplant patients because they are usually sicker.

Utilitarians see justice as creating the greatest years of life per donated organ. Under such constraints, UNOS should give first-time patients priority over retransplant patients.

But maximal years per organ is not the only value in play. Shouldn't medicine save those who are about to die? Shouldn't others, who are less sick, wait?

Transplant teams bond with patients and find it difficult not to save them. Consider a hypothetical 41-year-old Judy Rogers, a former bank teller now on dialysis and disability who suffers severe depression. This is understandable: the medical team has worked very hard—over many years—to save Judy's life, and when she rejects an organ, the team does not want to be forced by UNOS to watch her die. Medical staffs would see this as *patient abandonment*. More simply, nurses, medical students, and the surgeon know Judy personally, whereas new patients are abstractions to them.

But it is reasonable to ask why identified patients should take priority over new patients: a new patient may benefit more and be more meritorious. Moreover, if the medical teams are allowed to select who gets a new organ, patients who are better at forming relationships with transplant teams will be favored.[29]

Although transplant teams identify with retransplanted patients, others may identify with the patients who are waiting. Consider a hypothetical Max Loftin, a 53-year-old accountant with severe depression and a dialysis patient waiting for a kidney transplant. A new kidney might cure his depression. But if present patients in hospitals get all next month's available kidneys as second or third retransplants, Mr. Loftin goes on to miss his appointments and hence to die, a nameless victim.

An actual patient named Ronnie DeSillers in Miami, who received *three* liver transplants, caused bitter feelings among patients waiting for a liver. Because his father knew how to work the system, Danny Canal of Wheaton, Maryland, in 1998 received *three quadruple* organ transplants (the first due to multiple listing). Did 11 other people deserve never to get an organ so Danny could get 12?

The Rule of Rescue

The rule of rescue, named by bioethicist Albert Jonsen, refers to giving scarce medical resources to an identified patient, rather than to equally deserving and equally endangered anonymous people.[30] We can cite countless examples of this rule.

Frequently, the media identify the person. If television follows the plight of a small girl trapped in a deep well, thousands will send dollars for her rescue; meanwhile television doesn't cover the plight of another young boy in peril, he is not rescued, and he dies. Is this just?

In 1982, hospital administrator Charles Fiske interrupted a televised news conference to successfully plead for a liver donation for his daughter, Jamie. For over 25 years since, desperate parents have used such methods to save their children in organ failure. Belding Scribner illustrated it in rescuing Ernie Crowfeather.

From the perspective of distributive justice, why is the rule of rescue problematic? Why is it an unjust way to distribute organs?

First, television often identifies the rescued person, but who gets to live shouldn't be decided by who gets on television. Television favors people who look good on television, which means attractive, articulate people and families who know how to work reporters. But who gets to live shouldn't be decided by who is most photogenic.

The rule of rescue makes journalists and their editors the gatekeepers of life and death. The rule of rescue replaces the God Committee with the assignment editor ("Oh, we just did a child transplant story. Let's wait a month before we do another.").

And for every identifiable person who is saved, there are a dozen anonymous patients who are lost. If one life is worth the same as another, why is identification by a newspaper important?

When a physician admits a hypothetical Karen Smith to a hospital, Karen becomes identified and a candidate for rescue. Once inside, the medical team bonds to the smart, gregarious Karen. Once inside, physicians bestow a million dollars worth of publicly funded resources on her. Again, if there are many worthy candidates for a scarce medical resource, who gets to live shouldn't be decided by the likes of hospital staff or the whims of physicians in admitting patients.

Hospitals frequently set up rules and committees to prevent just this sort of thing. Left-ventricle assist devices (LVADs) can be bridges to heart transplants, but if hearts don't materialize, how long can a hospital keep patients on LVADs, especially if the patients have no coverage? The physician who initially admits his patient for an LVAD may feel like he's saved a life and is a hero, but he may be a villain to the hospital's administration, which must pay for the resulting care.

The rule of rescue is really a particular instance of the general conflict between impartial ethical theories and partial ones. On one side, we have Kantian ethics and utilitarianism, which treat everyone the same and which oppose the rule of rescue. On the other side, we have the Ethics of Care that values particular relationships. Our moral intuitions stem from both kinds of theories, which explains why they pull us in different directions.

It is precisely the pull of partialist theories that attracts us to rescuing the patient before us in the hospital bed. It is precisely that pull that impartial theories urge us to resist in seeking a more impartial way of deciding who gets into the hospital bed in the first place. Partial theories implicitly discount the value of unidentified people not in the circle of concern of the medical team.

Sickest First, UNOS, and the Rule of Rescue

As we have seen, utilitarianism clashes with the ethics of care over retransplants and the same clash looms larger in how UNOS allocates organs.

A utilitarian wanting to maximize human life in the lifeboat for the long row to Africa selects the strongest rowers, tosses the weak, sick, and elderly overboard, and eats the dog. Similarly, utilitarians wanting maximal years per organ allocate organs only to first-timers and allow no retransplants. For impartial ethical theories such as utilitarianism or Kantian ethics, one human life counts as much as another, regardless of whether that life is my father, my neighbor, my patient, my fellow citizen, or a complete stranger.

Piggybacking this logic on some facts leads to a surprising conclusion: giving organs to the sickest patients does not maximize the most years per life per organ.

Why? Because some patients are too near death. When they die, the organ has been wasted.

Therefore, the best way to get the most organs per life is to give the organ to moderately sick people just experiencing organ failure. In that way, with a limited supply, more people live longer.

Congress, many surgeons, and the families of many patients reject such an impartial system. As their loved one grows closer to death, they grasp for life. Even if it wastes an organ, they feel that after waiting for years on the list for an organ, they deserve their one chance to live.

So strong is this feeling that in the fall of 2000, Congress *mandated* that the UNOS allocate organs on the basis of *sickest first*. As the fact sheet on the UNOS website states: "For heart, liver and intestinal organs, patients whose medical status is most urgent receive priority over those whose medical status is not as urgent."[31]

Howard Eisen, head of Temple University Hospital's heart transplant program, disapproves. "What you're doing is giving hearts to people who will do less well with them. People are waiting longer, so they get sicker, and end up getting two operations when they would otherwise need one."[32]

Sickest first equates the rule of rescue to a standard of distributive justice. Is this fair to the others down the line who took better care of their bodies and therefore are not now as sick?

Living Donors

For many decades, an ethical bright line existed in transplant surgery of, "First, do no harm," which in part meant "Do not harm one person to benefit another." In 1954, Dr. Joseph Murray successfully transplanted a kidney from Ronald Herrick, a 23-year-old man, into his identical twin Richard, who was dying of kidney disease. Since the transplantation involved identical twins, immunological rejection posed no problem, and Richard accepted the transplanted kidney. Since no compatibility barriers existed, and since a brother's life was saved, the benefits of this surgery appeared to outweigh possible harms to the donor, and consequently ethical concerns were overridden. This precedent demonstrated the viability of live organ transplantation and paved the way for alternatives to cadaveric transplantation.[33]

As noted, half a century later a remarkable change occurred: in 2003, *the number of live donors has surpassed the number of cadaver donors* (brain-dead patients whose relatives consented to harvesting their organs).[34] In 50 years, transplant surgery had leapt from making one exception—an exception from a traditional rule in order to save a life—to a norm where the majority of organs today come from letting people volunteer to have surgeons risk harm to them to benefit another.

In 1989, the first transplant occurred from a healthy parent (a mother) to a daughter—from Teri Smith to Alyssa Smith. While he was removing the lobe of Teri's liver, surgeon Christopher Broelsch of the University of Chicago nicked Teri's spleen and had to excise it. Broelsch called the loss of Teri's spleen a "major complication," saying it gave him "the sickest feeling to have trouble with the first patient."[35]

Also in 1989, Marissa Ayala was conceived to provide stem cells for her sister Anissa, who had leukemia.[36] Preimplantation genetic diagnosis (PGD), the practice of analyzing artificially fertilized embryos, allowed Anissa's parents to choose an embryo that could serve as a compatible bone marrow donor for Anissa. Should Marissa have been conceived as a resource for Anissa, what is now called *a savior sibling*? Jodi Picoult's novel *My Sister's Keeper* brought to life the tensions in this scenario. Marissa's bone marrow was taken and given to Anissa, which saved Anissa's life, but does one happy result justify creating a thousand more children to serve as resources for dying siblings?

In 1993, transplant centers accepted and recruited adult relatives of children for organ transplants, and Nilda Rodríguez gave one-quarter of her liver to her sick granddaughter. In the same year, James and Barbara Sewell each donated part of a lung to their 22-year-old daughter, whose own lungs had been damaged by cystic fibrosis, a genetic disease that is typically fatal by age 30 (the patient usually dies from infection and collapse of the lungs). By 1997, as the practice became more accepted, California surgeon Vaughn Starnes had taken lobes from 76 donors for 37 recipients. One commentator in the same year noted that the practice was "ethically problematic," implying that a norm had not yet been established.

From 1990 to 2002, surgeons in St. Louis performed 207 lung transplants on 190 children.[37] All 190 children were under age 18; 121 were ages 10–18; and the most common reason for transplantation was cystic fibrosis. This means that surgeons took lung lobes from 207 healthy adults for these children. Italian surgeons reported similar results for 1996 to 2002, giving 55 people of mean age 25 years a lung transplant.[38]

Something similar happened with liver transplantation among relatives. From a few isolated cases in 1993–1994, such requests eventually became the norm: "There now exists an ethical imperative to develop this [live-donor donation of livers]," said Jean Edmond, M.D., director of liver transplantation at New York Presbyterian Hospital in 1999.[39] Between 1996 and 1999, surgeons performed over 70 transplants among adult relatives, with 45 in the first half of 1999, showing exponential growth.

In 1999, officials confirmed the first death from adult-to-adult liver donation and they estimated that two to three other adults had died from donating parts of organs to their children.[40] By 2003, at least five people had died.[41] Exact figures are unknown.

The surgical journal *Transplantation* reported in late 2002 that 56 people who had previously been living organ donors later required a kidney transplant.[42] Of the 56 people, only 43 received transplants, and of these, 36 worked. Of these 56 candidates, two died while waiting for an organ and one died after the operation.

Consider the sad case of Walter Wood, 45, who donated to his brother under the impression that kidney transplants were relatively safe and done only to save a life. Wood experienced an unexpected outcome during surgery: his abdominal muscles ruptured. He has since been in constant pain and unable to perform the simplest of tasks. As a result of his severe disability, Walter lost his job, had to sell his house, and approached bankruptcy, "I'm in constant pain from the surgeries I've had. I can't even move around in bed," Wood says.

Protecting patients such as Walter Wood is a problem in the system because the transplant team understandably focuses on the sick recipient of the organ, not the donor. Not only that, transplants occur only on people who have medical coverage, so the transplant team and its hospital gets paid for medical services to the recipient. In contrast, it receives nothing for caring for donors and gives such care at a financial loss. In sum, transplant teams have asymmetrical relationships to donors and to recipients.

After he donated part of his liver to his brother in 2002, newspaper reporter Mike Hurewitz of Albany, New York, died a gruesome death at Mount Sinai Hospital in New York City. Also, 69-year-old Barbara Tarrant from North Carolina disastrously donated a kidney to her mentally retarded son and wound up paralyzed on her left side and without coherent speech.[43]

Widely regarded as heroic in the popular media, living donor transplantation carries real dangers. Surprisingly, no one knows how many donors have ended up like Walter Wood, Mike Hurewitz, or Barbara Tarrant. Why? Because living-donor transplant centers have no obligation to report deaths or injuries to the UNOS, nor does UNOS have any legal obligation to monitor such deaths and injuries.

Amazingly, until recently, no hospital, transplant center, or medical department tracked deaths and injuries from live donors such as Walter Wood. Once donors leave the hospital, they are on their own—for medical care, for insurance, for follow-up—and no one has done a long-term study on their problems.

Given the lack of such studies, an obvious question arose: How could donors give *informed* consent about the risks of donation? After nearly a decade of uncertainty, a 2009 study at the University of Minnesota that mainly tracked white, middle-class donors found only slightly more problems with donors than nondonors, although nonwhite donors seemed to fare worse.[44]

Costs and the Medical Commons

The cost of a liver transplant for a child is on average about $146,000 for the operation and $6,000 a year thereafter; a kidney transplant costs $60,000 for the first year and $6,000 a year thereafter; dialysis costs $32,000 a year; an average heart transplant costs $91,000 the first year and $6,000 a year thereafter; a bone-marrow transplant costs $100,000. Figures like these give many people pause.

During the 1970s, the biologist Garrett Hardin discussed the *tragedy of the commons*, a situation in which no one reduces his or her consumption of some public resource until the resource becomes so ravaged that it disappears. The concept originated centuries ago in England, when pastures held in common were overgrazed: in each town, each shepherd increased his own flock until there were so many animals that the common could no longer support them. Point: unregulated pursuit of self-interest leads to destruction of public resources.

Former Colorado governor Richard Lamm agrees. He has emphasized that Americans cannot continue such extravagant policies and do well. In particular, as a matter of intergenerational justice, America cannot fund extravagant care for the elderly on the backs of the working young: "When a society faces fiscal reality and seeks to optimize its dollars, it not only starts on the road to financial sanity, but it also brings dramatic change to existing medical practices. Dialysis and transplantation will undoubtedly undergo major change."[45]

Lamm continues, "Dr. Thomas Starzl recently gave a liver transplant to a 76-year-old woman. It cost $240,000. Dr. Starzl should understand that with the average U.S. family making $24,000 a year, he has sentenced ten U.S. families to work all year so that he could transplant a 76-year-old woman."

This topic will be explored much more in the last chapter of this book, where questions of fairness are raised about the 40 million working Americans without medical insurance and their subsidies of those who have insurance. Most of these Americans work and have FICA and Medicare taxes taken from their paychecks—Medicare taxes that pay for dialysis and kidney transplants. Ironically, the only medical care they are entitled to is to be stabilized in emergency rooms and to all treatments, should their kidneys fail.

Non-Heart-Beating Organ Transplantation

The issue of exactly how a patient, whose body is a potential source of organs, gets declared dead, has simmered in the background of organ transplantation for nearly half a century. Between 1954 and 1967, organs for transplantation either came from living, related donors (e.g., a kidney from one twin to another) or by patients who were dead (cadavers). Physicians declared patients dead by cardiopulmonary criteria, that is, the hearts of patients stopped beating and the patients stopped breathing. These criteria were not ideal because when tissue no longer receives blood, damage occurs very fast, and such damage often occurs while the heart is stopping.

With the Harvard definition of brain death in 1967, declaration of death in cadavers switched to neocortical criteria, allowing retrieval of organs from cadavers who had their breathing and circulation maintained artificially by ventilators. Because obtaining organs from patients declared dead this way did not injure organs, and because all states passed neocortical brain-death laws, procurement of organs for transplantation switched almost entirely to use of the neocortical standard. After that, surgeons obtained organs in better shape for the receiving patient.

In recent years, improvements in automobile safety have reduced the pool of such bodies while burgeoning numbers of transplant programs have learned to transplant sicker people. Supply has dropped while demand has soared.

The University of Pittsburgh Medical Center in 1993 developed a protocol to start obtaining organs from patients who were declared dead by the old cardiopulmonary criteria. Their novel idea was to manage death in the small class of patients where the underlying illness causing death has not damaged the organ and where the patient or the family has signed a "do not resuscitate" order.

In this protocol, a patient on a respirator is moved to the operating room where his respirator is removed, breathing stops, the surgical team waits a few minutes for breathing to resume, the patient is declared dead, and then his organs are removed.

The official name of this protocol is the non-heart-beating (cadaver) donors (NHBD). This phrase is not felicitous, for it seems to be an oxymoron (can a cadaver be a "donor"?).

The NHBD protocol declares death after two minutes during which no pulse is detected and ventricular fibrillation, asystole, or electromechanical dissociation occurs. It allows drugs to be administered, such as vasodilators and anticoagulants, that are given solely to maximize health of organs to be transplanted. It declares that death occurs when there is irreversible loss of *cardiac function*, as opposed to the neocortical standard, which declares that death occurs when there is irreversible loss of *all brain activity*, including brain stem activity.

A 1997 study requested of the Institute of Medicine (IOM) by the Secretary of Health and Human Services distinguished between *controlled* and *uncontrolled* NHBDs. Before the Harvard, neocortical definition of death was adopted, patients died in "uncontrolled" ways as their hearts stopped beating and injured their other organs. In the Pittsburgh protocol, the IOM said, "the (deaths of) donors are controlled because the timing and thus the process of donation are controlled through the timing of (withdrawal of) life support." These patients generally suffer from severe head injuries or progressive neurological illness.

One aspect of the new protocol that some people have trouble accepting is that the judgment of irreversibility differs from the judgment about lack of neocortical activity. The only way to know if such changes truly are irreversible is to start cardiopulmonary resuscitation (CPR), but in the Pittsburgh protocol, of course, the family and/or competent patient must explicitly decline CPR.

This point must be stressed. Consent of the patient distinguishes physician-assisted dying from murder. If the family has not consented to the Pittsburgh protocol, staff might be charged with accelerating death to harvest organs.

Another point to stress here is that CPR on a dying or elderly patient is a brutal way to die and often involves breaking chest bones. It is a peculiar form of torture practiced today. Fewer than 15 percent of hospital patients who receive CPR ever leave the hospital.[46] If a family understands these facts, it might elect to forgo CPR and allow the Pittsburgh protocol.

Hence the essential idea of the NHBDC protocol: Because the family, the patient, and the physicians believe the patient is going to die soon, why not manage the death to create life for others? For the family, something good may come out of the death, the gift of life to another person.

A 1993 conference explored the ethical issues of the Pittsburgh protocol but did not achieve a consensus. Although all agreed that the dead-donor rule should continue—that is, that organs should be taken only from dead patients—they could not agree on whether families should be allowed to consent to organ procurement under the new protocol. "The Pittsburgh protocol gives an interpretation of irreversible that comes down to a low probability of auto-resuscitation and excludes the possibility of interventions that could restart the heart."

But what about the ethical issue where families consented but did not understand the issues? Critics object on Kantian grounds that the patient is not being treated as "an end in himself." Alan Weisbard argued that the Pittsburgh protocol indirectly brings about the death of some people to benefit others." Medical sociologist Renée Fox thought it "morally offensive" to ask families, nurses, and residents to be involved in this effort, and criticizes the "macabre" public policy of championing maximal organ transplantation.[47]

In April 1997, the controversy made national news in the worst way when a bioethics professor in Cleveland went to a district attorney, charging that transplant surgeons at the famous Cleveland Clinic were about to violate the law. The headline of the *Cleveland Plain Dealer* was "Murder, She Said" and a few days later, *60 Minutes* interviewed Mary Ellen Waithe and broke the story nationally. Other bioethicists criticized Waithe's elevation of a dispute in public policy to charges of illegal activities with overtones of criminal mischief.

The *60 Minutes* story on the Cleveland Clinic revealed that the University of Wisconsin Medical Center had been using a NHBD controlled-death protocol to harvest organs for over 20 years. During this show, a point of contention was whether the administration of heparin and regitine accelerated the death of donors. Heparin, a blood thinner, prevents clot formation, and regitine dilates blood vessels, keeping organs perfused with blood.

Surgeons at centers using NHBD hotly deny the claim that administration of heparin and regitine hastens death. The Institute of Medicine study vindicated such surgeons, noting the NHBD protocols across the country divided evenly between allowing the use at some stage in the donation process of one or both of these agents and expressly prohibiting or not mentioning them.

In most cases, the IOM report allows careful administration of these drugs. Nevertheless, because under certain circumstances in certain patients, there is a concern that these agents might be harmful, this report recommends case-by-case decisions on the use of anticoagulants and vasodilators and consideration of additional safeguards such as involvement of the patients' attending physician in prescribing decisions. The IOM also recommended waiting five minutes, rather than two, after life-support was removed, before declaring death.[48]

The God Committee, Again

It's easy to criticize. Critics of the God Committee probably couldn't do a better job. Problem drinkers like Ernie Crowfeather, immature people, and people with poor personal hygiene fare poorly on dialysis, and dialysis nurses often hate them.

Life on dialysis is not great. It has a high symptom burden, meaning that quality of life is low. As one nephrologist reports about daily life on dialysis,

> Insomnia is extraordinarily common and many [patients] experience severe muscle cramping and pains of different sorts. Itching is an equally common phenomenon, along with nausea, vomiting, and poor spirits. Our data indicates that among the roughly 300,000 patients undergoing dialysis in any given year, about 65,000 (or 23%) will die.[49]

Maybe the God Committee correctly considered which people had the strength to endure these procedures. Today, when everyone gets dialysis, many patients indirectly commit suicide by failing to comply with regimens or by missing appointments. The life expectancy for dialysis patients falls between one-eighth and one-third of the rest of the population, in part because too many patients who are old and sick get dialyzed.[50]

In 2006, a new form of home dialysis became available called *Rogosin dialysis* or *nocturnal dialysis*.[51] It requires a $13,000 dialysis machine at home and a $5,000 water purifier, but it can be done at home, six nights a week for eight hours each night. Complying with nocturnal dialysis means not needing to go to dialysis clinics three times a week for out-patient dialysis under nursing supervision.

Like out-patient dialysis, nocturnal dialysis requires cleanliness and personal hygiene. Pet hair may clog the machine, so people with pets are ineligible for the program. At present, patients with poor hygiene, or those who cannot part with pets, cannot use Rogosin dialysis. So history, and its ethical issues, repeats itself once again.

FURTHER READING AND RESOURCES

Renée Fox and Judith Swazey, *The Courage to Fail: A Social View of Organ Transplants and Dialysis*, 2nd ed. rev., Chicago, University of Chicago Press, 1974, 1978.

Institute of Medicine, *Non-Heart-Beating Organ Transplantation-Medical and Ethical Issues in Procurement*, Washington, D.C., National Academy Press, 1997.

René Fox and Judith Swazey, *Spare Parts: Organ Replacement in American Society*, New York, Oxford University Press, 1992.

Thomas Starzl, *The Puzzle People: Memoirs of a Transplant Surgeon*, Pittsburgh, University of Pittsburgh Press, 1992.

DISCUSSION QUESTIONS

1. In getting a transplanted organ that saves your life, which of the following should a just system of allocation consider: Whether the patent smoked; whether the patient drank alcohol extensively; whether the patient has medical insurance; whether the patient is rich and gets herself listed in several medical centers; whether the patient has already received one organ transplant.
2. Isn't it human nature to rescue the sickest first? To stave off death from someone you know? Do we want surgeons to be bureaucratic robots or to have a heart? What's wrong with the rule of rescue and caring for patients who are known?
3. Even if people have a small amount of free will, shouldn't the system act as if they had lots of it? By rewarding good behavior and punishing bad behavior, doesn't the system itself become a major causal factor in how people behave? On the other hand, if it rescues unhealthy behavior, doesn't the system undermine healthy behavior and reward unhealthy habits?
4. Who is going to pay for organ transplants if more and more people keep getting them? When 40 million Americans lack basic coverage, isn't this luxurious medicine for the well-off?
5. If you are a physician or a nurse and a patient doesn't want to cooperate—if he keeps smoking, eating five sausage sandwiches for breakfast each day, and drinking a bottle of wine with dinner each night—and his health gets worse and worse, are you justified in being angry with him? Or does getting mad at him just cause him to avoid coming back to see you? Is moralism a tool

for changing behavior or is it a primitive venting of feelings by the health provider?

6. Do families of the NHBD protocol understand what's going on? Do they believe that not every possible effort will be made to keep their son alive and that his death is being managed so that his organs can be transplanted in the best shape? Even if they don't understand all this, is that bad? If the patient is going to die anyway, isn't this a way of getting something good out of the process?

CHAPTER 12

Using One Baby for Another

Babies Fae, Gabriel, and Theresa, and Conjoined Twins

This chapter discusses the 1984 case of Baby Fae, who briefly lived with a baboon's heart; the 1987 case of Baby Gabriel, an anencephalic baby whose heart went to another infant, Paul Holc; the 1992 case of the anencephalic Baby Theresa, whose parents wanted to donate her heart to another baby; and a series of cases about separating conjoined twins. This chapter's key question concerns whether dying babies should be used in experimental medicine, even to help another dying baby.

EXPERIMENTAL MEDICINE AND BABIES

Baby Fae, 1984

Doctors delivered Baby Fae in Barstow, California, on October 14, 1984. Three weeks premature, she weighed five pounds. Noticing her pallor, the pediatrician transferred her to the more advanced Loma Linda Hospital, a Seventh-Day Adventist facility near Riverside, California, about 60 miles from Los Angeles. Physicians there diagnosed her with hypoplastic left heart syndrome (HLHS).

Affecting one in 10,000 babies, HLHS leaves the normally powerful left side of the heart and aorta underdeveloped and too weak to pump blood. HLHS almost always kills infants within two weeks.

Fae's mother, a 23-year-old, unmarried, unemployed Roman Catholic and her father, a 35-year-old laborer, had no medical insurance. The two had a son and had lived together for five years, but at Fae's birth, they separated.

At Loma Linda, doctors told the mother that Fae would soon die; they kept her overnight in the hospital and then released her. The mother had Fae baptized and took her to a motel to wait for death.

Surgeons call transplantation of an organ from one species to another a *xenograft*. In 1964, James Hardy implanted a chimpanzee heart into a 68-year-old man, who lived 90 minutes.[1] In 1977, Christiaan Barnard piggybacked a baboon heart next to the heart of a 25-year-old Italian woman, who lived 300 minutes; he later used the same technique to implant a chimpanzee heart in a 59-year-old man who lived four days. During the 1960s, Thomas Starzl and Keith Reemtsma performed six transplants each with simian kidneys and eventually abandoned the projects.[2] Baboon kidneys worked at best only two months. In 1975, a British cardiologist connected veins and arteries of a dying one-year-old boy to a live baboon, neither of whom lived through the operation.

Leonard Bailey, the 41-year-old chief of pediatric surgery at Loma Linda, had been aggressively pursuing heart xenotransplants for seven years. According to physician and critic Kenneth Stoller, during this period Bailey had performed about 160 xenotransplants, "mostly on sheep and goats, none of whom survived more than six months."[3] During the previous year, Loma Linda's Institutional Review Board (IRB) had been considering xenografts by Bailey, and it had recently granted him permission for five operations.

When Baby Fae's mother first came to the hospital and doctors discussed options with her, Bailey was away at a convention. When he returned on October 16, he called her to discuss a xenograft.

On October 19, he readmitted Baby Fae to Loma Linda and placed her on a respirator, and for several hours, discussed the operation with Fae's mother, father, and grandmother. They all also watched a slide show about the operation. Both parents then signed a consent form, which had been reviewed in great detail by the IRB; they later signed a second form.

Bailey's immunologist, Sandra Nehlsen-Cannarella, began antigen-typing tests to find the best match for Fae among potential baboon donors. These tests took six days. Using Fae's reaction to her own blood and tissue as a control, Nehlsen-Cannarella tested various beings for compatibility: Baby Fae's mother (finding a weak immune reaction), some lab workers (strong reaction), herself (strong reaction), three baboons (strong reaction), and three additional baboons (weak reaction). A baboon named Goobers, a nine-month-old female from the Foundation for Biomedical Research in Texas, had a "very, very weak" reaction, so she became the source of the xenograft.[4]

The fact that a baboon heart might be used at all indicates a common ancestor of humans and primates. Human blood strongly resembles primate blood, thus we might expect to find some close matches of blood types between humans and primates. Moreover, one-third of humans have a preformed antibody against tissue from other humans. About 70 percent of humans also have a preformed antibody against baboon tissue; Baby Fae was among the 30 percent who did not. Bailey gave this fact considerable weight, arguing that previous ignorance about human-baboon matching explained Hardy's earlier failures with xenografts.

Yet chimpanzees are closer to humans in evolution, so Bailey was once asked on a radio show why he had picked a baboon rather than a chimpanzee. He replied, "Er, I find that difficult to answer. You see, I don't believe in evolution."[5]

On October 26, the tissue-typing tests arrived, and Bailey said Baby Fae's heart was dying and her lungs were swelling with fluid. Whether Fae was dying at this precise point is important: According to the hospital's spokesperson, a baboon heart was used because there was no time to find a compatible human heart, so the transplant had to take place immediately.

Bailey placed Fae on a heart-lung machine that lowered her blood temperature to 68 degrees. Meanwhile, he sedated Goobers and excised her walnut-sized heart. He then removed Fae's defective heart and replaced it with Goobers's healthy one.

Over the next four hours, he connected the transplanted heart and arteries. Then the heart-lung machine raised Fae's temperature to 98 degrees, and Goobers's heart began to beat spontaneously inside Fae.

On October 29, nurses weaned Fae from her respirator. On November 5, Bailey predicted that the animal heart would grow with Fae, and that she might celebrate her 20th birthday.

Two other surgeons who had grabbed fame chimed in. Christiaan Barnard predicted that soon medicine would have baboon farms for simian xenografts. William DeVries, said, "I really have sympathy for what [Bailey and his colleagues] are going through."[6]

Two weeks after surgery, Fae showed the first signs of rejection of the donor heart. Soon she deteriorated and went back on a respirator.

On November 15, Fae developed heart blockage and renal failure; Bailey started closed-heart massage and dialysis. She then died, having lived 21 days with her baboon heart.

Bailey attempted no more xenografts, but other surgeons did. In 1992, Thomas Starzl at the University of Pittsburgh transplanted a baboon liver into a 35-year-old man with hepatitis B. He lived 70 days. The same year, a woman waiting for a human liver at Cedars Sinai Medical Center in Los Angeles received a pig liver as a bridge to a transplant, but she died 32 hours later. In 1993, a man with hepatitis B received a baboon liver at the University of Pittsburgh; he was 62 years old and he died during the operation. Since 1963, surgeons transplanted organs of baboons to humans in 33 operations, but none have succeeded.

Surgeons hope that transferring human genes into pigs will allow porcine xenografts, but none have worked to date. Even when drugs suppress immunorejection, a more lethal *hyperacute rejection* soon occurs in all xenografts.

ETHICAL ISSUES

Animal Donors and Animal Rights

Animal activists criticized Bailey: "This is medical sensationalism at the expense of Baby Fae, her family, and the baboon," said People for the Ethical Treatment of Animals (PETA).[7] Activists protested outside Loma Linda Hospital, claiming that Fae's life was not worth more than Goobers's. Philosopher Tom Regan claimed the operation had "two victims," Fae and Goobers.

Regan argued that beings who "have a life" have a *right* to life. He held that Goobers had a biographical life in that it mattered to her whether she would live or have her heart cut out: "Like us, Goobers was somebody, a distinct individual." Regan argued that all primates have equal moral value, so Goobers did not exist as Fae's resource:

> Those people who seized [Goobers's] heart, even if they were motivated by their concern for Baby Fae, grievously violated Goobers's right to be treated with respect. That she could do nothing to protest, and that many of us failed

to recognize the transplant for the injustice that it was, does not diminish the wrong, a wrong settled before Baby Fae's sad death.[8]

Regan argued that even if human beings had obtained benefits in the past from using animals, it was wrong to continue using primates this way as resources.

Other animal-rights philosophers emphasized that Baby Fae and Goobers, considering their youth and individual potential, differed more than Baby Fae and an anencephalic baby.[9] Anencephalic babies lack potential cognitive ability, whereas Goobers has more cognition, agency, and consciousness than such a dying human baby.

Some philosophers contemplated the large breeding facility from which Goobers had been bought and offered the image of a similar facility supplying anencephalic babies as sources of organs. If this image shocks, they asked, why do we tolerate such a facility for primates, especially when such primates resemble us more than severely retarded humans? Are we just in denial?

So why not use an anencephalic newborn as a donor? As we shall see, this logic prevailed in the later cases of Baby Gabriel and Baby Theresa.

Bailey retorted that, "People in southern California have it so good that they can afford to worry about this type of issue."[10] Moreover, he claimed, "When it gets down to a human living or dying, there shouldn't be a question" of using an animal to save that human.

The director of Loma Linda's Center for Christian Bioethics agreed:

On an ethical scale, we will always place human beings ahead of subhumans, especially in a situation where people can be genuinely saved by animals. That is the story of mankind from the very beginning. Animals, for example, have always been used for food and clothing.[11]

Of animal-rights activists, Fae's mother said, "They don't know what they're talking about."[12]

Alternative Treatment?

Was alternative treatment possible? One alternative to a xenograft for Fae was a human donor heart. Loma Linda claimed that the xenograft was necessary because Baby Fae was dying and no human heart was available. Bailey argued that it would be impossible to find a heart because the donor would have to be less than seven weeks old, and criteria for neonatal brain death were problematical ("You can have a flat EEG on a newborn, and yet the baby will survive.")[13]

Most neonatal transplants come from anencephalic babies; and Bailey maintained that most parents of such infants would refuse to accept the fact that their baby was brain-dead, and would not agree to donate the baby's organs in time. He described the baboon heart as Baby Fae's "only chance to live."

An associate surgeon at Loma Linda defended Bailey:

It would have to be the sort of case where an infant fell out of a crib and was declared brain dead but the heart was okay. Then all these tests would have to be done to insure a proper matching. With Baby Fae, we had five days to do those tests, getting the best possible [animal] donor. With a human heart, we might not have been able to keep the recipient alive.[14]

In his memoirs, surgeon Thomas Starzl describes Paul Teraski as a "symbol of integrity" in the transplant community.[15] Teraski, director of the Southern California Regional Organ Procurement Agency, said that an infant heart had been available *on the day* of Baby Fae's xenograft. Teraski added, "I think that they [the Loma Linda team] did not make any effort to get a human infant heart because they were set on doing a baboon."[16]

Bailey agreed that he didn't look for a human heart:

> We were not searching for a human heart. We were out to enter the whole new area of transplanting tissue-matched baboon hearts into newborns who are supported with antisuppressive drugs. I suppose that we could have used a human heart that was outsized and that was not tissue-matched, and that would have pacified some people, but it would have been very poor science. On the other hand, I suppose my belief that there are no newborn hearts available for transplantation was more opinion than data or science, but it is scientific to acknowledge that the whole area of determining brain death of newborns is very problematical.[17]

Another alternative existed. Pediatric surgeon William Norwood had developed surgery for HLHS that attempted to repair the left ventricle. He had performed his operation many times at Children's Hospitals in Philadelphia, with a success rate of 40 percent. Bailey claimed that children did not do well enough after the Norwood procedure to justify this operation for Baby Fae. But given Bailey's interest in xenografts, was he an impartial judge?

Babies as Subjects of Research

Critics objected to Bailey's surgery not because of risk or experimentation—after all, surgery can discover what is possible only by trying—but because Bailey used a baby, who could not consent. In the decades since the earlier attempts at xenografts, the only new developments had been the discovery of cyclosporin and better matching of tissue, but both could have been used in a consulting adult.

In addition to questions about whether using Fae made sense medically, a more general question is whether parents should volunteer children for experiments. Protestant theologian Paul Ramsey argued that it is always wrong for parents to volunteer their children for *nontherapeutic* research:

> If today we mean to give such weight to the research imperative, then we should not seek to give a principled justification of what we are doing with children. It is better to leave the research imperative in incorrigible conflict with the principle that protects the individual human person from being used for research purposes without either his expressed or correctly construed consent. Some sorts of human experimentation should, in this alternative, be acknowledged to be "borderline situations" in which moral agents are under the necessity of doing wrong for the sake of the public good. Either way they do wrong. It is immoral not to do the research. It is also immoral to use children who cannot themselves consent and who ought not to be presumed to consent to research unrelated to their treatment. On this supposition research medicine, like politics, is a realm in which men have to "sin bravely."[18]

Catholic theologian Richard McCormick demurred, holding that parents can volunteer children for "low-risk" nontherapeutic research.[19] Based on the Roman Catholic tradition of natural law, he argued that just as adults should volunteer for low-risk, nontherapeutic research, infants should be volunteered for the same kind of research.

Neither Ramsey nor McCormick used the utilitarian justification of the greatest good for the greatest number. To many people, though, utilitarianism offers the most natural justification. If no one volunteered for such research, progress would halt, so for the general good, both adults and babies should participate. Because HLHS is a congenital defect of babies, how can treatment for it advance unless some HLHS babies participate?

Informed Consent

Many people wondered whether Bailey had carefully described the Norwood procedure to Fae's mother. Was she informed that a human donor was available? Fae's mother had no medical insurance. Bailey offered her the xenograft for free. Fae's mother had no money for the Norwood procedure or for a human heart transplant. Costs for such a transplant can be a quarter million, with immunosuppressive drugs costing $20,000 a year for life.

Bioethicist and University of Southern California law professor Alexander Capron summed up this criticism:

> Doubts linger, not only about the adequacy of the information supplied to Baby Fae's parents but about whether their personal difficulties made it possible for them to choose freely, and whether the realization that their child was dying may have left them with the erroneous conclusion that consenting to the transplant was the only "right" thing to do.[20]

In most respects, the mother's poverty and lack of insurance rendered her consent meaningless. Faced with the death of her baby and no other realistic options, what else could she choose?

And was the mother informed about the probable outcome of the xenograft? Did Baby Fae's mother understand that Bailey's xenograft was a shot in the dark, unlikely to work, and a procedure that might merely extend her baby's dying?

Historically, lack of informed consent was always a problem with xenografts. Boston University law professor George Annas emphasized that in previous attempts to implant animal hearts in humans, patients were poor, vulnerable, and rarely consented.

In 1963, Keith Reemtsma at Columbia University implanted chimpanzee kidneys in a 43-year-old African-American man who was dying of glomerulonephritis. In 1964, James Hardy at the University of Mississippi implanted a chimpanzee heart into a poor deaf-mute man who was dying, was taken to the hospital unconscious, never consented to the operation, and survived for only two hours. These operations were experimental, were not therapeutic, and were characterized by exploitation and lack of consent. Annas saw Baby Fae's case as a continuation of such practices. Calling Bailey the champion of the "anything goes" school of experimentation, he concluded:

> This inadequately reviewed, inappropriately consented to, premature experiment on an impoverished, terminally ill newborn was unjustified. It differs from the xenograft experiments of the early 1960s only in the fact that there was prior

review of the proposal by an IRB. But this distinction did not protect Baby Fae. She remained unprotected from ruthless experimentation in which her only role was that of victim.[21]

The Media

This case drew an enormous amount of attention from the media. True, Loma Linda tried to protect the family's privacy and confidentiality, but it and Bailey withheld more than identifying details. Their account of events leading up to the surgery was confusing; hospital spokespersons gave occasional misstatements of fact; and Loma Linda refused to release a copy of the consent form which Fae's parents had signed. Journalists complained about secrecy and the public's right to know.

This situation formed an interesting contrast to the case two years earlier of Barney Clark's artificial heart. Just as many reporters came to Loma Linda as to Utah, but they got much less information. William DeVries had held daily press briefings; Bailey held fewer. Reporters accused Loma Linda of ineptitude and said that aspects of the case begged for clarification.

While journalists accused Bailey and Loma Linda of reticence, they also accused them of publicity seeking, self-promotion, grandstanding, and adventurism.[22] In contrast, Keith Reemtsma at Columbia University gave no news conferences until his patient had been discharged from the hospital and until he had prepared and submitted a scientific paper. Reemtsma argued:

> Science and news are, in a sense, asymmetrical and sometimes antagonistic. News emphasizes uniqueness, the immediacy, the human interest, in a case such as [Baby Fae's]. Science emphasizes verification, controls, comparisons, and patterns.[23]

Law professor Alex Capron argued similarly:

> There was a time when the public learned of biomedical developments after they had been reviewed by, and generally reported to, the researchers' scientific and medical peers [a procedure that protected everyone's dignity and meant that the public would learn only of genuine advances] rather than merely being titillated by bizarre cases of as yet unproven import.[24]

As we shall see below, this criticism also applies to separation of conjoined twins, which has almost never been done as part of a scientific protocol where results are carefully studied over decades and which is commonly done with great attention by television.

Therapy or Research?

Was Fae's xenograft therapy or research? Was alternative treatment available? Did the xenograft have a chance to help Fae, or was she just one sacrifice among thousands on the altar of medical research?

A *therapeutic* procedure offers a patient a reasonable chance of benefit; a procedure which offers little chance is *research* and *experimental*. This medical distinction can be expressed in Kantian ethics as the difference between treating people as "ends in themselves" and using them as "mere means." Essayist Charles Krauthammer wrote:

> Civilization hangs on the Kantian principle that human beings are to be treated as ends and not means. So much depends on that principle because there is no crime that cannot be, that has not been, committed in the name of the future against those who inhabit the present. Medical experimentation, which invokes the claims of the future, necessarily turns people into means.[25]

Was Bailey's best scenario possible? Was there a probability that Fae could have lived to age 20 with a baboon heart? At one point, Bailey phrased his claim differently, saying that Fae had a chance to "celebrate more than one birthday with her new heart."[26] Was this modest scenario possible?

Bailey claimed his operation had *therapeutic intent*:

> I have always believed it would work, or I would not have attempted it. . . . There was always therapeutic intent. My dilemma has been educating the university and the medical profession.[27]

He made these comments nine days after the operation, when Baby Fae was still alive and seemed to be doing well. He also said that xenografts might soon be preferable to human transplants.

Immunologist Nehlsen-Cannarella argued that, if a perfect match had been found with the best-matched lymphocytes, the operation could have been therapeutic. With such a perfect match, Fae could have accepted the heart.

Other surgeons castigated Bailey, rejecting the idea of *therapeutic intent* and saying that Bailey needed *therapeutic probability*. Almost any experimental surgery has a remote chance of being therapeutic, but that's not enough.

These surgeons also rejected Bailey's and Nehlsen-Cannarella's claim about tissue typing. In 1970, Paul Teraski had discovered that while tissue typing can improve transplants within families, it couldn't outside of families. Surgeons resisted Teraski's findings, but accepted the limitations his results suggested. Thomas Starzl wrote in 1992:

> Twenty years later the only controversy is whether matching under all circumstances means enough to be given any consideration in the distribution of cadaver kidneys. By exposing the truth, Teraski had made it clear that the field of clinical transplantation could advance significantly only by the development of better drugs and other treatment strategies, not by vainly hoping that the solution would be through tissue matching.[28]

Most transplant surgeons agreed. The American expert on pediatric transplants, John Najarian at the University of Minnesota, said of the Baby Fae case: "There has never been a successful cross-species transplant. To try it now is merely to prolong the dying process."[29] He also said that Fae's death on November 15 was "reasonably close to what could be expected," because three weeks was about how long it usually takes for rejection to do its damage.

In a review of this case, the editor of *Journal of Heart Transplantation* concluded:

> From the experimental data and past clinical attempts, there is nothing to indicate that a human infant will tolerate a primate heart for months or years using today's means to induce and control tolerance. The Loma Linda surgical team has not informed the medical community, as yet, of any new evidence that might suggest the contrary.[30]

The case against Baby Fae's transplant as "therapy" may be summed up as follows:

First, it had been known since 1970 that better antigen matches between donor and recipient would not improve transplants.

Second, even the best matches required long-term maintenance on cyclosporin. Bailey claimed that infants can be given larger dosages of cyclosporin than adults, but cyclosporin eventually produces toxic side effects.[31] The autopsy on Baby Fae indicated that her kidneys were probably poisoned by the massive dosages of cyclosporin she received.

Third, Bailey argued that since an infant's immune system is not fully developed, babies might initially tolerate xenografts. But this is not certain; and even if it were true, an initial success would be followed by failure as the baby's immune system developed and rejected the xenograft.

Fourth, only one heart xenograft had been tried previously, and this had a disastrous result.

Fifth, Loma Linda was a small medical institution. In their zeal to perform a xenograft and be famous, the staff was blind to their own limitations.

Sixth, Bailey himself was an amateur: He had never performed a human heart transplant, and he had never published about xenografts.

Taking all this into account, Baby Fae had no chance of surviving one year, let alone reaching her 20th birthday. Thus the surgery was not therapeutic but experimental. *Nature* concluded that "the serious difficulty over [Bailey's] operation . . . is that it may have catered to the researchers' needs first and to the patient's only second."[32] In his essay in *Time*, Krauthammer said that Baby Fae had lived and died in the realm of experimentation:

> Only the bravery was missing: no one would admit the violation. Bravery was instead fatuously ascribed to Baby Fae, a creature as incapable of bravery as she was of circulating her own blood. Whether this case was an advance in medical science awaits the examination of the record by the scientific community. That it was an adventure in medical ethics is already clear.[33]

In a review of the case, the American Medical Association and top medical journals criticized Bailey, concluding that xenografts should be undertaken only as part of a systematic research program with controls in randomized clinical trials.[34]

Baby Gabriel and Paul Holc, 1987

Like the Terri Schiavo case two decades later, the Baby Fae case received saturation coverage in the media, making Bailey and Loma Linda household names. When his xenograft program failed, Bailey tried to use his new fame to create a center for heart failure on infants with HLHS with donated hearts from anencephalic babies.

In 1987, surgeons and medical ethicists at a conference in Ontario, Canada, who were sympathetic to Bailey's goal (Bailey had been a resident in cardiac surgery in Ontario in 1974), created guidelines for using anencephalics as organ donors, guidelines called the *Ontario Protocol*.

The most important of its guidelines stated that an anencephalic baby could become a donor only after being pronounced dead by the classical criteria of brain death. Another guideline was that the potential donor could not be expected to live more than one week; this standard was meant to ensure that the donor was born dying. At birth, an anencephalic was to be put on a respirator to preserve its organs, then taken off every six hours to see if it could breathe on its own. If a baby failed to breathe for three minutes, it could be declared brain dead by three physicians independent of the transplant team.

It should be noted that the respirator is necessary in this protocol because the normal course of anencephaly is for the heart to stop beating gradually: this diminishes blood flow, so the organs become anoxic and start to deteriorate; by the time the brain stem is dead, the heart and kidneys are no longer useful for transplantation.

Because maintaining the brain stem may prevent a potential donor from becoming brain dead, the Ontario Protocol was ill-conceived.

UCLA pediatric neurologist Allan Shewmon severely criticized the Ontario Protocol. The leading authority on anencephaly, Shewmon held that anencephalic babies should not be used as donors at all, because there was no consensus in neurology about determining brain death in them.[35]

The Ontario Protocol was not applied to a case until February 1988, though it had been in the news for some time before that.

In October 1987, a Canadian couple, Karen and Fred Schouten, learned after eight months of pregnancy that their fetus was anencephalic. They decided to bring it to term and to donate its organs. When her heart began to fail after birth, the baby, a girl named Gabriel, was ventilated. The United Network for Organ Sharing (UNOS) was alerted, but no potential recipients were found in Canada or the northeastern United States.

Meanwhile, at Loma Linda Hospital, Bailey was working with another couple, Alice and Gordon Holc, also Canadian, whose eight-month fetus had HLHS and needed a heart transplant and who had come to Loma Linda because of the publicity the Holcs were receiving. The Schoutens and Gabriel flew to Loma Linda. There, the Holcs's baby, Paul, was prematurely delivered by cesarean section to get the donor heart. Three hours later, Gabriel Schouten's heart was excised and transplanted into Paul Holc's chest.

This was the first time a transplant from an anencephalic baby to another infant resulted in a baby who could grow up and lead a normal life. In gratitude to the Schoutens and to Bailey, the Holcs named their baby Paul Gabriel Bailey Holc. Karen Schouten later said that she felt good about her decision and how it had benefited Paul Holc: "Paul is very special to me because he has a part of our baby inside him. One day maybe I'll see him. I hope he comes to me when he's 30 years old and says, 'Hi. Guess what? I made it.'"[36]

In 1994, NBC aired a TV movie about the case, which ended by showing the real Paul playing in first grade and hugging the real Karen Schouten. Paul Holc, aka "The Incredible Holc," turned 13 in 1998 and was healthy and doing well.

Perhaps waiting too long for a consensus, Bailey never applied the Ontario Protocol in the Schouten-Holc case. Its first application came at Loma Linda in 1988 with Michael and Brenda Winners and their anencephalic baby. That case had a sad result: No recipients were found.

This was the first of 12 unsuccessful attempts by Bailey to transplant organs from anencephalic babies to other babies.[37] Of these 12 potential donors, 10 lived beyond the one-week limit, one could not be matched to a recipient, and in the remaining case the physicians decided against a transplant. In 1988, Bailey suspended his transplant program. There was a de facto moratorium on transplants from anencephalics until the 1992 case of Baby Theresa raised the issue again.

Baby Theresa, 1992

In 1991 in Fort Lauderdale, Florida, Laura Campo and Justin Pearson—who were not married—conceived a child. Like Fae's mother, Laura had no medical insurance and did not see a physician until her twenty-fourth week of pregnancy. During her eighth month of pregnancy, she learned that her fetus was anencephalic.

Anencephaly is a congenital neurological disorder characterized by absence of the cerebrum and cerebellum, as well as the top of the skull, resulting in exposure of the brain stem.[38] However, anencephaly "does not mean the complete absence of the head or brain."[39] Because there is a brain stem, an electroencephalogram can be taken, and autonomic functions such as breathing and heartbeat may be present. Anencephalics do not meet the Harvard criteria of brain death.

Anencephaly is perhaps the most serious of all birth defects, because the baby essentially lacks the higher brain necessary for personhood. Anencephalics are born dying. There is no hope of growth into childhood or adulthood. The open skull is vulnerable to infection, and most anencephalics die within one week, though in rare cases some have lived for one year.[40]

Anencephalics are the major potential source of donor organs for other babies born with congenital defects. When the recipient is an infant, a donor organ must be very small, and so an infant donor is needed. However, few infants are involved in accidents that leave them brain dead but with healthy organs. Babies who die as a result of abuse or from sudden infant death syndrome usually have damaged organs that are unsuitable for transplantation.

Because the diagnosis of anencephaly was made so late in Laura Campo's pregnancy, and because Laura's health was not in danger from the fetus, no legal abortion could be performed. Like most mothers of anencephalic fetuses, Laura said that if she had known the diagnosis earlier, she would have aborted.

After hearing a talk show about organ donation from anencephalic babies, Laura decided to bring the fetus to term to serve as a source of organs.

Anencephaly occurs in one in 500 pregnancies. Over 95 percent identified prenatally are aborted. Of those carried to term, 60 percent are stillborn. Since an anencephalic is likely to have a swollen head (hydrocephalus), vaginal delivery may kill it, and Laura had a cesarean delivery to keep the organs healthy for transplantation.

In the United States, 2,000 babies a year need organ transplants; this number includes 600 babies with HLHS, about 500 with liver failure, and another 500 with kidney failure. About 300 anencephalic babies are born alive each year.

Since 1968, it has been technically possible to use anencephalics as organ sources. A few days after Christiaan Barnard's transplant, Adrian Kantrowitz transplanted a heart from an anencephalic baby to another infant, who died six hours later.[41] Kantrowitz had almost performed a transplant 18 months earlier, but he had to wait for the anencephalic donor's heart to stop beating, and then restart it, which proved impossible.

In 1992, Laura Campo had a baby girl named Theresa Ann Campo Pearson. Pictures of Theresa showed a beautiful baby wearing a pink knitted cap that covered the top half of her head. Removing the cap revealed the brain stem inside a partial skull.

Under Florida law, before Theresa's organs could be donated, she had to be brain dead. Like most states, Florida used the Harvard standard. Unless Baby Theresa was brain dead, no one would remove her organs.

The parents asked Judge Estella Moriarty to rule Theresa brain dead. But Judge Moriarty correctly ruled against the couple: "{I am}unable to authorize someone to take your baby's life, however short—however unsatisfactory—to save another child. Death is a fact, not an opinion."[42]

The couple appealed to Florida's District Court of Appeals, which affirmed Judge Moriarty's decision. The baby then began to experience organ failure. At this point, the neonatologists said, "We had to tell the parents [that] all they were doing was prolonging the baby's death."[43] They removed the respirator and Theresa died the next day. By then, surgeons couldn't use her organs.

The next day, the parents appeared on television to plead for a change in Florida's laws regarding brain death. Laura Campo was upset and depressed and shouldn't have been allowed to be on the show. A calm, eloquent surgeon joined them and discussed the need for donor organs.

Even though Baby Theresa died, Florida Supreme Court decided *not* to change the law and that anencephalic newborns should *not be* considered dead for organ donation.[44]

ETHICAL ISSUES: INFANTS AS "DONORS"

Terminology

The cases of Babies Fae, Theresa, and Gabriel raise ethical questions about using one infant as a source of organs for another. One argument against using infants as organ donors is their vulnerability. In general, the more vulnerable people are, the less defensible it is to do something to them without their consent, and babies are some of the most vulnerable humans.

In this regard, a question of terminology arises. When an infant's organ is used as a transplant, who is giving what as a "gift"? Terms like donation and "the gift of life" seem to be inappropriate in this situation; since no baby ever consents to donate his or her organs, a baby cannot really be described as providing a gift.

More accurate terms are: "organ salvage," "organ transfer," "organ recovery," "organ reassignment," and so on. Such terms seem cold, and this connotation suggests why people resist using infants' organs as sources for other infants and why organ procurement agents prefer phrases such as "gift of life."

On the other hand, one possible argument in favor of using infants' organs for transplants would be analogous to McCormick's argument: Parents should choose for a child as the child ought to choose in adulthood. Another possible argument is utilitarian: Infants' organs should be used for transplant if that resulted in the greatest good for the greatest number and if otherwise the organ would be wasted.

Anencephalics and Brain Death

One vital question in the debate over anencephalics as donors has to do with brain death. Shewmon argued that there are no good criteria for brain death in infants, and whether or not this is true, brain death in anencephalic infants is unclear.

Anencephaly is a medical term describing a range of gross congenital brain deficits, all of which entail no chance of normal brain function but some of which do not entail immediate brain death.[45] The fact that most babies do not die the first week—and thus could not be donors under the Ontario guidelines—illustrates this problem, because some kinds of anencephaly are similar to persistent vegetative state (PVS); therefore, with maximal supportive care, some anencephalic infants could survive indefinitely. One critic said, "I have an uneasy feeling that what lurks behind the anencephalic issue is the vegetative state issue."[46]

If neurologists misdiagnose some patients in PVS, then misdiagnosis of anencephaly-leading-to-organ-transfer could also occur.

Some commentators have suggested creating a new category of legal brain death, or an exemption from the usual legal criteria of brain death, to allow for transfers of organs from anencephalic babies. Such a new category or exemption is needed for organ donation because anencephalic infants are neither dead nor about to die quickly enough, and allowing them to die naturally could destroy their organs.

So the question boils down to this: Should we change our criteria of brain death for infants to get more organs from other dying infants? Disability advocates agreed: "Treating anencephalics as dead equates them with 'nonpersons,' presenting a 'slippery slope' problem with regard to all other persons who lack cognition for whatever reason."[47]

Two physicians considered a proposal to adopt a system used in Germany, where anencephalics are considered "brain-absent" and therefore brain-dead. They rejected this proposal for America:

> Not only are the brains of such infants not completely absent, but there is also a remarkable heterogeneity of morphologic and functional features in the infants considered anencephalic. . . . The causes of the neural-tube defects, including anencephaly, are complex and multiple—a fact that confounds the issue and supports the concept that the condition is quite variable. It is worrisome, but not surprising, that the diagnosis of anencephaly is occasionally made in error. Indeed, too many errors have been made for the diagnosis to be considered reliable as a legal definition of death. We conclude that anencephalic infants are not brain-absent and that the condition is sufficiently variable that the establishment of a special category is not justified.[48]

Another problem is that diagnosis of anencephaly, even as a range, is often problematic. Diagnosing brain size or brain function at birth is controversial (see Baby Jane Doe case). Will overzealous physicians and parents, wanting to bring some good out of a tragedy, declare babies anencephalic when they have some lesser defect—say, microcephaly? These media sometimes report cases of retarded children allegedly diagnosed as anencephalic and who now function well.

A slippery slope might occur here: If borderline anencephalics can become a source of organs, there might be a tendency to use infants with closely related disorders such as atelencephaly (incomplete development of the brain) and lissencephaly (unusually small brain parts). It has been argued that "the slippery slope is real, because some physicians have proposed transplants from infants with defects less severe than anencephaly."[49]

Judge Moriarty wrote in her medical review for her decision, "There has been a tendency by some parties and *amici* to confuse lethal anencephaly with these less serious conditions, even to the point of describing children as 'anencephalic' who have abnormal but otherwise intact skulls and who are several years of age."[50]

Some critics have asked whether less was being done for anencephalic babies when these babies were seen as potential organ donors. Alex Capron described the situation as follows: "By far the most fundamental problem . . . was trying to sustain an anencephalic's liver, heart, and kidneys without temporarily giving life to its brain stem, the one organ that needed to die for transplant to begin."[51]

According to the Ontario Protocol, a potential anencephalic donor is to be maintained on a respirator, but periodically removed from the respirator to see if independent breathing will occur. Is this removal in the best interest of the infant? Is the anencephalic infant really being seen as a patient? Or as an organ source? (The Pittsburgh Protocol raises the same questions.)

A counterargument here is that with anencephaly, birth is not morally relevant. That is, most fetuses diagnosed as anencephalic are aborted (indeed, anencephaly is one of the best reasons for aborting a fetus during the second term), and the birth of an anencephalic does not make a moral difference. If abortion is appropriate in anencephaly, why should it be considered immoral to do less to prolong the life of an anencephalic who is a potential organ donor? It might be argued, along these lines, that since anencephalics almost always die a few days after birth, why not allow physicians to kill anencephalics painlessly and transplant their organs at the optimal time?

Another question concerns keeping an anencephalic fetus alive to be a later source of organs, a neonatal version of the non-heart-beating donor protocol. There seems to be a real distinction between keeping a fetus alive for this purpose and simply using the organs of a baby who has accidentally become brain dead or who has unexpectedly been born anencephalic. Some critics say we shouldn't cross this line.

So how many anencephalic organ sources are we talking about? Most anencephalics are identified in utero and most are aborted. Of the approximately 650 anencephalics brought to term each year in the United States, about 60 percent will be stillborn. Of the approximately 300 anencephalics who are born alive and survive immediately after birth, about half will be possible donors of hearts, kidneys, and livers; the others will be unacceptable for various reasons, including organ malformation, low birth weight, and lack of consent by family. The number of possible donors would be further reduced after blood and tissue matching. Taking all this into account, one study estimates that *only about 30 recipients a year* would benefit from using anencephalics as sources of organs.[52]

Given that serious problems exist about using anencephalics as organ sources, is this figure—30 babies a year—large enough? Would it justify changing our criteria of brain death? Most ethicists and doctors decided negatively: The numbers were too small for so big a change.

Costs and Opportunity Costs

In the Baby Fae case, many critics questioned whether so much money should be spent on a single case when the same amount of money could have done so much good for so many others. Although Loma Linda never revealed the cost of Fae's surgery and the associated treatment, it probably cost at least $500,000. Would it make sense to perform a thousand such operations a year, at a cost of maybe $1 billion, while thousands of babies are born deformed because their mothers could not afford prenatal tests like amniocentesis and sonograms?

In the case of Baby Gabriel and Paul Holc, the surgery alone cost $140,000; in addition, there were costs of flying everyone to Loma Linda and, for the Schoutens and the Ontario hospital, the cost of keeping Gabriel Schouten alive for a week. Consider that thousands of pregnant women in the United States get no prenatal care and as a result, many babies are born with preventable defects. Isn't the system biased in favor of dramatic surgical cases and against these anonymous women and their children?

CONJOINED TWINS: THE ETHICS OF SEPARATION

What about costs of separating conjoined twins in 14-hour operations with dozens of surgeons? Millions of dollars can easily be spent on one case. Why is so much free care given on these dramatic cases, while other babies are ignored? How many poor women with babies with HLHS go to motels to wait for their babies to die?

Separation of conjoined twins also raises issues about use of babies in risky surgery and about surgeons seeking fame. On any given day in any major children's hospital, surgeons operate on two desperately ill infants and no one notices. Spectacular surgery occurs, teams spend weeks nurturing each child back to health, but the public is indifferent.

Now make one change and have the two infants enter the hospital as conjoined twins, connected at the head, sternum, or pelvis, and everyone takes notice. Why is that?

Philosopher Alice Dregger argues that it's a modern freak show, the kind of thing that people once paid to see in exhibits.[53] In the eighteenth century, physicians paid such people to exhibit themselves. But as this philosopher and historian of science argues, at least back then such people got paid and were allowed to exhibit their bodies with dignity. Today, the only message they get is: "You're abnormal. We can surgically normalize you, even at risk of killing you. Be grateful."[54]

Separating conjoined twins, especially adults, may often be a reach for fame by the hospital and by the surgical team, saying, "Hey. We can do this and nobody else can! We're the top dogs!" More charitably, it may be just another version of the rule of rescue: We can separate these two conjoined babies, give them separate lives, and feel good about doing so.

In lionizing these cases and their surgeons, the media often describe twins undergoing separation as "brave little fighters," the surgeons as "heroes," and the hospital as performing operations that are "medically necessary" But is this really so?

Johns Hopkins's Ben Carson became famous in 1987 for successfully separating seven-month-old German craniopagus twins (joined at the head and sharing part of the same brain). Since then, he has written several best-selling books about his surgeries on conjoined twins and his life.[55] In 1994, he and his team tried to separate seven-month-old South African craniopagus twins, who both died during the operation. In 1997, he traveled with a 50-member team to successfully separate two Zambian craniopagus twins facing in opposite directions, who did not share any organs.[56]

In 2003, he joined the team of surgeons separating Ladan and Laleh Bijani, the adult Iranian women who both died during the operation. Dregger criticizes what Carson said he told the twins in obtaining consent, that a 50 percent chance existed that one of them would die or be disabled from the surgery:

> But as a leading expert in the field, Carson surely knew of the most comprehensive study of craniopagus separations, which had concluded that "mortality and morbidity after surgical separation of craniopagus twins is horrendous: of the 60 infants operated on, 30 died, 17 were impaired, 6 were alive but ultimate status unknown, and only 7 were apparently normal."[57]

As Dregger points out, at their advanced age, experts agreed that their skulls had thickened and hardened, their brains had matured and were less resilient, thus making their chances of success even worse than the above dismal statistics.[58] Dregger wonders whether these women were given true information about the dismal prospects of the surgery.

In 2004, Carson attempted to separate the German craniopagus twins Lee and Tabea Block. His surgery was only partially successful, as Tabea died during the surgery.[59]

Like Leonard Bailey, Carson, a self-described Christian evangelical, does not believe in evolution: "I don't believe in evolution . . . [it] says that because there are these similarities even though we can't specifically connect them it proves that this is what happened."[60]

Conjoined children can live and grow into late adulthood while conjoined. Eng and Chang lived into their 70s, each married and fathered several normal children.

But don't conjoined twins do better when separated to live separate, independent lives? This is like the problem of other minds seen with involuntary commitment of homeless people with mental illness: from our point of view, they'd be better off in institutions, but they may not agree (see next chapter). Also, "conjoined twins almost invariably state that, from their point of view, they don't need to be separated to be individuals, because they are *not* trapped or confined by their conjoinment."[61]

Perhaps the most spectacular issue here is how little is known about long-term survival for conjoined twins who were separated and about their subsequent quality of life. As Dregger notes, the one extant study merely asked whether separated twins were later alive or dead, with no other questions asked. How can surgeons get informed consent without real data? The assumption always is: anything is better than living like this.

But is it? What is the resulting quality of life for survivors? In retrospect, what do the separated twins think of the operation? Would they do it for their own children, if they were conjoined? How many mourn the loss of a twin killed in the operation?

Some adult conjoined twins claim surgeons and parents are prejudiced against life as conjoined adults, thinking that their quality of life is so low that likelihood of death for one during surgery to free the other is preferable.[62] Dregger calls these *sacrifice surgeries* and argues that they pose the most challenging ethical questions. Surely they raise the most controversial assumption of all: that a chance of normalcy for one is worth the death of the other.

In discussing separation of the conjoined twins Angela and Amy Lakeberg in 1993, Dregger writes, "Yet no matter how justified the ends, it is troubling to see surgeons actively cause the death of a child like Amy—who was obviously conscious and as entitled to the conjoined heart as her sister."[63]

In 2002, UCLA surgeons separated one-year-old Guatemalan craniopagus twins in a 22-hour operation. The story received saturation coverage nationwide, illustrating the rule of rescue. In 2006, Dr. Carson announced he would separate 10-year-old craniopagus twins from Delhi, India.

CONCLUSION

There is an old saying, "Beware the surgeon with one case." That summarizes the ethics of the cases in this chapter. As Alice Dregger states, "Unlike drugs and many nonsurgical medical procedures, surgeries, at least in the United States, are largely exempt from systematic review. There is little tradition or regulation in support of rigorous systematic review."[64]

When experimental surgery is done, it should be in a well-conceived research design. One surgeon grandstanding for fame should not be allowed. Should Loma Linda be proud of Leonard Bailey and what happened there? Should Hopkins boast of separating conjoined twins? What's the opportunity cost of all this famous surgery?

FURTHER READING AND RESOURCES

George Annas, "Baby Fae: The 'Anything Goes' School of Human Experimentation," *Hastings Center Report* 15, no. 1, February 1985, pp. 15–17.

Alice Dregger, *One of Us: Conjoined Twins and the Future of the Normal*, Cambridge, MA: Harvard University Press, 2004.

"Baby Fae: Ethical Issues Surround Cross-Species Organ Transplantation," Scope Note 5, Washington, D.C., Georgetown University, Kennedy Institute of Ethics,

Denise Breo, "Interview with 'Baby Fae's' Surgeon," *American Medical News*, November 16, 1984.

Charles Krauthammer, "The Using of Baby Fae," *Time*, December 3, 1984.

Thomasine Kushner and Raymond Belotti, "Baby Fae: A Beastly Business," *Journal of Medical Ethics* 11, 1985.

DISCUSSION QUESTIONS

1. Was Baby Fae used as a guinea pig to advance a medical experiment? Did she have a chance to live to age 20?
2. Was it right to treat Goobers as a thing when a human donor heart was available?
3. Should anencephalic babies born dying be allowed to be used as heart donors for babies who might live?
4. How can separating conjoined twins be seen as good for the parents and the surgeons but not good for the twins themselves?

CHAPTER 13

Involuntary Psychiatric Commitment

The Case of Joyce Brown

This chapter describes a homeless woman living on the Upper East Side of Manhattan whom psychiatrists committed against her will for treatment for schizophrenia. Defended by the ACLU, her case raised issues about paternalism, political psychiatry, rights of mental patients, and compassion.

This chapter's key discussion question concerns whether people with mental illness who are unlikely to harm others should be committed for their own good.

JOYCE BROWN

In the 1980s, mentally unstable, homeless people overwhelmed Manhattan; mental health professionals and the public wanted something done. In 1987, New York City started Project Help to assist such needy, homeless people, but they resisted. Could Project Help seize them anyway, for psychiatric evaluation and involuntary commitment? Or should they just be left (as some defenders of Project Help criticized) "to die with their rights on"?

The first person picked up was Joyce Brown, a 40-year-old African-American woman. For eighteen months, she slept outside a Swensen's ice cream parlor on Second Avenue and 65th Street, near Gracie Mansion, where Mayor Ed Koch lived. During the day, she panhandled for money to buy food, cigarettes, and toilet paper. Mayor Koch spoke to her on the street sometimes and Project Help chose her as a testcase.

Controversially, Project Help broadened its standards for involuntary commitment beyond the standard, legal requirements of mental illness and dangerousness. It added two new criteria: "self-neglect" and a "need to be treated for mental illness."

Joyce's physical appearance suggested mental instability. Her teeth needed care; she tucked her hair under a bulky, white, knit cap. She looked disoriented, muttering to herself as she panhandled. She sometimes sang, "How much is that doggie in the window?" When residents of the block threw her money, she tossed it back. One neighbor described her as "full of rage." She cursed approaching black men, but liked babies. She sometimes defecated and urinated in gutters. On bitterly cold nights, police tried to take her to shelters, but she resisted.

Project Help forcibly brought her to the emergency room of Bellevue Hospital, where psychiatrists injected against her will with five milligrams of Haldol, an antipsychotic drug, and with two milligrams of Ativan, a fast-acting, short-term tranquilizer. They then took her to a new 28-bed, locked psychiatric unit on the nineteenth floor.

The Legal Conflict

After psychiatrists evaluated Joyce Brown at Bellevue, they informed Mayor Koch that she was neither sufficiently insane nor sufficiently dangerous to legally commit without her consent. Although schizophrenic, Brown did not pose danger to herself or others. New York state law allowed involuntary injections only in emergency rooms; and in the psychiatric unit at Bellevue, Joyce Brown refused further drugs.

Once police bring people to a psychiatric facility, their release rarely happens until a judge holds a hearing. For her hearing before Judge Robert Lippman, Joyce called the American Civil Liberties Union (ACLU). If she would waive confidentiality and agree to publicity about her case to help other homeless people, which she did, the ACLU agreed to represent her.

Her three sisters from New Jersey testified at the hearing. Married, working, and middle class, they had been searching for Joyce for 18 months. All four girls grew up in Elizabeth, New Jersey, well-churched daughters of a Methodist minister.

They described Joyce as a "bright, attractive, and happy-go-lucky child." She had graduated from both high school and business school and had held several jobs at Bell Laboratories. During these years, she had been a "big, healthy girl" who wore nice clothes and jewelry and "always drove around in a new Cadillac."

They said that Joyce had started taking heroin in her twenties, and later cocaine. She worked for ten years as a secretary for the New Jersey Human Rights Commission (HRC). In 1982, her mental health and her job performance plummeted. In 1985, at age 38, because of absenteeism and use of drugs, the HRC fired her. She then left her family and went to a shelter in Newark, but after she assaulted someone there, the shelter expelled her.

Her sisters then tricked her into a voluntary commitment in the psychiatric ward of East Orange General Hospital in New Jersey. When she was diagnosed as psychotic, psychiatrists forced antipsychotic drugs on Joyce. She resisted and attendants put her in an isolation room. Altogether, she spent two weeks locked up there, after which she fled to East 62nd Street in Manhattan, living under various aliases and avoiding shelters for the homeless, considering them dangerous for unattached women. She shunned her sisters, fearing they would commit her again.

At her hearing, Brown spoke well, called herself a "professional street person" and answered probing questions:

Q: Why had she torn up paper money given to her? A: "I only need $7 a day to live on. I tore up additional money given to me to prevent being robbed of it at night."[1]

Q: Why did she defecate on herself? "I never did," she replied, although she had used the streets because no local restaurant would let her use its restroom. "I offered to buy something and they still refused."

Four psychiatrists testified for the city that Brown suffered from schizophrenia, should be treated in an institution, and, if left on the street, would deteriorate. They denied that this was "political psychiatry" and stated that Joyce Brown's "self-neglect" was "so severe" that she should be helped against her will. They noted that schizophrenics are often bright and have periods of rationality.

Three psychiatrists testified for the ACLU that she was not psychotic, not dangerous, not unreasonable in her answers, and not incapable of caring for herself on the streets. In his summation, an ACLU attorney said the city had not proved that Brown showed danger to herself or others: "The only evidence the city had is that she goes to the bathroom in the streets. I see that in New York City every day, because there's a lack of public restroom facilities."

In her rebuttal, the city's attorney replied: "Decency and the law and common sense do not require us to wait until something happens to her. It is our duty to act before it is too late."[2]

Judge Lippman ordered Joyce Brown freed. He had found her "rational, logical, and coherent" throughout her testimony;[3] he said that she "displayed a sense of humor, pride, a fierce independence of spirit, [and] quick mental reflexes"; and he noted that she met none of the conditions set forth in *O'Connor v. Donaldson*.

Even if all psychiatrists had considered her psychotic, he stressed that the city had not proven her dangerous to others or herself:

> I am aware that her mode of existence does not conform to conventional standards, that it is an offense to aesthetic sense. [Nevertheless] she copes, she is fit, she survives . . . [s]he refuses to be housed in a shelter. That may reveal more about conditions in shelters than about Joyce Brown's mental state. It might, in fact, prove she's quite sane. [Also] there must be some civilized alternatives other than involuntary hospitalization or the street.[4]

After the hearing, Brown's sisters called the judge's decision "racist" and "sexist." They argued that if his own wife or mother were sleeping on the streets, "he would not stand for it." They insisted that Joyce needed treatment.

The sisters then revealed that after Joyce had been hospitalized, they had gotten her declared mentally disabled and she had accordingly received $500 a month in Social Security disability payments, which they had been holding for her. Brown had refused the money, rejecting the "lie" that she was mentally disabled.

After her victory, Brown and her ACLU lawyers held a press conference, where she said, "I didn't want to play the game before, but now I am. . . . I am going to get an apartment, go back to work, and get my life together." She criticized the city for spending $600 a day on her care: "I could be living at Trump Tower."[5]

Why did Brown appear so different at her hearing than on the streets? Her psychiatrists claimed she had improved rapidly in the hospital. She dismissed their claim, asserting she had never been crazy. She resented being taken into Bellevue like "cattle" and affirmed that living on the street was a rational choice. Her sisters dismissed this assertion: "You might be able to survive one winter, or even two, but you can't survive that way forever."

Mayor Koch blasted Judge Lippman's decision: "If anything happens to that woman, God forbid, the blood of that woman is on that judge's hands." Reminded by a reporter that Lippman had found Brown lucid, Koch replied, "This woman is at risk. When she lay on the ground in the rain, in the snow, uncovered—was that lucid?"[6] When asked if Brown's commitment was "political psychiatry," Koch asked, "*Who* would claim that?" When told that it had been Brown herself, he replied, "*That alone* proves she's crazy."[7]

The city and Koch appealed to a five-member New York State Appellate Court, before which the ACLU argued that Brown would not return to the streets but would live in a supportive residence for the homeless. The city argued that where she would live was irrelevant: "She was not hospitalized because she was living on the streets [but because] three psychiatrists said she needed medical and psychiatric help."

The appellate court reviewed the testimony of a social worker who said she had observed "fecal matter" on the sheets in which Brown wrapped herself. The appellate court reviewed the testimony of another psychiatrist who said that Brown had told him she often defecated and urinated on herself. It found that "the evidence presented in this case clearly and convincingly demonstrated her past history of assaultive and aggressive behavior."[8]

The appellate court overruled Judge Lippman, saying he had placed too much emphasis on Brown's testimony instead of that of the psychiatrists. Surprisingly, the majority noted that this case required the high standard of proof of "clear and convincing evidence" rather than the weaker one of "preponderance of evidence," and that the city had met that higher standard.

After the appellate decision, Koch said, "Up until this moment, the only treatment has been a loving safe environment. Now we will seek to treat her medically." But New York state law required the city to get a court order to medicate her against her will. In 1988, a state judge ruled against forced medication. Bellevue Hospital then released her, saying there was no point in still holding her.

After being held for 84 days and then released, Brown said:

> I was incarcerated against my will. . . . [I was] a political prisoner. The only thing wrong with me was that I was homeless, not insane. You just can't go around picking everyone up and automatically label them schizophrenic. I'm angry at Mayor Koch, the city and Bellevue. They held me down and injected me. . . . They took my blood against my will. . . .
>
> I need a place to live; I don't need an institution. . . .
>
> People are treated differently just because of your economic status, [because of] what you look like and where you live. . . .
>
> I was mistreated, mentally abused, and I will never, ever, forget this.[9]

The Aftermath

Released to live in a hotel for women run by a nonprofit agency, Joyce worked temporarily as a secretary in the ACLU office. In early 1988, she became a celebrity. She received half a dozen offers for books and movies, and dined at Windows on the World, a restaurant atop the World Trade Center. She appeared on *The Donahue Show* and *60 Minutes*. She loved the attention.

She lectured to law students at Harvard on "The Homeless Crisis: A Street View." She observed, "It looks like I have been appointed the homeless spokesperson."

Then things worsened. Her roommate at the hotel said Joyce had "a lot of anger inside." While walking to work, she muttered racial slurs and obscenities to herself. By March 1988, Joyce began begging in Times Square, shouting obscenities at passersby. Asked about herself, she insisted, "I'm not insane."[10]

In September, police charged her with possession of heroin and two hypodermic needles in a Harlem housing project.[11]

During 1989, Joyce lived in a supervised residence for formerly homeless women in Manhattan. Unconfirmed reports indicated that she entered and left psychiatric hospitals between 1989 and 1994. After a decade of interventions, her physicians discovered that addiction to drugs was her main problem, not schizophrenia. At last report, she had thrown off drugs and was living on her own, and attending a daily support group for former drug users.

Thus she may never have been a true schizophrenic, and hence never met the commitment standards of *O'Conner v. Donaldson*.

Ideology and Insanity

Early humans believed that the voices characteristically heard by schizophrenics came from the gods. Psychologist Julian Jaynes claims that the first humans to have identifiable thoughts experienced them as terrifying internal voices; he argues that the human brain evolved as bicameral to control them.[12]

Hippocrates held that mental disorders had natural causes. Plato thought an imbalance between parts of the mind caused insanity. Roman physician Galen continued this naturalistic concept.

The Middle Ages abandoned this naturalistic approach, substituting demonic possession and exorcism. The insane sometimes were forced to live on a *ship of fools*, which sailed from port to port to take on food and water, but which never was allowed to disembark its human cargo.

From the fifteenth to the eighteenth centuries, the public saw the insane as possessed by demons, or as witches, and often killed them.

The sixteenth century saw the founding of Bethlehem Royal Hospital in London, based on naturalistic principles. It had more patients than it could handle, and hence, a slurring of its name lies behind "bedlam."

The French physician Philippe Pinel (1745–1826), head of the Bicàtre Hospital for the Insane in Paris, unchained his patients, used compassion, and looked for natural causes, all with therapeutic results.

In the nineteenth century, Quaker institutions practiced "moral treatment," allowing patients to roam the grounds, work in gardens, and to live in a homelike atmosphere.

In the twentieth century, psychiatry embraced pharmacological treatments. Psychiatry then faced two related, ethical issues: commitment for political or social deviance, and patient rights against involuntary treatment.

Patients' Rights

If one accepts that the insane need therapeutic help rather than criminal justice, then they need no trial to commit them for treatment. In a benevolent system, committing psychiatrists act in the best interests of patients.

In the 1960s and 1970s, movies such as *King of Hearts* (1966) and the Oscar-winning *One Flew over the Cuckoo's Nest* (1975) attacked such benevolent commitment as unjust. Lawyers who defended patients' autonomy argued that psychiatric diagnoses were biased, that large public mental institutions abused patients, and that psychiatry needed checks and balances. These lawyers eventually battered down the locked doors of psychiatric wards.

In this battle, psychiatry saw itself as benevolent and argued that liberal lawyers had deprived the insane of necessary treatment. It emphasized that biochemical imbalances caused schizophrenia, which could be rectified pharmacologically. However, some people with schizophrenia had to be forced to take their medications or they would fare poorly.

Thomas Szasz, a famous gadfly in psychiatry, saw no problem with patients who voluntarily sought help, because psychiatrists properly should help them. He criticized forcing psychiatrists on people like Joyce Brown—people who did not see themselves as mentally ill and who resisted intervention. Szasz held that such involuntary commitment rarely benefited the patients and politically existed to rid society of strange people.

Szasz essentially argued that a physical disease, such as AIDS or cancer, has a physical cause. Some mental illnesses have a physical cause in the brain, and these mental illnesses are real. But pseudo-mental illnesses have no physical cause and merely result from problems in living. A mental illness with no physical cause, Szasz famously held, is a *myth*, not a disease. (Szasz did not claim, as some critics say, that most mental illness is a myth.)

Szasz concluded that psychiatry could not be objective, or value-free, in social cases. He held that it is "much more intimately related to problems of ethics than is medicine in general."[13] Consider that interpersonal relations—relationships between wife and husband, between the individual and the community, among colleagues, among neighbors—inevitably involve stress, conflict of interests, and strain. Much of this disharmony has to do with incompatible values, and to pretend that psychiatrists can offer value-free approaches to resolving them is ludicrous: "Much of psychotherapy revolves around nothing other than the elucidation and weighing of goals and values—many of which may be mutually contradictory—and the means whereby they might best be harmonized, realized, or relinquished."

Szasz wonders who truly defines norms of "correct" and "psychotic" behavior. He opposed classification of personality disorders as mental illness. According to him, psychiatry presumes that love, continued life, stable marriage, kindness, and meekness indicate mental health, whereas hatred, homicide, suicide, repeated divorce, chronic hostility, and vengefulness indicate mental illness. These presumptions are evaluative, not factual.

A famous study by D. Rosenhan, "On Being Sane in Insane Places," figured famously in movements for rights of patients. In this study, several sociologists, psychiatrists, and others voluntarily entered mental hospitals, saying they heard voices—a major symptom of schizophrenia.[14] Once committed, they acted normally and no longer mentioned their voices. Because of the label "schizophrenic" in their medical charts, the staff continued to see them as schizophrenic. Ironically, although the staff did not see through the sham, several of the genuine mental patients did.

Legal Victories for Psychiatric Patients

In 1972, in *Wyatt v. Stickney*, Alabama federal judge Frank Johnson ruled that a committed mental patient must either receive treatment or be released. Johnson's decision specified the institutional conditions necessary to ensure minimal treatment: at least 2 psychiatrists, 12 registered nurses, and 10 aides for every 250 patients. Even in 2000, many states for years had not met this minimal standard.

Johnson required state mental institutions to provide individualized treatment plans, to allow patients to refuse invasive electroconvulsive therapy and lobotomies, and to establish the least restrictive conditions necessary for treatment.

Johnson's ruling prefigured the *O'Conner v. Donaldson* decision by the United States Supreme Court in 1975.[15] In 1943, at age 34, Kenneth Donaldson got into a fight with coworkers over politics and someone knocked him out. His parents considered him crazy and petitioned a Florida judge to commit him. Committed, he underwent 11 weeks of electroshock treatment and was then released.

In 1956, while he was visiting his parents in Florida, his father asked for a sanity hearing for Kenneth, saying that his son had a persecution complex. The judge then committed Donaldson to the Florida State Mental Hospital, where he was held against his will for 15 years. During those years, he constantly petitioned the courts for a new hearing. All the while, he rarely saw a physician and never received treatment. Inside the institution, staff presumed him insane and—like Rosenhan's impostors—he could not prove otherwise. In 1971, when his case was about to be heard, officials released him.

A lawyer then helped Donaldson sue for damages against the superintendent of the institution, J. B. O'Connor. The case reached the Supreme Court, which decided for Donaldson, ruling that he should not have been held against his will, even if he was mentally ill, unless he had been dangerous to himself or others and had no means of existing outside the institution.

O'Connor v. Donaldson established two necessary conditions for involuntary commitment:

1. Suffering from mental illness (being "insane")
2. Being dangerous to others or being dangerous to oneself

Note that both conditions, insanity and danger to oneself or others, must be met for involuntary commitment. Judges later interpreted dangerousness as imminent risk to life or imminent risk of bodily harm; "imminent" means within days or hours. Two psychiatrists arbitrate. Evidence of dangerousness to oneself can consist of attempted suicide, threats of suicide, and gross neglect of basic needs.

With these legal changes, the courts moved from a medical model of civil commitment, which had been used in the early 1960s, to a patient's rights model in the 1970s.

In the 1990s, many states added a third requirement for involuntary commitment:

3. Provision of the least restrictive environment by the institution.

Conditions 1 (mental illness) and 2 (dangerousness) applied in all states, since the Supreme Court had established them; two-thirds of the states also applied condition 3 (least restrictive environment).[16]

In some states, the *O'Connor* criteria have been interpreted to mean that a person must commit an *overt act* before a hearing occurs for involuntary commitment. This interpretation is controversial and has been opposed by relatives, who can often perceive a pattern of threats and hostility and do not want to wait until someone is injured or killed before a hearing takes place. At present, courts and legislatures are struggling with the implications of this "overt act" requirement.

Deinstitutionalization

These legal decisions entailed the release of many mental patients from large state institutions, because such institutions often could not provide individualized treatment (as required by *Wyatt*) and they were not the least restrictive environment for patients.

Other factors also contributed to *deinstitutionalization*. New psychotropic medications allowed more outpatient treatment. The Kennedy administration advocated small, community-integrated facilities rather than large, impersonal state institutions. In the words of President Kennedy, "Reliance on the cold mercy of custodial isolation will be supplanted by the open warmth of community concern."[17] Other factors pushing deinstitutionalization in the 1970s included tight budgets, psychiatrists who sought lighter workloads, and a general distrust of authority.

All these factors emptied American mental institutions. By 1980, state institutions released 50 to 75 percent of their mental patients. In 1955, nearly 560,000 patients lived in state mental institutions; in 1988, only 130,000 did so. All levels of government saved money, this pleased the ACLU, and mental patients flooded into communities.

But the "warmth of community concern" envisioned by John Kennedy did not appear. Communities rejected halfway houses. Mental patients scraped by on warm-air grates more often than in group homes. Bag ladies suddenly appeared on city streets. Charities set up soup kitchens for hungry street people. In the 1980s, Reaganites hailed soup kitchens as proof that the homeless didn't need government housing rather than seeing it as a band-aid.

Deinstitutionalization failed to help people with mental illness because governments never allocated funds for community homes; because communities rejected halfway homes; because mental health services were fragmented between county, state, and federal agencies; because housing was scarce; and because the legal pendulum had swung toward patients' rights.[18]

During the month psychiatrists released Joyce Brown from Bellevue, under its expanded criteria, Project Help helped 466 homeless mentally ill people. It estimated that 800 to 1,000 such people still lived on Manhattan's streets.

When New York City officials planned Project Help, they assumed that people such as Joyce Brown would stay for a few weeks in psychiatric hospitals and would then be moved into community facilities, where they would live under supervised conditions. When Project Help picked up these people, however, they were far sicker than had been expected. Many more places were needed in psychiatric hospitals than had been expected.

Violence and the Mentally Ill Homeless in the Cities

In 1977, Juan Gonzalez, a homeless man suffering from symptoms like Joyce Brown's, went berserk on the Staten Island Ferry and with a sword, killed two people. As a result, the public clamored for incarceration of potentially dangerous mentally ill people.

The concept of potential danger soon came to be used to justify holding someone temporarily for a cool-down observational period. Gonzalez had been picked up for just such a period just before the killings and diagnosed as a paranoid schizophrenic, but as he wasn't considered imminently dangerous to others, he had been discharged.

In 1991, Keven McKiever, a homeless man who had gone to Bellevue Hospital seeking care and had been turned away, stabbed to death Alexis Walsh, a former Radio City Rockette. In 1993, Christopher Battiste, a homeless mentally ill drug abuser, allegedly murdered an elderly woman in the Bronx on a Sunday morning as she came home from church.

Larry Hogue, a homeless, mentally ill African-American Vietnam veteran, sometimes lived peacefully on a street corner on the Upper West Side of Manhattan, but when he took illegal drugs, he became hostile, violent, and what *60 Minutes* called the "wild man of 96th Street." A state judge ruled that he could be involuntarily committed against his will for detoxification, but that he would have to be released "as soon as he decides to seek outpatient care."[19]

In 1999, two schizophrenic men not taking their prescribed medications pushed innocent people in front of oncoming subway trains in New York City, killing a young woman named Kendra Webdale and leaving the other victim without legs. Both men had a history of violence. In previous years, similar events had occurred:

> Reuben Harris, who suffered from paranoid schizophrenia, had 12 hospitalizations and a history of violent behavior, pushed Song Sin to her death in the same manner in 1995. Jaheem Grayton, who also had a history of violence and severe mental illness, pushed Naeeham Lee to her death after struggling to steal her earrings in 1996. Mary Ventura pushed Catherine Costello into the path of a subway train in 1985, three weeks after being discharged from a psychiatric hospital.

These cases resulted in passage in New York in 1999 of *Kendra's Law*, where a psychiatrist or relative can force hospitalization for a mentally ill person who has been hospitalized within the last three years, who has a history of violence, and who will not take his medication. At least 41 states passed laws implementing such Assisted Outpatient Treatment programs, where outpatients can be forced to take medications and remain under supervision (California, Maine, Maryland, Massachusetts, New Jersey, Pennsylvania, and Rhode Island have not).[20]

The courts and the general public have come to expect psychiatrists to be able to predict dangerousness among the mentally ill, but can they? To assess the potential for violent behavior, emergency-room psychiatrists simply ask patients about their own tendencies toward violence and their own past acts of violence.[21] This is not a sophisticated tool, although in practice this question seems to work better than any other test.

The famous legal decision *Tarasoff* should be noted here.[22] In this case, Prosenjit Poddarin 1969 confided to his psychotherapist at the University of California that he planned to kill Tatiana Tarasoff, which he did. Tarasoff's parents sued the therapist and claimed the university should have broken confidentiality and warned the girl and parents of Poddarin's threat. The actual decision has been misinterpreted to say that therapists must breach confidentiality to warn potential victims when life is at stake. In fact the 1976 decision merely said that, in such situations, therapists have a duty to take "reasonable steps" to protect potential victims, such as notifying police or seeking involuntary commitment of the person making the threat.

ETHICAL ISSUES

Paternalism, Autonomy, and Diminished Competence

Paternalism in medicine is treatment of adult patients as incompetent children who do not know their own best interests. Under which conditions might paternalism be justified? One condition is *temporary incompetence*, followed by a return of competence. In these situations, if patients later agreed with paternalism, for example, where people prevented from committing suicide later agreed that they were glad to be alive, it could be justified.

Questions about patients' competence underlie any discussion of paternalism. In this regard, one question has to do with the basic concept of competence. The American legal system tends to treat mental patients as if they were either totally competent or totally dysfunctional and thus subject to involuntary treatment. Many observers argue that this is a false dichotomy. Competence is not an either-or capacity, but a matter of degrees on a gradient.

Another question concerns proof of competence and incompetence. This issue is not necessarily clear-cut: the psychiatrist Virginia Abernethy argues, for instance, that "disorientation, mental illness, irrationality, [and] commitment to a mental institution do not conclusively prove incompetence."[23]

Abernethy describes the case of "Ms. A," a highly intelligent, independent woman who lived alone in a large house with six cats, in an unheated garbage-strewn room.[24] After a fire in her house, Ms. A was hospitalized but found competent and released. As winter came, a concerned social worker investigated; he found her feet were black, ulcerated, and bleeding. When he tried to get her to go with him to a hospital, she chased him away with a shotgun. The police later came and forcibly hospitalized her. At the hospital, her feet were diagnosed as gangrenous, and surgeons wanted to amputate; when she refused, psychiatrists began to evaluate her.

It turned out that Ms. A's feet had blackened once before, a few years earlier, and she had recovered. She now hoped for another recovery, but the psychiatrists interpreted this as "psychotic denial" and tried to get her to say that she wanted to live, so that they could amputate. She refused, avoiding their questions. Ms. A was faced with a dilemma: either she had to let the surgeons amputate, or she had to let the psychiatrists conclude that she was in denial and therefore psychotic. It might seem unfair to present a patient with such a choice, and trying to avoid the choice would seem to be reasonable. Amazingly, according to Abernethy, "Her rejection of the two-choice model became the grounds, finally, for concluding that Ms. A was not competent to refuse amputation."

Abernethy analyzed the psychodynamics of this process. First, a false aura of medical emergency "pervaded the psychiatric consultations and judicial process." Second, "Ms. A herself was quick to anger and regarded most interactions with medical personnel as adversarial." Third, Ms. A's anger created anger in those evaluating her competence: "Professionals who think of themselves as altruistic, or at least benevolently motivated, may be particularly sensitive to hostility because they feel deserving of gratitude." Abernethy says that psychiatrists are outcome-oriented and cannot tolerate a patient's self-destructiveness, even in the name of autonomy and even when self-destruction results from an underlying disease that they cannot stop. Abernethy emphasizes that "hope is not a criterion of psychotic denial."

In some ways, Joyce Brown resembled Ms. A. Like Ms. A, she rejected her diagnosis, hoped that she was sane, and thought she could take care of herself. Like Ms. A, she saw psychiatrists as enemies. Acknowledging her to be generally competent, psychiatrists claimed both women had a *focal incompetence,* a specific incompetence to make decisions about their own treatment. Abernethy notes, "The criterion of a focal delusion is dangerously liable to error because a patient can easily be seen as delusional in an emotionally charged interchange, when in other circumstances he addresses the same issue appropriately." Abernethy sums up: "Competence is presumed and does not have to proved. Incompetence has to be proved."

Homelessness and Commitment

What really mattered in the Joyce Brown case—insanity or homelessness? The ACLU, noting that Joyce Brown did not want to leave the street and had never been proven dangerous, argued that her presence embarrassed the rich people in her neighborhood. New York City had thousands of people like her, so why was there no outcry about others? Why did no one write letters to the *New York Times* about the Joyce Browns in the Bronx? Once Brown was gone, how many of her former neighbors on the Upper East Side inquired about her?

Norman Siegel, executive director of ACLU, extended this argument to Koch and the city as well: "In sweeping up the homeless, the Mayor is attempting to place these people out of sight and out of mind and hide the crisis from the public consciousness." Siegel claimed that Project Help targeted areas seen by tourists and inhabited by the rich.

Mayor Koch emphasized that homeless people were picked up for treatment, not to remove them from public places. Homeless people gravitated to rich areas because they were safer there and such places offered them better opportunities for begging.

Koch claimed that Brown's insanity was the true issue and her homelessness merely a side issue. Her ACLU lawyers disagreed: "The Joyce Brown story has captured the issue of the homeless that a lot of people have been trying to deal with for years."[25] Koch's goal, the ACLU implied, was to get homeless people off the streets, not to treat the mentally ill; Koch didn't seem worried about schizophrenics who camped out in bad neighborhoods.

The ACLU suggested reinstituting public baths (which had been widely available in the city during the depression) and using condemned housing as temporary shelters. Incarcerating the homeless "for their own good" was cheap; building homes for street people costs much more.

No one could deny that affordable housing was rare in New York City. The problem of creating permanent housing for the city's homeless had frustrated many good minds. The city maintained thousands of families in squalid welfare hotels at exorbitant rates. Critics feared that providing rented housing would encourage more people to depend on such government handouts. They also pointed out that the city was one of the most expensive places in the United States in which to subsidize public housing.

Psychiatry and Commitment

During this case, ACLU lawyer Robert Levy and psychiatrist Robert Gould, both of whom testified for Brown, emphasized the political dangers of involuntary roundups, handcuffing, forcible injections of medication, and confinement in locked wards. Levy and Gould said that Brown had been examined at least five times previously and had been found "not to require involuntary hospitalization." They claimed that nearly half of the 215 people brought to emergency rooms by Project Help did "not require involuntary hospitalization." They argued that to allow "preventive detention based solely on nebulous predictions of future self-destructive behavior" would invite abuse. They warned of "totalitarian regimes" using psychiatry for control of dissidents.[26]

When confronted with arguments like this, Mayor Koch replied, "This is not political psychiatry! This is not Russia! We're trying to *help* this woman!"

On the other hand, how broadly should standards of commitment sweep? In cases like Brown's, how many people might be forced into mental hospitals by relatives? (Isn't this what Barbara Streisand portrayed in *Nuts*?) How many psychiatrists might use medication, time-out rooms, restraints, and continued commitment not as treatment but as punishment for patients who thwart their will?
Part of the debate about Brown's case concerned the ability of psychiatry to help schizophrenics. Judge Lippman noted that the four city and three ACLU psychiatrists had disagreed dramatically, and concluded, "It is evident that psychiatry is not a science amenable to the exactness of mathematics or the predictability of physical laws."

Most psychiatrists objected. They pointed to schizophrenics who were dysfunctional but who gained years of ability after being forced to take medication. They said that such patients stabilize and become free from delusions and that many patients, if they take their medication regularly, can return to life outside institutions. The psychiatrist Paul Chodoff defended limited involuntary commitment as follows:

> Is freedom defined only by absence of external constraints? Internal physiological or psychological processes can contribute to a throttling of the spirit that is as painful as any applied from the outside. The "wild" manic individual without his lithium, the panicky hallucinator without his injection of fluphenazine hydrochloride and the understanding support of a concerned staff, the sodden alcoholic—are they free? Sometimes, as Woody Guthrie said, "Freedom means no place to go."[27]

In fact, many people suffering from paranoid schizophrenia can be improved by treatment. The big issue here is whether some must be forced to be so improved.

Suffering and Commitment: Benefit and Harm

Columnist Ellen Goodman argued that the ethical questions in this case boiled down not to whether people like Joyce Brown would harm themselves, but to whether they suffered. Brown should be taken off the streets, she argued, before she dies there "with her rights on."[28]

But was the matter so straightforward? To say that commitment is justified to end suffering assumes first that a person is really suffering, and second that involuntary psychiatric commitment will stop that suffering.

Consider the first assumption, that the person suffers. When someone like Joyce Brown protests that she does not need or want help, it can be asked—as Thomas Szasz asked—who determines—other than the patient herself—that she is "suffering" enough to be locked inside a psychiatric ward? Who bears the onus of proof, the patient or the psychiatrist?

With regard to the second assumption, that involuntary commitment can help, it is important to consider the nature of involuntary commitment. What Brown feared most was another commitment to an inpatient unit like the one at East Orange Hospital. Would she really be helped by involuntary psychiatry, involuntary medication, and involuntary therapy in a locked unit within a large public institution? In another time-out room?

Brown's court-appointed psychiatrist found that she suffered from "serious mental illness" and would benefit from medication—but that she would suffer more from forced treatment than from the mental illness itself. In such a situation, she might harm herself while trying to resist the administration of antipsychotic medications and tranquilizers. Also, commitment might destroy her fierce independence; and if it did not—if she continued to resist—she might end up with a lobotomy, like McMurphy in *One Flew over the Cuckoo's Nest*.

Moreover, the long-term side effects of antipsychotics of this period were as bad as the original disorder: administered over years, they created tardive dyskinesia in 10–25 percent of patients. This condition impairs voluntary movement, is untreatable, and when the medication is stopped, persists in two-thirds of the affected patients.

It can also be argued that the potential benefits of involuntary treatment cannot be defined objectively. Most psychiatrists think that people such as Brown benefit from living on medication and by losing their inner voices. But aren't benefit and harm, above the level of basic needs, defined by each person's own self-concept and life plans? As three lawyers write:

> When faced with an obviously aberrant person, we know, or we think we know, that he would be "happier" if he were as we are. We believe that no one would want to be a misfit in society. From the very best of motives, then, we wish to fix him. It is difficult to deal with this feeling since it rests on the unverifiable assumption that the aberrant person, if he saw himself as we see him, would choose to be different than he is. But since he cannot be as we, and we cannot be as he, there is simply no way to judge the predicate for the assertion.[29]

Isn't it a shaky application of paternalism to say that Joyce Brown had to be treated so that she could obtain someone else's idea of a benefit? Psychiatrists imply that mentally ill patients suffer internal pain, but if that is so, why don't all patients want to get rid of it? Isn't it illogical—isn't it begging the question—for psychiatrists to explain that patients don't want to get rid of this pain because they're crazy?

What makes us go round-and-round on this issue is that schizophrenia *is a disorder of thought*. So some people with such disorders of thinking will in fact fail to understand their obvious best interests.

Housing for the Mentally Ill as an Ethical Issue

Recently, the term"homeless" has been attacked by a new wave of critics as inappropriate for the wandering mentally ill; instead, "substance abusers who lack housing" has been substituted. Critics challenged the ACLU's view that people like Joyce Brown are primarily victims of a greedy or indifferent society which failed to provide affordable housing; they say there is evidence that as many as 85 percent of panhandlers are alcoholics, substance abusers, or mentally ill—and that all of these need treatment.[30] These new critics advocate mandatory treatment and police intervention to prevent panhandling. They urge people not to give money to beggars, saying that those who do give money are "enablers of addiction."

Supervised group homes remain an elusive ideal, except in a few enlightened states like Vermont and New Hampshire. Whether we are discussing severely physically disabled people like Larry McAfee, welfare reform, or the mentally ill homeless, the best living facility for many people is a supervised group home. Living in such a home is much better than being warehoused in a large institution or being left to fend for oneself. Supervised group homes in safe neighborhoods are the perfect compromise between institutionalization and independence.

Deinstitutionalization has continued. In 1993, in New York, 2,400 new group home beds had been planned in preparation for the release of 1,000 more people with mental illness from large institutions in 1994, but the number of new beds was later cut to 800. When New York's highest court ruled in 1993 that the city must provide housing for homeless mentally ill patients discharged from city hospitals, the city estimated that it would cost $300 million to do so and disputed the ruling.[31] Nine years later, a study by the *New York Times* exposed widespread failings in the city's adult homes for mentally ill people, "allowing some of its most vulnerable citizens to be exploited in a system plagued by inept, wasteful and fraudulent services."[32]

Many cities emulated New York City's mayor Rudolph Giuliani, who forced homeless people off the streets in the 1990s and into city-funded shelters away from tourists and the affluent. Cities such as Sacramento, Seattle, and Atlanta forced homeless people to move out and did not build new shelters.

When cities tried to build group homes, fights ensued. Residents on Earle Street in Greenville, South Carolina, one of its oldest neighborhoods, sued in 1994 when charities tried to open a sixth group home there. In Alabama, Birmingham's Southside, Forest Park, and Avondale neighborhoods had too many group homes, while surrounding, affluent suburbs had none. All around the country, certain neighborhoods in each city became categorized as the preferred area for group homes, where too many were built. Such identification made other neighborhoods passionately resist having even one such home there, lest more follow.

In the twenty-first century, lack of housing remains a problem for mentally ill homeless people, who are often also plagued by drugs, dysfunctional families, and poverty.

FURTHER READING AND RESOURCES

Alice Baum and Donald Burnes, *A Nation in Denial: The Truth about Homelessness,* Boulder, CO, Westview Press, 1993.

Paul Chodoff, "The Case for Involuntary Hospitalization of the Mentally Ill," *American Journal of Psychiatry* 133, no. 5, May 1976.

Saul Feldman, "Out of the Hospitals, onto the Streets: The Overselling of Benevolence," *Hastings Center Report* 13, no. 3, June 1983.

Charles Krauthammer, "How to Save the Homeless Mentally Ill," *New Republic,* February 8, 1988.

J. Livermore, C. Malmquist, and P. Meehl, "On the Justification for Civil Commitment," *University of Pennsylvania Law Review* 117, November 1968.

Paul Chodoff, "The Case for Involuntary Hospitalization of the Mentally Ill," *American Journal of Psychiatry* 133, no. 5, May 1976.

The video "Brown vs. Koch" from *60 Minutes* may be available for purchase for a reasonable fee.

DISCUSSION QUESTIONS

1. "The easiest way to become homeless in America is to lose your job, lose your medical insurance, and be unable to afford housing. It can happen to anyone." Is this true, or do people usually screw up, say, by using drugs, when they lose their jobs and places of living?
2. "When faced with an aberrant person, we think he would be happier if he were as we are. . . . But since he cannot be as we, and we cannot be as he, there is simply no way to judge the predicate for the assertion.[33] This "problem of other minds" in psychopathology has its limits. Shouldn't some crazy people be helped for their own good?
3. Are most problems of psychotherapy, as Szsaz says, problems of values, about which psychiatrists have no special training or insight and, for having different values, people shouldn't be involuntarily committed, should they?
4. During his administration as mayor of New York City, Rudy Giuliani used heavy-handed police tactics to rid Times Square and other touristy areas of Manhattan of homeless people. Was he justified in doing so by the greater good? Today, you see maybe 1 percent of the number of homeless people that one saw in Joyce Brown's time on the streets.
5. Has deinstitutionalization worked for the best interests of people with mental illness, especially as community centers never came about?

CHAPTER 14

Testing in Advance for Genetic Disease

This chapter discusses ethical issues in presymptomatic testing for genetic diseases, in other words, testing for diseases whose symptoms may take decades to appear. It discusses Huntington's disease, breast cancer, type 2 diabetes, and Alzheimer's disease. Its essential questions for discussion focus on how much individuals with positive tests can be held responsible, if at all, for developing genetic disease, and whether they should take such predictive tests.

GENETIC DISEASES

Case 1: Nancy Wexler and Huntington's Disease

Clinical psychologist Nancy Wexler, born in 1945, graduated from Radcliff College in 1967. After a ten-year deterioration and catatonia, her mother died of Huntington's disease, a devastating, fatal neurological disease lacking cure or treatment. Because the Huntington's gene is dominant, Nancy and her sister Alice each had a 50 percent risk of inheriting the disease. Because the average age of onset is 36, victims usually have children before learning they are affected.

A severe, progressive neurological disease, Huntington's causes neurons in the caudate nuclei region of the brain to rapidly shed. Although age of onset varies, the gene is completely *penetrant* by age 65: the gene affects everyone with the disease.

Huntington's progresses through several stages (each about five years long). First comes loss of muscular coordination and changes in personality, making victims angry, hostile, depressed, and sexually promiscuous. Next comes slurred speech, distorted facial expressions, constant muscular jerkiness, and staggering and falling. The third stage brings incontinence, dementia, and dependence on others, usually in an institution. In the last stage, victims are vegetative.

At present, 25,000 Americans have Huntington's, and about 100,000 Americans have an afflicted parent. Most victims are white. People at risk of Huntington's constantly wonder if each stumble augurs onset of the disease.

Unlike others at risk for genetic disease, Wexler helped both to discover the gene for Huntington's and to develop a predictive test for it. Around 1800, a European sailor with Huntington's jumped ship around Lake Maracaibo in Venezuela. He had 14 children, and because families there were large, by 1981 he had 3,000 descendants. Of these, 100 had Huntington's and another 1,100 were at risk. In 1981, Nancy led an expedition there to obtain blood samples from these descendants and to test them to find a genetic marker for Huntington's. Coresearcher James Gusella found such a marker in 1983.

In 1987, though the gene had not been discovered, Gusella developed a *linkage test* for Huntington's, meaning he could test for a batch of genes that tended to be inherited (or "linked") together. The test allowed people such as Nancy to know their risk, for example, 5 percent versus 80 percent. In this way, this linkage test (versus a direct test for the gene itself) prefigured today's genetic tests where people can know that they have an 80 percent risk of hereditary breast cancer or little risk but do not get a simple yes-or-no answer.

In 1986, before the linkage tests, Nancy Wexler taught as a professor of clinical neuropsychology at Columbia University. She then said she would like to take the test when it became available. However, she later changed her mind, famously deciding *not* to take the test.

The implications of her decision stunned people in medical genetics because a leading advocate for testing, who carried a 50 percent risk, had decided at the last minute not to know her risk. And she had spent a decade helping to develop this very test. Moreover, she was a clinical psychologist who should have known her own heart.

Indeed, not only did Nancy not take the test, but she also became an advocate for others not to take it. To people who want to be tested so that they could decide to go to law school, she said: "Go to law school! Develop your mind! What are you going to do if you're positive? Spend the rest of your life waiting to be a patient?"

In 1983, James Gusella discovered a marker for Huntington's and thought that finding the actual gene would take a few years, but in fact, it took *ten* years. Over the next decade, other researchers discovered single genes for muscular dystrophy, cystic fibrosis, neurofibromatosis ("elephant man" disease), colon cancer, ataxia, and sickle-cell anemia. In 1993, six laboratories discovered the exact location of the Huntington's gene.[1] Now at-risk people could test directly for it.

By then, Nancy Wexler had become even more convinced that people should not take it. In 2008, at age 63, she led the successful fight to get the FDA to approve tetrabenazine, the first drug that can ameliorate Huntington's symptoms.[2]

Background: Basic Genetics

The gene is the basic unit of heredity. It consists of DNA, an organic molecule. Packed inside each of the 46 chromosomes in humans is a complicated strand of interwoven DNA, the famous double helix. The number of genes varies on each chromosome.

The pattern of the four nucleotide bases (A, C, T, and G) in the 46 double helices makes up a person's genetic code. Between 30,000 and 40,000 sequences of these 138 billion pairs of bases are genes.

The Human Genome Project, one of the greatest projects in the history of science, began in October 1993 with the goal of mapping which parts of human

DNA were genes. Costing $3 billion, it finished in 2003 after having mapped all the human genes.

Knowing which parts of DNA are genes, and where they are, begins genetic knowledge. In the next steps, scientists must identify what genes do, with what other genes, and through which mediating proteins (proteinomics). In addition, some genetic diseases stem from variants in standard genes, or from nonfunctioning genes, so the causes of disease are complex.

Of great importance, varying environmental inputs determine how genes express themselves. Exposure of the fetus to drugs, nutrition in childhood, and use of tobacco affects how genes control bodily characteristics. In genetics, this is called the *norm of reaction*.[3]

Genetic diseases are inherited disorders. Some genetic diseases are caused by a dominant gene, e.g., Huntington's disease, where just one copy of the bad gene is needed to get the disease. However, most of us carry genes for recessive genetic diseases but are not affected by them. We are *heterozygous*, having a dissimilar pair of genes for an inherited recessive disease.

Heterozygotes of recessive traits may not experience a disease, but can pass the gene for it to their offspring. If two parents who are heterozygous for a disease both bequeath the gene for the disorder to an offspring, that person will be *homozygous* (have an identical pair of genes) for the disorder. Homozygotes always express the disease.

Case 2: Genes for Breast Cancer

Breast cancer is more complicated than Huntington's. Most breast cancer is not caused by a single gene, has both preventive and curative treatments, and is not uniformly fatal.

Joan is a 50-year-old woman who had breast cancer at age 45 and had the affected breast removed, followed by radiation and chemotherapy and a maintenance course of tamoxifen. In high school and college, she smoked one to two packs of cigarettes a day, and for a decade in college and graduate school, used oral contraceptives. Cancer in females is associated with smoking and the pill, especially both together.

Joan blames herself for her cancer, but because her mother and aunt had breast cancer at the same age, wonders if she might have hereditary breast cancer. If she does, her daughters might take precautions. Moreover, if she does have the gene, her smoking and use of contraceptives might not have given her breast cancer.

Is most breast cancer caused by one gene? Despite the conventional wisdom, it is not. In fact, 95 percent of breast cancer is not caused by a single gene. But the 5 percent that is caused by a gene is one center of controversy.

In 1990, Mary Claire-King discovered a single gene, BRCA1 (BReast CAncer1) causing one form of breast cancer and ovarian cancer; its exact location was identified in 1994. Alan Ashworth in 1995 discovered another gene, BRCA2. In 2002, researchers discovered a third gene, CHEK2. Mutations in any of these genes cause breast cancer. Women in families expressing mutations in these BRCA1 or BRCA2 run an 80 percent risk of developing breast cancer in their lives, compared to a 9 percent risk for other women. Both BRCA1 and BRCA2 are autosomal dominant genes. By 2009, some researchers believed that four genes and one DNA region "expose the genetic underpinnings of the disease in about one-third of patients."[4]

The Eugenics Movement

Before genetics became a science, a number of ill-founded ideas about heredity abounded. American pragmatist philosopher George Santayana famously said, "Those who cannot learn from history are doomed to repeat it." Knowing the mistakes of the eugenics movement helps us spot mistakes in public policy about today's genetics.

One mistake, *phrenology*, claimed that the inherited size and shape of the head determined intelligence and character. Although it seems ludicrous now, physicians then palpated the skull to assess character and IQ.

Other misconceptions stemmed from crackpot versions of Charles Darwin's theory of evolution by natural selection, especially his concept of "survival of the fittest." Darwin used fittest simply to mean "best adapted," so "fit" referred to the adaptation between an organism and its environment. Unfortunately, many people misunderstood "fit" to apply to social positions.

This misconception, *social Darwinism*, saw evolution in terms of group competition in human societies. Elitist, white social Darwinists held that social advantages implied biological superiority; therefore upper classes would prevail in any competition. They claimed that the fittest races would prevail in struggles for existence, so they predicted that blacks (whom they saw as biologically unfit) would not survive into the twentieth century.

Social Darwinism can most charitably be described as unsophisticated. Not based on any understanding of evolution, it failed to take into account the vast numbers of organisms involved in attempts to survive, the enormous length of time over which these attempts evolve, or the ongoing role of adaptive mutations.

The *eugenics movement* flourished from 1905 to 1935 and hoped to improve hereditary characteristics through voluntary, selective breeding. Charles Darwin's cousin, Francis Galton, coined the term "eugenics" in the late 1880s.

Eugenics popped up worldwide: in Germany, Austria, Scandinavia, Italy, Japan, and South America, but as historian Daniel Kevles writes, "the center of this trend was the American eugenics movement. Its headquarters was at Cold Spring Harbor on Long Island, New York. . . ."[5]

This point bears emphasizing: Although many people identify modern eugenics with German Nazis, Americans—with their heterogeneous population—most passionately championed eugenics. American politicians, popular media, and scientists espoused it, advocated "eugenic marriages" and sterilization of the unfit, and declared that the American gene pool had declined through interbreeding with unfit races.

At the beginning of the twentieth century in the United States, a few prominent families—largely of English, Swiss, German, and Dutch ancestry—exercised enormous wealth and power; they controlled many newspapers, magazines, and even universities. They obsessed about breeding and feared that the purity of Americans would be contaminated if their children bred with Irish, Italians, Turks, Jews, Asians, and African Americans. Watching the many progeny of Irish, Italian, and Greek immigrants, they saw Malthusian doom approaching. They thought the unfit had no right to bear children.

A prominent New York urologist, William Robinson, proclaimed about people with mental retardation: "It is the acme of stupidity to talk in such cases of individual liberty, of the rights of the individual. . . . They have no right in the first instance to be born, but having been born, they have no right to propagate their kind."[6]

Social Darwinism and eugenics contradicted each other: if the white race would emerge triumphant, why worry about excessive breeding among other races? If the lower classes were so unfit as to be destined to die out, why prevent them from breeding?

Eugenics enjoyed popularity because of a pervasive bigotry (the same climate in Germany led to the rise of Hitler, anti-Semitism, and the Holocaust). The newspaper magnate William Hearst and Theodore Roosevelt thundered against "yellow niggers" who had invaded America from Asia. When Henry Ford ran for president in the 1920s, he promised to rid the country of the "Jew bankers," whom he accused of having caused America to enter World War I; later, he would accuse Jewish bankers of causing the Depression.[7]

The eugenics movement affected critical legislation in the United States. While the Nazis famously sterilized 225,000 "mental defectives," the United States also practiced large-scale involuntary sterilization. In 1907, Indiana first required sterilization of the retarded and criminally insane; 30 other states soon followed. California led the nation in sterilizations, accounting for nearly a third of the national total; Virginia was second and Indiana third.[8] By 1941, physicians had sterilized over 36,000 Americans against their will, often for the vague condition of "feeblemindedness" or because victims had been born into large families on welfare. Some states did not reverse their sterilization laws until the 1960s.

The eugenics movement lay behind the famous (1927) *Buck v. Bell* decision by the United States Supreme Court. Supposedly retarded like her mother, Carrie Buck had been committed at age 18 to a state mental institution in Virginia. Pregnant when committed, Carrie gave birth to a daughter inside the institution.

Harry Laughlin, an influential geneticist who worked at Cold Spring Harbor, concluded that Carrie Buck's retardation was hereditary. He based this conclusion not on his own examination but upon reading a written report of a social worker, who said Carrie had a"feeble look" about her. Laughlin then declared that Carrie Buck "lived a life of immorality and prostitution," and that all the Bucks belonged to the "shiftless, ignorant, worthless class of anti-social whites of the South."

The U.S. Supreme Court upheld in *Buck v. Bell* the legality of the Virginia law permitting Carrie Buck's sterilization. Justice Oliver Wendell Holmes wrote the majority opinion:

> It is better for all the world, if instead of waiting to execute degenerate offspring for crime, or to let them starve for their imbecility, society can prevent those who are manifestly unfit from continuing their kind. The principle that sustains compulsory vaccination is broad enough to cover cutting the Fallopian tubes. (He concluded that) "Three generations of imbeciles are enough."

The legacy of eugenics included the *Immigration Restriction Act of 1924*. Triumphantly hailed by eugenicists, it assumed the inferior genes of Asians, Africans, Greeks, Irish, Poles and Italians, and the superior genes of the English, Dutch, Scotch, Scandinavians, and Germans. President Calvin Coolidge enthusiastically signed the act into law. As vice president he said, "America must be kept American. Biological laws show . . . that Nordics deteriorate when mixed with other races."[9]

This Immigration Act established quotas according to countries of origin. Based on how many people from a given country were already in America, such quotas denied entry to people from "inferior" countries.

Indeed, America as a "melting pot" originally poured scorn on immigration. Similarly, the Statue of Liberty today symbolizes freedom, but after 1924, thousands of the world's "huddled masses" had only a glimpse of freedom before their boats were sent back.

Eugenicists assumed many false statements, including:

1. *The reductionist assumption* that each trait identified by morality or social distinctions was caused by a gene in a one-to-one relation. Prostitution, retardation, poverty, and criminality were each supposedly caused by a single gene.
2. *The reductionist assumption* that genes cause diseases in a simplistic, one-gene-to-one-disease way. A few genetic diseases, such as Huntington's and sickle cell, do work this way, but most do not.
3. *Ignorance about recessive inheritance.* Two unaffected carriers can each pass a gene for a recessive trait to a child, who will then be homozygous for the trait.
4. *Ignorance of environmental effects on expression of genes.* How a gene, or a combination of genes, is expressed depends in part on what happens during gestation, in early childhood, and in the overall environment. Genes have a fan-like range of expression (their norm of reaction), and which point on the fan manifests in a particular person depends on what happened in his or her environment.
5. *Naiveté about the ease of controlling reproduction* in couples. Humans are driven to have sex, and if they aren't careful, children result. When informed of risk of a child with genetic disease, few humans can or will prevent birth of children, especially without access to contraception!
6. *Ignorance of mutations and chromosomal breakage.* Not knowing about these aspects of genetics, eugenicists mistakenly believed that if all retarded people could be prevented from reproducing, retardation could be eliminated from the gene pool.
7. *Ignorance of population genetics.* Eugenicists hoped to perfect humanity through selective breeding, but population genetics have since shown that there will be a regression to the mean. *Regression to the mean* is the inherent tendency in stable populations to return to an average value over time; in population genetics, the underlying causes creating a mean value in a population will eventually normalize any deviant values.

After 1935, the eugenics movement declined in the United States. Geneticist Hermann J. Muller said that eugenics was "hopelessly perverted," a cult for "advocates for race and class prejudice, defenders of vested interests of church and State, Fascists, Hitlerites, and reactionaries generally."[10] Another leading geneticist, J. B. S. Haldane, said at the time of the sterilization programs that "many of the deeds done in America in the name of eugenics are about as much justified by science as were the proceedings of the Inquisition by the Gospels."[11] Advances in population genetics prompted Haldane to remark, "An ounce of algebra is worth a ton of verbal argument."[12]

Case 3: Testing for Diabetes

Maria Lopez, a 30-year-old woman, has type 2 diabetes and struggles to control it.[13] Her extended family in East Harlem in New York City includes many older diabetic relatives. At 5 feet, 6 inches, Maria weighs 267 pounds and considers herself overweight. She has always fought to control her weight, finding it hard to exercise, and loves French fries and soft drinks. Diagnosed with diabetes at age 15 after she was hospitalized for spells of fainting, she once lost 100 pounds, but has since gained it back.

Diabetes mellitus is a disease of high blood sugar levels (hyperglycemia) caused by insufficient secretion or function of insulin, a hormone produced by the pancreas. *Type 1 diabetes,* once called juvenile onset diabetes or insulin-dependent diabetes mellitus, has low or no secretion of insulin. In *type 2 diabetes,* once called adult-onset diabetes, obesity-related diabetes, or non-insulin-dependent diabetes mellitus, the body's cells are resistant to insulin.

Diabetes may soon reach epidemic proportions: The Centers for Disease Control estimates that 21 million Americans suffer from diabetes and another 41 million are prediabetic.[14] One of three Americans will become diabetic at some point in their lives. As they adopt Western diets high in fats and processed corn sugars, more people worldwide succumb each year.[15] Americans of Chinese, Korean, and Japanese ancestry develop type 2 diabetes at a rate 60 percent higher than whites.[16]

In 2006, epidemiologists discovered that over 800,000 of its citizens in New York City, more than one in eight, had type 2 diabetes.[17] This incidence in this city is a third higher than in the nation. In East Harlem, as many as one in five people has diabetes.[18]

Maria Lopez says her diabetes makes her miserable. "I have never wanted this disease to control my life." Since first diagnosed, she has denied her disease and that it could lead to her death. "I'm a traditionally built woman from a culture of strong, big women," she says. "I eat what I like. To hell with needles and machines."

Diabetics must monitor their blood sugar several times a day. In the past, they did so by drawing blood with real needles, but new, small kits allow miniscule, almost painless sticks to do the same, greatly reducing the hassle of monitoring one's blood sugar. Nevertheless, Maria used to find it embarrassing to use such kits around other teenagers, so she sometimes faked numbers on her daily sheets.

Diabetics should give up beer, cokes, French fries, potato chips, pies, cakes, and "everything else that tastes good," Maria says. But many diabetics in East Harlem live in poverty, stress, with easy access to junk foods.

Public health educators urge Maria to exercise daily and to eat a low-fat diet high in fresh fruits and vegetables. "That's not so easy to do," she says. "And my two daughters (aged ten and eight) like to go to McDonalds." Blood sugar monitoring consumes time and requires effort.

Uncontrolled diabetes leads to kidney failure, retinal damage and blindness, gangrene (especially in legs, leading to amputation), damage to nerves, and heart failure.

In public health, diabetes is "the Rodney Dangerfield of diseases," says the director of a diabetes center, "a stealth epidemic."[19] Research to cure diabetes gets far less money than cancer or AIDS. Most medical care for diabetics merely manages crises rather than trying to prevent the disease and its crises.

In 2006, scientists at DeCode Genetics discovered a gene for type 2 diabetes. The head of DeCode explained:

> If you have one copy of this variant, which 38 percent of people do, your risk of developing type 2 diabetes is increased by 40 percent," Stefansson, who is chief executive officer of DeCode, says. "Seven percent have two copies and have a 140 percent increase in risk."[20]

In understanding this result, it is important to distinguish between *absolute and relative risk*. In a population of a thousand, suppose 10 people are expected to have type 2 diabetes. If everyone in this population had one copy of this gene, then we would expect 14 people to develop this kind of diabetes, and for those with two copies, 24 people. So if the absolute risk of diabetes is low, say, in Africa, then having one or two copies of this new gene doesn't mean that huge numbers of people will get diabetes. As a 2009 survey of prediction of risk of disease from genetics remarked, "the great majority of the newly identified risk-marker alleles confer very small relative risks, ranging from 1.1 to 1.5."[21]

How then to explain the growing epidemic of type 2 diabetes in the developed world? Two answers: first, genetic studies reveal that most genetic conditions, such as type 2 diabetes, result from combination of several genes; second, such combinations produce diseases in combination with specific environmental causes, such as Western diets high in saturated fats and sugar.

Case 4: Testing for Alzheimer's Disease

By 2009, researchers had discovered that a specific group of genes may account for up to half of cases of Alzheimer's disease.[22] Studying 815 subjects, they compared 300 subjects carrying one and two copies of the gene with 500 people who did not. Subjects who had two copies of this allele had "accelerated neuropsychological decline in their early 60s" and "early amyloid deposition in frontal cortexes" (i.e., build-up of plaque in the part of the brain called the amygdala, responsible for memory of emotional responses). Some carriers of the allele also showed signs of mental decline in their 30s and 40s.

Alzheimer's creates fear in most people because it strikes at their identity. Consider Roy Smith, a 61-year-old male whose mother died of Alzheimer's disease and who worries that his memory isn't what it used to be. Could he have Alzheimer's, like his mother?

Preliminary evidence suggests that drinking alcohol accelerates the decline that accompanies Alzheimer's. If Roy tests positive for the gene, should his wife and son criticize him when they see him drink a few beers? What if Roy replies, "If you had my results, you'd want to drink some beers, too." If his family is going to get moralistic about his drinking, would it be better for Roy if he hadn't taken the test?

ETHICAL ISSUES

Responsibility, First Take

One philosophical question we want to consider in this chapter is this: when a disease has a genetic basis, how responsible, if at all, are people who get their diseases?

One thing we notice right off is that for some genetic diseases, no matter what people do, they will get the disease. Huntington's is like that, because it is autosomal dominant and with time, fully penetrant. That means that everyone with the gene who lives long enough will suffer the disease.

However, and this is very important, most diseases with genetic underpinnings are not like Huntington's. To think so would be to repeat the simple, reductionistic mistakes of the eugenics movement. For free will and responsibility, wrongly inferring that all diseases with genetic components are like Huntington's would encourage fatalism about many of these diseases that is scientifically incorrect.

As said, over their lives, women with BRCA1 or BRCA2 run an 80 percent risk of developing breast cancer, compared to a 9 percent risk for women without these genes. Both BRCA1 and BRCA2 are autosomal dominant genes. These genes seem like Huntington's in that, even if women live the most healthy lives, they will still get breast cancer. For such women, double mastectomy may be one of the only actions they can take to reduce their chances of getting breast cancer.

Things are more complex for diabetes. Consider whether Maria is *responsible* for getting diabetes. Normally, we recoil at this question because we realize that if we hold her responsible, she can be blamed for her disease. It's bad enough to have diabetes, why add to that by being moralistic?

Using the Golden Rule, we imagine what it would be like to get a diagnosis of diabetes ourselves: Do we want a moralistic physician saying, "You should have eaten better! Now you have nobody to blame but yourself."

But if type 2 diabetes is genetic, then isn't such blame incorrect? Wouldn't Maria have gotten diabetes anyway, no matter how she ate? In the words of the debate over free will, isn't it false that she "could have done otherwise"? Even if her disease is partly environmental and due to poor diet, didn't something cause her to *crave* bad foods? So isn't blame about diabetes just stupid?

Isn't lack of blame much more clear with Roy and Alzheimer's? Given Roy's two copies of the APOE 4 gene, there isn't much he can do to avoid Alzheimer's, right? Well, yes and no. Evidence suggests that drinking alcohol accelerates the decline of people with this gene. Moreover, taking cognitively enhancers such as donepezil may prevent onset of severe symptoms of Alzheimer's by six months. Moreover, the most significant way to maintain brain activity is by increasing blood flow, and the best, safest way to do that is through exercise. If we discovered that Roy had done nothing to prevent his Alzheimer's, couldn't we say that he could have delayed some of it?

Recall that, when a person has two copies of the gene rather than one (is homozygous rather than heterozygous), risk of developing type 2 diabetes jumps 100 percent from 40 to 140 percent above normal. A large amount of evidence in genetics suggests that this *one-hit, two-hit model* explains many things. If you have two "hits" or copies of BRAC1, your chances of getting breast cancer jump from low to high. It is the same with diabetes and Alzheimer's. If there is a gene for being gay or lesbian, then the same may be true: two copies and you're attracted to members of the same sex at an early age, but with only one copy, it varies.

Most people with genetic components of conditions will have only one gene or one copy of a genetic variant. That means that what happens in their environment, or how they behave, will play a major role in whether or when they develop the condition. This one-hit-two-hit model has major implications for personal responsibility, motivation to be healthy, genetic fatalism, and presymptomatic testing.

On the other hand, a person with two copies of genes for diabetes, Alzheimer's, or any other genetic disease is much more likely to get the disease. Still, it's not as bad as Huntington's, where everyone who lives long enough gets it, because 80 percent is not 100 percent.

Testing as Self-Interest

Testing for genes for breast cancer may benefit the woman affected. Even with surgery, radiation, and chemotherapy for breast cancer, about 20 percent of women will still die from it. For this reason, significant percentages of women testing positive for breast cancer or for the genes BRCA1 or BRCA2 decided to remove both breasts in hopes of living to old age.

This is a significant ethical issue whose pedigree requires some explanation. In the 1960s, many women under 50 with breast cancer elected to have a bilateral mastectomy to remove both cancerous and precancerous tissue from their breasts.[23] In the 1970s and 1980s, studies showed that for most women with breast cancer, those getting a lumpectomy fared no worse than women getting bilateral mastectomies. Because significant percentages of women experienced loss of femininity and self-esteem after their mastectomies, sparing them this surgery was thought to be a benefit.

However, the current view is that women with the breast cancer genes have an 80 percent chance of developing breast cancer during their lives, so for them bilateral mastectomy holds out a chance to prevent the cancer from starting at all.

Even before clinical trials finished, large numbers of women testing positive for BRCA1 and BRCA2 had preventive bilateral mastectomies. In 2002, a clinical trial proved that, five years after surgery, women with a BRCA1 or BRCA2 mutation undergoing prophylactic bilateral mastectomy have a statistically significant lower risk of breast cancer.

However, if there is any lesson in the ethics of genetic testing, it is that everything is complicated. Later studies suggested that the figure of 80 percent risk was exaggerated. Women with breast cancer initially recruited for studies of the two breast cancer genes came from families with breast cancer in grandmothers, mothers, daughters, and sisters, resulting in a selection bias.[24] So, based on biased data showing their high risk of breast cancer, some women had their breasts removed.

Now add another twist. Besides the three mutations of BRCA1, BRCA2, and CHEK2 that cause breast cancer, hundreds of variant mutations now are known, each conferring a different degree of risk. Moreover, the risk of each variant may vary with the peculiarities of each family. Conveying all this information accurately requires sophistication by patient and genetic counselor.

But the history of genetics shows that sophistication and understanding of subtle, complex issues are not strengths of public policy or among the public. Women are likely to think, "I have the breast cancer gene" and fear death in a few years from breast cancer.

If a woman has BRCA1, BRCA2 or CHEK2, the benefits of knowing early are that taking birth control pills reduces risk of ovarian cancer by 60 percent and taking the drug tamoxifen reduces risk of breast cancer by nearly half. More radically, prophylactic bilateral mastectomy increases longevity. These same benefits apply to men, who account for about 2 percent of all cases of breast cancer.

Similarly, testing for the gene for type 2 diabetes could lead to benefits for Maria Lopez, especially if she could adopt a healthy lifestyle. For Maria and especially her daughters, it will be important to eat a low-fat, low-processed-sugar diet and to exercise to keep their weight normal. In some cases, a positive test for the type 2 gene could be a wake-up call to adopt a healthy lifestyle.

Testing for Alzheimer's could lead to some benefits, even for people with two copies of the gene. Knowing she will need someone to take care of her in old age, a woman might become very loving toward her spouse and children. She might avoid all alcohol and take donepezil (trade name, Aricept). She might exercise daily to maximize blood flow, the primary preventive of early dementia.

Testing Only to Hear Good News

When people take genetic tests, do they really understand what they're doing? One genetics counselor says, "When people say they want this test to find out if they have the gene so they can make decisions, they really want to find out that they don't have it."[25]

Yet half of people at risk for Huntington's will have the gene, and some people will have two copies of genes for diabetes, Alzheimer's, and cancer. And there's no way to prepare them for this terrible news.

In the first study of presymptomatic tests for Huntington's, most people at risk originally said they would take the test, but after counseling, some changed their minds.[26]

The same study reported that "[p]articipants found to be probable gene carriers reported being surprised or shocked by the test result."[27] They had not expected to have the lethal gene.

Another consideration is that self-knowledge is seldom perfect. As the SUPPORT study showed, many people simply cannot predict how they will react to bad news, here testing positive for a terrible genetic condition.

Since Huntington's or Alzheimer's cannot be cured or ameliorated, a positive test will tell someone that she is going to die an early, terrible death. Not everyone can deal with such knowledge. As Nancy Wexler says, for some people, especially teenagers and young adults, such knowledge could be a toxic burden, warping their lives.

Moreover, when little treatment is available, is it wise to give people such a diagnosis? Perhaps people should not be burdened with more truth than they can bear.[28]

On the positive side, testing for genes for breast cancer or diabetes allows intervention at an early stage. In one family, one of two sisters at hereditary risk worried about developing breast cancer and had planned to have her breasts removed as a preventive measure; she took the test for breast cancer genes, which turned out to be negative, and she canceled her surgery. Her sister did not think she was at risk and had refused mammograms but discovered she had the BRCA1 gene. A previous examination of her breasts had found nothing, but a reexamination found a minuscule node, and a biopsy determined that cancer had already begun, so a radical mastectomy was performed. Without the genetic test, this second sister might not have discovered her cancer until many years later.

Testing also allays fears of women who are incorrectly certain they have such genes when they do not. Also, for some women, a mysterious, random turn of fate becomes testable and predictable. Although all women who test positive dislike the news, and although some who tested negative felt guilty, almost all think it's better to have a way to know.

Testing as a Duty to One's Family

Knowing one's likely genetic fate isn't just a concern of individuals. People are not atomistic; they come embedded in families, with children and parents, brothers and sisters.

The major argument favoring testing for serious genetic disease concerns childbearing. Nancy Wexler did not have children for fear that one might inherit Huntington's, yet perhaps her decision was misguided. If she had taken the test and been negative, she could have had children unaffected by Huntington's.

On the other hand, people who test positive should not have children or should test embryos and implant ones lacking the Huntington's gene. Why is that? Because parents should want the best lives for their children, and such lives start with freedom from genetic disease. No parent should willingly inflict a serious genetic disease on his or her child.

A second argument for testing concerns spouses and caretakers. Consider the following example. A man who was at risk for Huntington's (he could have just as easily been at risk for Alzheimer's) but had decided not to take the test discussed his reasons before a large medical class. His reasons were greeted with respect; but as the class ended and the students started to file out, a woman cried out from the back of the room, "What about me and the kids? What about my view about testing him?" It was the man's wife.

She wanted to be able to plan for the future. If her husband were positive, she would be taking care of him. She might also have been thinking of money:

if her husband was positive, he would eventually need custodial care, and they would have to start saving up for that or, if possible, arrange for life or health insurance. Moreover, when these neurological diseases strike, the family as well as the victim will suffer emotionally; they should prepare themselves for this. Finally, they might try to make the most of whatever time remains before onset.

Besides a strict duty to one's family, compromises are possible. For instance, middle-aged people who do not want to know may feel that they have escaped the disease and that they can now take the test as a gift to their children. Another compromise is to have blood samples taken and stored for later testing.

Testing One's Family by Testing Oneself

In any genetic testing, testing one family member has inevitable implications for other members of the family. In more ways than one, the results of testing affect the entire family.

In one family where a woman tested for hereditary breast cancer, confidentiality was very difficult to maintain among the women of the extended families. It was hard for a woman to resist her family and not discover her status: in testing a middle-aged woman for some genetically dominant conditions, one is also telling her mother and her daughters their risk of developing breast cancer.

It is important to keep in mind that in testing for dominant, single-gene diseases, such as Huntington's and the breast cancer genes, there is no such thing as testing only a fetus or testing only a parent: a positive fetus reveals a positive parent; a positive parent reveals that any children are at risk.

Helping families understand genetic testing is difficult. Hayes notes, "Many medical professionals have difficulty viewing genetic issues in a family context. . . . Most researchers cannot possibly know what it is like to grow up in a family haunted by a genetic disease. . . . "

Testing may tear families apart. Consider the right to know. Even in a life-or-death situation, judges have ruled that relatives cannot be compelled to be tested for compatibility as bone marrow or organ donors. Such decisions indicate that judges will not force genetic tests on relatives.

If a person tested positive for Alzheimer's and concealed it from a prospective spouse, could that be grounds for annulment? Does a prospective spouse have a right to know about such a test? Or does marrying "for better or worse" cover such questions?

Can one parent have a child tested in order to find out if the other parent is affected? Suppose that a father tests positive for Huntington's and refuses to tell his teenage daughter, Laura. Suppose that a genetic counselor is aware of the father's result. When Laura gets married, what should the counselor do? Recommend general genetic tests to her? Suppose she refuses. If she knew that her father was positive, would she agree to testing? If so, should the counselor violate the father's confidentiality? To many people, the good of preventing another child with Huntington's outweighs the harm of violating privacy, especially where there is a strong sense that the affected parent had an obligation to reveal his result in the first place.

One advocate for families afflicted with genetic disease believes that:

> First and foremost, genetic testing must be viewed as a family issue, not an individual one. The person who enrolls in a testing program should be strongly encouraged to involve other family members, within reason. Testing one member of a family will affect other members. Persons who refuse to involve their families may not have considered fully the consequences for other members or for themselves.[29]

Personal Responsibility for Disease

Let us return to the question of the responsibility of Roy, Joan, and Maria for their diseases. Of course, the positive side of this question is whether Roy, Joan, and Maria can do anything to *prevent* getting these diseases.

The answer may be, "Yes and no." We can approach the question of responsibility in a less moralistic way by taking a different approach. Suppose Joan, Roy, and Maria each have teenagers and that all three parents want to reduce the chances that these children will suffer these diseases. The crucial question is then: *Can these teenagers avoid these diseases?*

Put this way, we are not being moralistic. Instead, we are doing conceptual, preventive work. Assume good education, maximal free will, and good familial support for good eating. Then ask, "Under such ideal conditions, if Maria's daughter inherits her genetic risk, can they avoid diabetes? Can Joan's daughter avoid breast cancer? Can Roy's son avoid Alzheimer's?"

These questions can be asked at different levels. First, metaphysical: does free will exist? Second, moral: are patients partly responsible for their diseases or good health? Third, clinical: how much change toward healthy lifestyles can physicians expect of at-risk patients?

Type 2 diabetes is an especially good candidate for prevention because we know that many Asian people do not get diabetes until they adopt Western lifestyles. (Similarly, for Asian men immigrating to North American, incidence of prostate cancer jumps from 1 per 100,000 to 70 per 100,000.[30]) The prevailing view about preventing diabetes is this:

> What is especially disturbing about the rise of type 2 [diabetes] is that it can be delayed and perhaps prevented with changes in diet and exercise. For although both types are believed to stem in part from genetic factors, type 2 is also spurred by obesity and inactivity. This is particularly true in those prone to illness.[31]

So are 21 million Americans "failures" in personal responsibility because they have diabetes? Are another 10 million "successes" because they staved off genetic predisposition?[32] Perhaps.

In 2007, researchers followed 91,000 women and discovered that those who drank one or more cans of soft drinks a day, compared to those drinking less than one can a month, were twice as likely to develop type 2 diabetes. If nothing else, women who carry genes for diabetes can stop drinking soft drinks.

Let us take a larger perspective with cancer. Cancer occurs when tumor-suppressing genes or DNA repair mechanisms cease to work, resulting in wild, uncontrolled growth of cells. Diabetes occurs when the body fails to allow cells to take up glucose from the blood.

Both diseases occur when environmental inputs trigger potential in an inherited genetic template. At the very least, avoidance of the inputs can delay onset of disease and perhaps avoid it altogether (people with genetic dispositions to alcoholism do not become alcoholics in countries where alcohol is banned). As a person ages, his or her immune system and organs deteriorate, and mutated cells in her body accumulate, making her more vulnerable to cancer and diabetes, so many people, despite healthy lifestyles, will eventually succumb to their genetic risk.[33]

Society can exert some control over how many carcinogens people ingest: it can ban tobacco in schools and hospitals, forbid smoking in public, and steeply tax tobacco. Similarly, it can ban junk foods and sodas from schools. Individuals at risk for cancer and diabetes can eat low-fat diets high in fiber, fresh fruits, and vegetables. In this way, both societies and individuals can reduce the incidence of cancer and diabetes.

But what if a daughter gets cancer or diabetes anyway? Should she be blamed? Answer: probably not. To say that these diseases can be partially preventable by healthy living is not to say that some cases aren't, like Huntington's disease, genetically inevitable. Second, other factors in a person's life may have prevented healthy living such that a person truly could not have done otherwise. In these cases, blame would be wrong.

Testing and Sick Identities

Nancy Wexler rejects an attitude she found dominant among the medical community about testing, which might be expressed as: "Come on! Take your knowledge like a man and don't be a sissy."

This attitude benefits the medical community and family more than the individual affected. If there is no cure for Huntington's or Alzheimer's, what's so good about knowing?

Nancy Wexler thinks that people who test positive for a disease, long before they experience any symptoms, may adopt a *sick identity* about it. If you're going to get Huntington's, she argues, you will in fact get it, so there's nothing you can do about it. Why burden yourself being self-identified as sick long before you are actually sick?

Moreover, some people are highly suggestible. People who are concerned about suicide often focus on the consequences of testing teenagers—a population that is already highly suicidal. Youngsters merely at risk for Huntington's, breast cancer, or diabetes already agonize about going to college and spending their parents' money, and those who learn for certain that they have these genes may be even more vulnerable.

Should girls under 18 years of age be tested for these genes if these genes run in their families? At first glance, the answer seems no, for a positive answer might take away the fun of childhood and adolescence. Moreover, great danger exists of developing a sick identity as a "woman with breast cancer" or a "woman who will get diabetes." On the other hand, eating junk food and smoking start early in many teenagers, so early testing might be beneficial.

Preventing Suicide by Not Knowing

Because 25 percent of people with Huntington's consider suicide and 10 percent carry it out,[34] scientists have debated whether tests for such diseases should be given. Nancy Wexler said, "We have to understand that the day you tell someone he has this gene, his life and view of himself change forever. We're worried about the potential for suicide."[35]

Is suicide an adequate reason for not testing? Even if some percent commit suicide, most will not. Nancy Wexler says, "Suicide is not unreasonable. It's not so awful that we can't discuss it or consider it." She observes, "For some of my friends who have Huntington's, knowing that they can commit suicide gives them a certain sense of control. They want to feel that if it gets too bad, they can have a way out. They can do something."[36]

Some scientists argue against paternalism: "I think we can trust people to make these decisions. I'm not so convinced we researchers should be dictating how the technology gets used."[37]

Testing Only with Good Counseling

Many people who are not absolutely opposed to testing—and even people who generally favor testing—argue that testing should be offered *only with good counseling*. Especially because the results will be probabilistic for most people (not "You don't have the gene," but "You have a 90 percent chance of not having the gene.").

This is, of course, paternalistic. However, it is true that some of those who test positive will wish they hadn't taken the test and some may develop emotional problems, and that counseling can help such people. As a matter of public policy, should people simply be allowed to buy their own test results through their private physicians, or should counseling be required?

The President's Commission on Bioethics (1983) emphasized that counseling should be guaranteed: "A full range of prescreening and follow-up services . . . should be available before a program [of genetic testing] is introduced."[38] Note, though, that the recommendation here is for making counseling available, not mandatory.

This is not a realistic policy. First, 44 million Americans lack medical insurance and would need to buy genetic counseling, an expensive proposition. Second, just finding a trained genetics counselor is not easy, and many people do not live near a major medical center that has such a skilled counselor. Even for people with good medical coverage for physical illnesses, most policies today do not provide good coverage for genetic counseling.

Nevertheless, this issue will not go away, especially in North America and England where commercial companies aggressively market direct-to-consumer genetic testing. Although such companies say genetic counseling is available after they test people, this seems like the wrong time to offer such testing, for the reasons stated above, namely, that after good counseling, many people decided *not* to be tested. But the commercial companies surely won't pay counselors to give that kind of advice to prospective clients. We discuss such companies more below.

Genetic Testing and Insurance

Genetic testing raises financial issues. For example, when one woman who tested positive decided to have a preventive radical mastectomy, she didn't want to tell her insurance company the reason for her decision because she was afraid her company would cancel her policy or raise her premiums, and perhaps even do the same for her daughters. Because her insurer didn't know anything, it thought she was being irrational and wouldn't pay for her surgery.

An important issue about genetic testing and medical insurance concerns confidentiality. Several national companies (such as Medical Information Bureau of Boston) inform insurance companies about applicants who are risks.[39] For people who take presymptomatic genetic tests and test positive, insurers could raise premiums for families. Worse, they could consider the result evidence of a preexisting condition and exclude that disease from future coverage.

For this reason, it is crucial to control the distribution of test results: that is, to decide who should and should not receive them. Many large institutions, such as the military, universities, and large companies, self-insure themselves and pass their losses along to employees through increased premiums. Moreover, some employers may not keep test results confidential, especially if key employees are involved; consequently, a positive result may keep an executive off the fast track. Violation of confidentiality might also keep a physician out of a medical group, a student out of a university or graduate school, and so on.

Congress in 2008 finally passed GINA, the *Genetic Information Nondiscrimination Act*. This federal law bans insurers from using knowledge about a person's genes (or the genes of her family) to determine eligibility for insurance or rates of premiums, or employers from using the same as a basis for hiring, firing, or assigning jobs.[40] Because of likelihood of adverse selection, GINA does not apply to people applying for life insurance or for coverage for disability or long-term care.

Genetic testing reveals the gaps in America's national, medical *nonsystem*. If everyone who tests positive for genetic disease can get expensive medical coverage, while those who test negative are allowed to opt out, insurance companies will quickly go bankrupt. As genetic testing stresses this stopgap system, inequities of future health that it reveals may force us to adopt a national, single-payer system (for more on this, see the last chapter).

Diabetes and genetic testing for it exposes similar problems. Almost no money is spent by medical centers for education and counseling to prevent diabetes because doing so generally loses money. In contrast, waiting until crises develop and then amputating gangrenous legs produces profits (because insurance reimburses physicians well for doing surgical procedures, not for talking to patients).[41] Similarly, insurance companies curtail benefits to diabetics to discourage them from enrolling in their plans: "In a 2003 survey, 87 percent of health insurance actuaries . . . said that if they were to improve coverage [for diabetics] with richer drug benefits or easier access to specialists, they would incur financial problems by attracting the sickest, most expensive patients."[42]

Premature Announcements and Over-simplifications

Almost every week, someone announces discovery of a gene for a disease. Yet almost all such reports mislead us into thinking the genetic revolution has come. For example, in 2007, researchers identified a gene that was a "risk factor" for heart disease.[43] Yet for previous announcements of 85 factors in 75 genes, when scientists examined the proof that they caused heart disease, they concluded that exactly zero "of the genes were more common in heart patients than in healthy people."[44]

In 1987, researchers retracted an earlier claim that manic depression was linked to a gene on the X chromosome.[45] By this time, earlier claims about genetic causes of schizophrenia and alcoholism had been retracted.

Today, geneticists believe that psychiatric disorders such as schizophrenia will not be found to be single-gene disorders. According to one leading researcher, common forms of mental illness may be caused by three to five genes acting together, probably with environmental cofactors.[46]

Like eugenics, much of the news about genetics in today's mass media is simplistic, alarmist, reductionistic, and premature.

The movie *Gattaca* (a good movie to watch relating to this chapter) illustrates these misconceptions, scaring us about, without GINA, the uses to which presymptomatic testing could be put. *Gattaca*'s real theme is about the power of labeling and the effects of such labeling on a family, individual, and society. Like being labeled "schizophrenic," being labeled "precancerous" or "precardiomyopathy" may so powerfully affect a person that it cripples his ambition and makes him a quasi-patient decades before he has any symptoms. And how horrible such toxic labeling would be if it were based on mistakes, such as assuming a variable genetic disease was fully penetrant.

Caveat Emptor: Making Money from Genetic Testing

In 2002, Myriad Genetics of Salt Lake City expanded its sales force from 85 to 600 agents to market BRCA1 testing directly to doctors and their patients. The tests, which cost between $750 and $2,750, would benefit only the 5 to 10 percent of people with breast cancer caused by these genes.

Unfortunately, BRCA1's discovery offered hope of a screening test only for women with hereditary breast and ovarian cancer—not for the 90 to 95 percent of women who develop nonhereditary breast cancer.

In some ways, marketing such tests is a win-win situation for Myriad Genetics. For the people who test positive, they get their money's worth and advance news. For the people who test negative, they get relief and will not complain about the money spent. The ethical issue arises when thousands of people seek relief who are really not at risk: they waste their money in getting a negative result. But it would be patronizing to say they can't spend their money as they choose, even irrationally.

Note that similar tests could be offered for genes for prostate cancer or diabetes, where only a small percentage of which is caused by a single gene. For most people, such testing would be a waste of money.

The hot item today in commercial genetics is a thousand dollar test to sequence a citizen's personal genome. Supposedly, this kind of test at this cost is just around the corner (although journalists have made this claim for about seven years now and the cost is still about $9,000 away).

For some people, such sequencing may give good information, especially if genetic cofactors of disease are accurately identified. For them, learning that they have two genes for type 2 diabetes may cause them to keep their weight in check, to eat healthfully, and exercise. But as Angela Trepanier, president-elect of the National Society of Genetics Counselors, says, many people are genetic fatalists and will say, "To hell with it. I'm doomed anyway. Where's the cheesecake?"[47]

The other great danger of such an overall test is contained in the aphorism, "Be careful what you wish for." A person buying such a test may expect a certain kind of news, but he may get unexpected news that is traumatic; for example, that one of the people he believed to be his parent is not really his biological ancestor. Or he may test to rule out cancer and heart disease, but discover he carries two copies of powerful genes for schizophrenia or Alzheimer's. Obviously, buyers should study these issues and carefully discuss their emotional intelligence, i.e., whether they can carry unexpected, genetic bad news without being aroused or agitated.

Blame and Responsibility: Final Thoughts

Genetic testing may lead each of us to think more carefully about causes of gene-associated diseases. Presymptomatic testing may give some people a small window of preventive control. People at risk for cancers of the breast or prostate may be able to avoid smoking or being around secondhand smoke (exposure of children to the latter among smoking parents is strongly associated with later development of diabetes when children grow up[48]).

Previously, three standards of evidence were discussed that are used in the law: preponderance of evidence, clear and convincing evidence, and beyond a reasonable doubt. These standards can be used to make a point. We know beyond a reasonable doubt that no one with Huntington's disease can do anything to prevent this disease from destroying their brains and killing them. We also know that, for people with single genes for breast cancer or Huntington's, or with two genes for Alzheimer's, diabetes, and other cancers, 80 percent of them will develop the disease.

This brings us to people with one gene for a disease like diabetes. Probably the best chance that prediabetics have to prevent diabetes is as children and adolescents, before they become overweight and have high levels of blood sugar. If they enter young adulthood overweight and accustomed to eating lots of processed sugars, the probability that they will develop diabetes is high.

Does that mean they should later be blamed for their disease? No. To hand out blame, we would need to know, at least with clear and convincing evidence, that they could have acted otherwise and eaten/exercised differently. It may be true that they could have, just as it may be true that the presumption of innocence allows some of the guilty to go free.

Also, people who do not have genes for type 2 diabetes cannot really know what it's like to crave fats and sugars and to be tormented by these cravings. Yes, everyone is tempted, but some are tempted so much more intensely and continually than others! Until we have evidence that prediabetics could have acted otherwise, we should not blame them as individuals or in public policy. We would need evidence beyond a reasonable doubt to do so, evidence we are unlikely to ever have.

Nevertheless, as with the hero of *Gattaca*, we should educate the young to think they can transcend their genetic dispositions. We want to give people hope. At the same time, when they turn out to be less-than-ideal, we don't want to condemn them.

Responsibility exists on a gradient, corresponding to an upward slope of free will. Two people with the same genes, placed at birth in different families (like Dickens's *The Prince and the Pauper*) may have differing degrees of free will and responsibility for their health or disease. This makes sense. Even so-called identical twins are identical for disease only 60 percent of the time, proving that having a specific DNA sequence doesn't doom one to a disease.[49]

Responsibility also exists on a social gradient. Poor people from dysfunctional families with no medical insurance, with genes predisposing them to diabetes or cancer, and little education, have less free will than well-educated young adults from loving, well-off families with good medical coverage who are blessed to have inherited good genes.

Finally, we need to avoid both a simplistic genetic fatalism ("I've got a gene for X, so I'm doomed!") and also a simplistic moralism ("You could've done X and prevented this!"). Neither attitude seems compatible with emerging facts. The history of eugenics shows that we always oversimplify issues in public policy. We will do so again.

FURTHER READING AND RESOURCES

Catherine Hayes, "Genetic Testing for Huntington's—A Family Issue," *New England Journal of Medicine* 327, no. 20, 1993.

Daniel Kevles, *In the Name of Eugenics: Genetics and the Uses of Human Heredity*, New York, Knopf, 1985.

Lenny Moss, *What Genes Can't Do*, Cambridge, MIT Press, 2004.

Matt Ridley, *Genome: The Autobiography of a Species in 23 Chapters*, New York, Harper Collins, 2000.

DISCUSSION QUESTIONS

1. How could some presymptomatic testing be considered toxic for the individual testing, especially testing at an early age?
2. Are couples testing their embryos or fetuses for Down syndrome, with the possibility of abortion, practicing eugenics?
3. To what degree, if any, are prediabetics like Maria Lopez and her daughters responsible for getting diabetes?
4. How do most claims about genetics oversimplify complex kinds of causation?
5. Why will most people taking genetic testing not get good value from their money?

CHAPTER 15

Preventing the Global Spread of AIDS

This chapter emphasizes prevention of the spread of acquired immune deficiency syndrome (AIDS) around the world as a challenge for bioethics. Such prevention may be the ultimate classic case because, by the end of 2007, over 58 million humans have already become infected or died of human immunodeficiency disease (HIV).[1] Millions more become infected each year, raising the question of how to slow this scourge.

The heart of the chapter discusses four approaches to stopping AIDS. As it explains, part of our problem stems from conflicts between these approaches. The chapter's essential question for discussion is: what role should ethics play in stopping the worldwide spread of HIV?

The chapter also discusses past epidemics, medical facts about AIDS, scandals about HIV infection of the blood supply, Kimberly Bergalis's case, homosexuality, contact tracing, mandatory screening, and needle-exchange programs.

BACKGROUND: EPIDEMICS, PLAGUES, AND AIDS

Throughout human history, epidemics have terrified humans. The bacterial disease known as the *Black Death* or simply, the *plague,* erupted in 1348 in Europe. It had two forms: *bubonic plague,* the most common and classic, characterized by inflamed swelling of the lymphatic glands in the groin and armpits, and was transmitted by fleas. Rats and other small mammals carried fleas to humans, and flea bites transmitted plague to humans. The bacillus *Yersinia pestis* causes bubonic plague. Untreated bubonic plague killed 50 percent of its victims. Today, antibiotics treat its earliest stages.

A virulent complication of untreated bubonic plague, *pneumonic plague,* involved the lungs. Easily transmitted by coughing, the microbe killed almost universally. Because of it, many physicians of the fourteenth century abandoned their profession.

In the same century, astrologers claimed that plague resulted from the conjunction of Saturn, Mars, and Jupiter; others claimed it resulted from sulfurous fumes released by earthquakes. Clergy taught that God had sent it to punish humans for great sins.

Historian Barbara Tuchman tells us that during medieval epidemics, "Organized groups of 200 to 300 . . . marched from city to city, stripped to the waist, scourging themselves with leather whips tipped with iron spikes until they bled. While they cried aloud to Christ and the Virgin for pity, . . . the watching townspeople sobbed in sympathy."[2] In so marching, they spread infected fleas.

The fearful ignorance of the times required *scapegoats* (in the Bible, goats were sacrificed to atone for bad things and as sacrifices to ward off worse things). So people accused Orthodox Jews, with their distinctive dress, of poisoning wells and spreading the plague. When atonement processions reached cities, they often attacked the Jewish quarter, trapped Jews inside, and set the area on fire. When plague followed, Jews were blamed, not the procession (which had brought the fleas).

Leprosy, cholera, and syphilis also terrified people. Leprosy, or Hansen's disease, creates lesions on the skin and kills slowly over years. Twentieth-century medicine learned that people get infected only through exposure over many months through the skin or mucosa. Before then, society banished lepers and forced them to live in isolated colonies, if they walked outside, lepers were required to ring cowbells to warn people of their presence.

Great epidemics of cholera from infected water also created fear of its victims. During the epidemic of 1813, Americans blamed those who fell ill, especially wanton prostitutes, drunken Irish, lazy blacks, and the dirty poor who lived along creeks used for both drinking water and defecation. Ministers praised God for cholera for "cleansing the filth from society."

In 1854, physician John Snow realized that cholera broke out only in the district that received water from the Broad Street pump in London. He discovered that infected water spread cholera and that clean water could prevent it. Nevertheless, many Americans stubbornly believed that sin and being Irish caused cholera, so many more died in the third great cholera epidemic of 1862.

Not until acceptance of the germ theory of disease after 1900 did public health prevent epidemics of cholera. In other words, it took a half a century for a medical insight to be translated into public policy to save millions of lives.

Victims of syphilis were also blamed for their disease. As discussed earlier, moralists blamed vice for the disease whereas scientists blamed spirochetes. (Chapter 10 on the Tuskegee Study discusses syphilis.)

A Brief History of AIDS

The first proven case of HIV came from a blood sample collected in 1959 from a man in Kinshasa, Democratic Republic of Congo. Genetic analysis of his blood suggests that HIV-1 may have stemmed from a virus that existed in the early 1940s or even the late 1930s.

Researcher Beatrice Hahn and her team at University of Alabama at Birmingham (UAB) proved in 1999 by DNA sequencing that the virus spread to humans from wild chimpanzees in southern Cameroon; HIV infected the blood of hunters there through catching, killing, and cutting up these chimps for bushmeat.[3]

Around 1978, gay men in the United States, Sweden, and Haiti begin to show signs of what would later be called AIDS. Between 1979 and 1981, Kaposi's sarcoma and *Pneumocystis carinii* pneumonia (PCP) unexpectedly showed up in gay males in Los Angeles and New York.

On June 5, 1981, the Centers for Disease Control (CDC) announced the discovery of a mysterious "gay-related infectious disease" (GRID) that had killed 3 gay men; only a month later, 108 cases of GRID were reported and 46 gay men were dead.

Three months after the first report of GRID in the summer of 1981, CDC announced that babies of drug-dependent women in New York City also had the disease; GRID was changed to AIDS.

In 1982, when physicians in New York and California had already seen hundreds of cases of AIDS, they still did not know its incubation or causative agent. CDC guessed that incubation could be many years and that many thousands of people could be infected. No one then diagnosed with AIDS had ever lived more than two years, so the disease frightened everyone.

In 1983, Luc Montagnier and the Institut Pasteur in France discovered that a virus, HIV, caused AIDS. Today this virus is called HIV-1. In 1986, scientists discovered a second form in West Africa, HIV-2, where it may have been infecting residents for decades. HIV-2 seems to develop more slowly and to be milder than HIV-1 but to be more easily transmitted heterosexually (the United States has reported few cases of HIV-2).[4]

As early as 1982, the CDC warned that donated blood could carry the agent causing AIDS. Blood then could have been screened for hepatitis, thereby indirectly screening for HIV, but officials deemed this too expensive and unfortunately did not do it.

In 1984, the FDA approved the enzyme-linked immunosorbent assay (ELISA) test for antibodies to HIV. Now blood donated or otherwise obtained could be tested for HIV. However, authorities running blood banks did not immediately test blood using the ELISA test. Why?

First, various groups politicized every fact about HIV and AIDS. A little historical background shows how this occurred. This background may predict what would occur if severe acute respiratory syndrome (SARS) or a lethal bird flu became epidemic.

AIDS and Ideology

By the end of 1981, CDC epidemiologists realized that gay men were being killed by a new kind of infectious disease of unknown nature and transmission. CDC postulated that sex among gay men might be spreading the disease, especially sex with anonymous partners in bathhouses in cities such as New York and San Francisco.

These bathhouses constituted what epidemiologists call an *amplification system* for the spread of a disease. Because some of the men had many anonymous sexual partners, some of whom, in turn, traveled to other places for sex with many numbers of partners, the virus could spread quickly. Another such system was easy, cheap travel by jet around the world. At one point, CDC identified a gay airline steward as Patient Zero, the first person to bring HIV from Africa to the United States and to introduce it to gay bathhouses, but later admitted that Patient Zero was an artifice, as HIV came to America from many different infected people.[5]

Sharing needles and syringes to inject drugs constitutes another amplification system. Blood withdrawn from a user's vein mixes both with a drug in the syringe and with viral particles from previous users.

A community's blood supply constitutes another amplification system. Blood banks pool both plasma and clotting factor for hemophiliacs from many sources. So one infected donation can infect many recipients.

The CDC called upon federal and state governments to fund studies to see if a new lethal disease had appeared in the blood system, but none responded. At the time, medical experts believed that all lethal infectious diseases had been discovered, so no one expected a new one to emerge.

By 1981, gay men and lesbians had won some freedom from historical prejudice against them: resistance against oppressive police round-ups began in June 1969 at a bar called the Stonewall Inn in Greenwich Village in New York City. Gay men there resisted the harassment by police in an event known as the Stonewall Riots, which fostered a new pride and encouraged gay men to come out of the closet (of shame and secrecy in which they had been hiding their sexual identity).

In North America and Europe during the 1970s, sexual freedom spread among heterosexuals, fueled by birth control, permissive attitudes toward nonmarital sex, Woodstock, mind-altering drugs, and rebellion against authority. So gay men and lesbians rode the crest of a larger fire of sexual change burning through traditional society. In medicine, psychiatrists removed homosexuality from their list of psychiatric illnesses.

But many people still despised gay men. Reverend Jerry Falwell, who founded Moral Majority, a religious political organization, blamed gays for AIDS. In 1982, the secretary of Moral Majority, Greg Dixon, wrote, "If homosexuals are not stopped, they will in time infect the entire nation, and America will be destroyed—as entire civilizations have fallen in the past."[6] This attitude persists. In 2001 when the World Trade Center was destroyed, Reverend Falwell and Minister Pat Robertson blamed gays and atheists for the event, saying it was God's punishment on America, echoing earlier clergy who had scapegoated Jews for plague and the Irish for cholera.[7]

The head of the Southern Baptist Convention said that God had created AIDS to "indicate His displeasure with the homosexual lifestyle."[8] Monsignor Edward Clark of St. John's University in Queens, New York, claimed that, "If gay men would stop promiscuous sodomy, the AIDS virus would disappear from America."[9] Politician and media commentator Patrick Buchanan decried, "The poor homosexuals—they have declared war on nature and now nature is exacting an awful retribution."[10]

Reverend Falwell, who died in 2007, advocated shutting down bathhouses where gay men engaged in anonymous sex. Owners of such bathhouses countered with ads in gay newspapers extolling freedom and lambasting Falwell as a bigot. When gay activist Larry Kramer argued that shutting down bathhouses would save gay men's lives, gay men attacked him as a prude.

Between 1983 and 1987, conservative politicians and clergy sparred verbally about AIDS with liberals and gay people. French philosopher Michel Foucault asserted that HIV did not cause AIDS and that HIV was not spread sexually. Foucault himself patronized bathhouses in the 1970s and died of AIDS in 1984, becoming perhaps the only philosopher in history to have his views empirically refuted by the manner of his own death.

In the *New York Review of Books,* contributing editor Jonathan Lieberson, a graduate student in philosophy at Columbia University, wrote several influential articles about AIDS in the mid-1980s. In one long article in 1986, he claimed that irrationality about AIDS was running wild, that only 10 percent of HIV-infected people would ever get AIDS, and that contact tracing should never be used to track down sex partners of HIV-infected men, even to save lives, because the newly won freedom of gay men and their sex lives was too important to sacrifice.[11] Around 1989, Lieberson himself died of AIDS (this periodical never apologized for these inaccurate pieces or to giving so much editorial power to an ideological graduate student).

Transmission of HIV

Despite many rumors to the contrary, HIV is transmitted in only three ways: through blood, through semen, or to babies during birth or breast-feeding.

Without treatment, HIV causes a progressive weakening of the immune system and hence, decreasing ability to resist normal infections. Without antiretroviral drugs, the average time between HIV infection and full-blown AIDS in 2005 was 9.5 years, and 9.2 months between AIDS and death.

Cells called T4 lymphocytes (or simply T4 cells) indicate the health of the immune system: the lower the number of cells, the worse it is doing. When the count of T4 cells drops below 200, a person with AIDS usually gets *opportunistic infections* such as Kaposi's sarcoma, PCP, a fungal infection called oral thrush, or cervical cancer.

Testing Blood, Again

In the midst of many controversies, authorities in 1984 weighed whether to test America's blood for hepatitis as an indirect test for HIV. Those *against* testing won.

Encouraged by Foucault and the *New York Review of Books*, some vocal gay men argued that their donations of blood should not be "quarantined" and that HIV had not really been proven to cause AIDS. Blood banks worried that, if they screened blood, they might lose income (although they do not technically charge for blood, they make money classifying, transferring, and storing blood).

In May 1984, Stanford University started screening blood for HIV. Two months later, defending a national decision *not* to screen, Health and Human Services Secretary Margaret Heckler said, "I want to assure the American people that the blood supply is 100 percent safe. . . ."[12]

Joseph Bove, M.D., who chaired the FDA's committee overseeing the safety of the nation's blood, said the "overreacting press" was causing hysteria about blood.[13] In March 1984, when the CDC counted 73 cases of deaths from AIDS caused by transfusion, Bove dismissed this danger: "More people are killed by bee stings."[14] Six months later, 269 people had died of AIDS from tainted blood.

In so assuring Americans, Bove and Heckler either lied, were incompetent, or both. In March 1985, most American blood banks began using the ELISA test to screen blood, a full year after they should have begun testing. Because of this lag, thousands of Americans and most hemophiliacs became infected with HIV. One of them was Ryan White, a hemophiliac who died at age 18 in 1990.

In 1985, a woman who was a prostitute and intravenous drug user tested positive for HIV. Now that Ryan White and she had the disease, AIDS seemed to be no longer just a gay disease. Now it had infiltrated heterosexuals and was in the blood supply.

Until 1986, people had hoped that most HIV-infected people would not die. Then that changed dramatically when researchers predicted that, without treatment, almost all the HIV-infected would get AIDS and die.

The same year, a few gutsy people founded ACT-UP to help people with AIDS. Its demonstrations forced the FDA to shorten by two years its process for approving new drugs and in 1987, AZT (zidovudine) became the first anti-HIV drug.

A decade later in 1996, scientists discovered protease inhibitors. These drugs block the protease enzyme needed to create new, mature particles of HIV. These drugs allowed people with AIDS to live somewhat normal lives.

At the start of AIDS, 25 percent of women born of infected mothers became infected. AZT blocks such *vertical transmission* to less than 1 percent.

Protease inhibitors plus AZT can cost $10,000 a year and cause severe complications. Because they require an obsessive attention to daily regimens, they do not cure HIV infection, but provide a way to survive it. The author knows professors, physicians, and administrators who were infected in the early 1980s, got these drugs early, and are still alive and working today.

In 2001, about 65,000 Americans over 50 lived with HIV, but in 2006, that number nearly doubled to 116,000.[15] At the National Institute of Health (NIH), the Mult-Site AIDS Cohort Study has been following the health of 2,000 subjects for the past 25 years. Although alive, many people with HIV in their late 50s suffer from Parkinson's or dementia, end-stage liver disease, diabetes, depression, and bouts of pneumonia. Despite these problems, as one person says, having them as a result of escaping AIDS is "better than the alternative."

Kimberly Bergalis's Case

In December 1987, David Acer, a dentist in Jensen Beach, Florida, extracted two molars from 21-year-old Kimberly Bergalis, a junior at the University of Florida in Gainesville. After graduating in 1990, Kimberly tested positive for HIV.

A young white male in his early 30s, Dr. Acer admitted to having had sexual relations over the previous decade with 100 to 150 men. In September 1987, he developed Kaposi's sarcoma. In July 1989, he sold his practice, sold his tools, and destroyed his records. In September 1990, he died of AIDS.

When his former patients tested themselves for HIV, six others tested positive. By using DNA sequencing, CDC proved that Dr. Acer was the source of infection in all his infected patients.

All the patients felt betrayed by the health profession. Kimberly Bergalis died publicly and painfully. In 1991, with little hair and weighing only 70 pounds, she testified before Congress, urging it to pass a law making it a felony for HIV-positive health professionals to interact with patients without revealing their HIV status. The law never passed and Kimberly died in December 1991 at age 23.

Exactly how or why Dr. Acer infected his patients remains a mystery. Some people believe that he deliberately infected heterosexuals so that Americans would no longer see AIDS as a disease of gay men. The truth will never be known for sure.

In some ways it is better if Dr. Acer deliberately infected Kimberly. Why is that? Because if he did, then she did not get infected through unsafe dental/medical practices, and hence, no reason existed to test dentists/physicians for HIV.

Retrospective analysis of cases of HIV+ dentists, surgeons, and internists reveal virtually no cases of accidental infection of patients. In general, probability of infection varies with amount of blood injected, how deeply the injection goes, and how much virus the blood contains. Also, the same procedures (double-gloving, masking, and no reuse of needles) that protect patients from infection also protect physicians and dentists.

THREE ETHICAL ISSUES IN STOPPING THE SPREAD OF AIDS

Homosexuality

Some people believe that teaching gay men how to practice safe sex condones sex between men. Although similar objections can be made to teaching safe sex, some people feel that sex between men, or sex between women, should not be tolerated.

Homosexuality has existed for thousands of years. In ancient Greece, bisexuality among men was popular, and leading Greek men such as Socrates preferred male lovers. Gay figures include Roman emperor Hadrian, King Frederick the Great of Prussia, playwright Tennessee Williams, and novelist Gore Vidal. According to the late Yale historian John Boswell, Christianity tolerated homosexuality more before the twelfth century than in later centuries.[16]

Although some people see homosexuality as a choice, most medical researchers believe that sexual orientation is biologically determined. In 1991, cancer researcher Simon LeVay published a paper in *Science* asserting that a specific region of the X chromosome in 40 pairs of gay men was associated with their sexual preference for men. The media dubbed this "the gay gene." Some people believe that if a person has one copy of this gene, he or she may or may not become gay, depending on the person's experiences. But if the person gets *two* copies of the gene, it is inevitable that the person will be gay. (A similar one copy/two-copy theory of cancer genes may explain why some people get some kinds of hereditary cancer so quickly whereas with others, it depends on environmental cofactors. See the previous chapter.)

The lived experience of gay men and lesbians testifies to this biological view. Virtually every gay man and lesbian reports fighting against his or her inner sexual attraction as children and teenagers and trying to accept into the norm of heterosexuality in advertising and culture. Because teenagers want to fit in, most gay and lesbian teenagers resist being attracted to members of the same sex and date heterosexually. Their sexual orientation appears a resisted discovery rather than a choice.

Many people harbor the false belief that state or federal laws protect sexual orientation. Only if Congress, a state, a city, or a county passed such a law would it be illegal to evict or fire someone because of homosexuality. Currently, except for San Francisco and two cities in Colorado, it is legal to do so almost everywhere.

Indeed, in *Bowers v. Hardwick*, the U.S. Supreme Court in 1988 allowed Georgia to keep a law making forms of anal and oral intercourse illegal between members of the same sex. Ironically, a footnote to the decision did *not* allow the state to criminalize the same behavior among heterosexuals. Obviously, this decision violates Mill's harm principle and cries out for an explanation of why such sexual behavior between members of the same sex is a crime, but not a crime between members of different sexes.

Five years later in 2003, the U.S. Supreme Court admitted in *Lawrence v. Texas* that it had made a mistake, that the issue was not (as the *Bowers* court said) whether the Constitution conferred upon "homosexuals a right to engage in sodomy" but whether the Constitution conferred a liberty interest to all Americans broad enough to allow consenting sex among adults.[17]

As we will see below, worldviews collide over homosexuality and stopping AIDS. Is conceptualizing homosexuality as an evil lifestyle *homophobia*? Part of the problem of stopping AIDS? Or is tolerance of homosexuality, drugs, and other "immorality" a root cause of the spread of AIDS?

Needle Exchange Programs

Needle exchange programs (NEPs) prevent the spread of HIV by giving drug users a clean needle and syringe each time they inject drugs, eliminating the need to share a possibly contaminated syringe. One study in New Haven, Connecticut, achieved a 33 percent reduction in HIV transmission by giving out clean needles to at-risk persons. A 1992 study by the CDC of 23 NEPs seemed to show no increase in drug usage by giving out clean needles.

But do such NEPs encourage nonusers to try hard drugs? If using such drugs had no risk of disease, might not more people use them?

Public health officials worry about *the exposure rate*. In most populations, a small percentage of people will always become addicted after exposure to an addictive drug, be that alcohol or heroin. If the same, say, 2 percent of people always become addicted, it matters a lot whether the population exposed is 20,000 or 20 million.

Prohibition kept alcohol's rate of exposure low, as it is in dry counties. Similarly, keeping cocaine and heroin illegal keeps their exposure rate low.

HIV Exceptionalism

In the first decade of AIDS, authorities in public health bowed to pressure from AIDS activists and did not pursue contact tracing the way they had with other sexually transmissible diseases. Because of prejudice against gay men, they feared that tracing those exposed to HIV might lead to some people losing their medical insurance or jobs. Besides, until AZT arrived in 1986, authorities could offer no treatment, so the benefits of identification were scant. So authorities made an exception for contact tracing for HIV.

Today, with AZT and protease inhibitors, early notification can save lives by helping the infected get prompt treatment.

Now if a HIV+ person knowingly practices unsafe sex, he can be charged in many states with a crime. In 1997 in New York, Nushawn Williams knew he was HIV+ and infected 28 teenage girls; he went to jail for doing so. In this case, contact tracing prevented even more girls from becoming infected.

HIV exceptionalism is now generally regarded in public health as a mistake. It succumbed to pressure from gay activists and may have cost some of them their lives.

In 2006, the CDC recommended routine testing of all patients by doctors for HIV. Of course this created controversy. Conservative religious groups retorted that no reason existed to test people in traditional marriages. In 2009, medical leaders repeated the call to make HIV-testing part of routine medical exams.

STOPPING THE WORLDWIDE SPREAD OF HIV: FIVE VIEWS

It seemed shocking that by 1987, 60,000 Americans had died of AIDS, more people than had died in the Vietnam War, and researchers guessed that in 1990, 10 million people might be infected worldwide. In 1992, Larry Kramer wrote:

> When I first became aware of this disease, there were only 43 cases in the United States; now there are 12 million people infected with AIDS around the world; within the next eight years, this figure could rise to 40 million. From 43 [people] to 40 million should be enough not only to cause some level of panic, but also to make everyone ask: how is this plague spreading so quickly? Indeed, 1 million new people worldwide were infected with the AIDS virus last year alone.[18]

Eighteen years after Larry Kramer wrote this, and after a quarter century of AIDS, we have little more wisdom on how to stop AIDS. Meanwhile, the number of victims of AIDS in the world has ceased shocking people.

By 2001, AIDS had killed nearly a half a million Americans, but in America, HIV infection had become a chronic infection with which you could live. American HIV-infected patients could even get married or become parents, but where most people lived, in the developing world, AIDS seemed unstoppable.

In 2001, when the virus had killed 20 million people and infected another 40 million, Secretary-General Kofi Annan of the United Nations called for new efforts. Singer Bono pressured America to give more aid, which under the George W. Bush administration, it did. Politicians aimed at universal access to treatment, costing $20 billion a year, and $10 billion of that idealistic number was actually donated.[19] In 2008, Bush created one positive legacy by signing PEPFAR (President's Emergency Plan for AIDS Relief), committing $48 billion over the next five years.[20]

Five years later in 2006, Kofi Annan lamented that, despite other progress, AIDS was "the single greatest reversal in the history of human development."

Why was he so gloomy? Because *25 years after Americans first heard of it, AIDS had killed 25 million humans.* Progress meant that "only" 35 million people worldwide had then been infected, 5 million less than 5 years before (although 5 million of the previous 40 million had since died).

Cumulative Deaths from AIDS

Year	Living HIV-Infected	Cumulative Deaths[21]
1981	600	200
1990	10,000,000	1,000,000
1999	30,000,000	10,000,000
2006	35,000,000	25,000,000
2008	33,000,000	29,000,000

The urgent issue now in medicine concerns stopping the spread of AIDS. Incorrect answers affect more people's lives than any other issue in bioethics, because, over the next 50 years, HIV could infect a billion people. Stopping the spread of HIV could save more lives than surgery, drugs, hospitals, and vaccinations combined.

From this perspective, *global bioethics* clamors for attention. Even domestic questions about resources at the end of life seem related: How can Americans spend so much at the end of life when so many millions in the world die of preventable diseases?

If moral actions create the greatest good for the greatest number of humans, then moral people will now be fighting AIDS. If past trends continue in the next decade, the 40 million people infected in 2006 could pass HIV on to another 50 million people.

Over the last 30 years, AIDS has changed whom it infects, from a disease of gay men and drug users to today, a disease of women and children. Women compose half of the world's HIV-infected population, 60 percent in sub-Saharan Africa. Young people under age 25 get half of all new infections worldwide.

The part of Africa south of the Sahara Desert has the greatest pool of HIV-infection, 26 million. South Africa alone has 5.5 million infected.

China and India cause concern because of amplification systems there. China's blood supply has been infected, which its officials deny. Migratory laborers and truckers in India acquire HIV from prostitutes and pass it along to their wives and then, to newborn children. In 2006, India surpassed South Africa as the country with the largest sheer number of citizens with AIDS, 5.6 million versus South Africa's 5.5 million. Altogether in 2006, Asia had 8 million infections.

Eastern Europe and Central Asia (the Ukraine, Kazakhstan, etc.) with large numbers of intravenous drug users, in 2005 had 1.6 million infected, up from 1 million in 2000.[22]

So how do we stop the spread of HIV around the globe? Part of the answer involves ethics. Should we: attack behaviors or the microbe? Use nonmoralistic education or moralistic condemnation? Spend money in developing countries on education? Buy cheap anti-AIDS drugs when the numbers infected keep doubling? When many lack clean water? Should we triage hopeless countries with masses of infected people, concentrating where we can save the most lives? These questions concerns will be discussed in the remainder of the chapter.

The following section sketches four views of how to stop AIDS, including exchanges between proponents of the different views.

Educational Prevention

Ultimately, nonmoralistic education is humanity's only hope of preventing HIV. Self-interested humans can learn to protect themselves against HIV by negotiating safe sex, using clean needles, avoiding infected blood, and taking drugs to prevent infection of newborns.

Prevention outranks cure, especially because AIDS has no real cure. An ounce of prevention is worth a pound of cure, i.e., it costs much less, in money and lives.

Cynics deride education, but it has worked. Between 1990 and 2010, new infections declined in the developed world. Blood became safe, people used condoms, and mothers stopped HIV from infecting their babies.

In the late 1980s, Thailand modeled how to arrest HIV. With a national campaign for 100 percent use of condoms, it advertised on television, hired outreach workers, ran testimonials by its royal family, and educated its sex workers, drug users, and citizens in preventing HIV infection. It allowed free access to testing and counseling and protected the infected against discrimination. It gave out free AZT and allowed production of generic anti-AIDS drugs for the poor. Over the next decade, new infections dropped 80 percent, preventing 200,000 HIV infections.[23]

Similar efforts worked in Uganda during the 1990s. Led by President Yoweri Museveni, Uganda ran testimonials on television by famous Ugandans diagnosed with HIV. Infection rates among Uganda's youth dropped dramatically, and in rural areas, by half, and by two-thirds among urban, pregnant women.

Brazil shows surprising success in using education to prevent HIV infection. Like Cuba, Brazil has a large commercial sex industry for both its citizens and tourists, so in 1990 its large cities had high rates of HIV infection. In 1996, the Brazilian government funded universal access to the best anti-AIDS drugs, resulting over the next decade in the creation of a national system of: out-patient centers, local manufacture of generic anti-AIDS drugs, and sophisticated labs and record keeping. As a result, Brazilian deaths from AIDS dropped in half and rates of infection in São Paulo and Rio de Janeiro dropped 54 and 73 percent, respectively.[24]

Brazil's huge population means this program is a great success. Although both Brazil and South Africa have similar middle-class economies, Brazil's efforts at educational prevention fared much better. Given the will and funding, education and prevention do work. One country fought AIDS head on; the other denied that HIV caused AIDS.

Feminism

The key to stopping AIDS is to empower women to prevent themselves from getting infected by HIV. The key to that is to empower women to vote, to earn money, and to reject domestic violence, so that they are empowered to negotiate safe sex.

A noted physician-fighter against AIDS concluded his 2006 review of this disease over 25 years with these words: "The prime mover of the epidemic is not inadequate antiretroviral medications, poverty, or bad luck, but our inability to accept the gothic dimensions of a disease that is transmitted sexually. Only if we cease to dodge this fact will effective HIV-control programs be established. Until then, it is no exaggeration to say that our polite behavior is killing us."[25]

The "gothic dimensions of AIDS" include the fact that reckless behavior by men around the world infects millions of women and children, that soldiers use mass rape as a weapon, that women and children are sold into sexual slavery, and that poor, powerless women cannot refuse sex from their more powerful, infected husbands. The only name for this behavior is *evil*.

This evil is the kind caused by human decisions. AIDS is not a punishment from God, but a way that sin manifests itself. Consider the case of 13-year-old Rhaki in Rajasthan, India:

> From a poor, rural family, Rhaki had an arranged marriage at age 13 to a 23-year-old man who worked in the distant city of Mumbai for 11 months of the year. Once a year, her husband returned for a month, during which time he had sex with her. While he lived in Mumbai, he had sex with prostitutes and became HIV+. At age 19, she learned that she and her 2-year-old son were HIV+.
>
> Despite the fact that she remained faithful to her husband and used no drugs, she was blamed for bringing shame into her family. She feared she would be ejected from the family and forced to become a prostitute in a distant city.[26]

In Namibia, one study found that 95 percent of a thousand women were forced in their first sexual encounter.[27] A third of the women in Sierra Leone reported the same. In sub-Saharan Africa, which had two-thirds of the world's HIV infections in 2006, 60 percent of those infected were women.[28] Of those newly infected and aged 15 to 24, a whopping 77 percent are women.

Dark reasons exist for this pattern. African men perceive that sex with a young girl is unlikely to infect them with HIV and some believe that sex with a virgin will cure HIV. These practices ensure that many teenage females will become infected.

In South Africa, India, and around the world, an amplification system exists that involves truck drivers, mobile soldiers, and commuting workers. South Africa's migratory pattern built up over a century, with millions of men traveling to distant mines and there housed in dormitories. Such patterns dramatically increase nonmarital sex. In Abidjan, the richest city in the Ivory Coast, migrants compose 40 percent of the city's population, and Abidjan has the highest incidence of HIV in West Africa.[29]

Despite efforts of the United Nations and Christians to stop it, human slavery still exists in parts of northern Africa. In India, Eastern Europe, Mexico, and Korea, young women are tricked, kidnapped, and sold into distant brothels, where they become sex workers, living like slaves.

In Bosnia-Herzegovina, soldiers raped as many as 50,000 women to make them pariahs. In East Timor, the Congo, Rwanda, Azerbaijan, and Uganda, rape became not only a spoil of war, but also a weapon in it. In Somalia and Darfur, marauders raped thousands of women and expelled them from their homes.

These are terrible human acts. To face a problem, you must name it. This is the human face of evil. To deal with it, you must confront it. This means that moral condemnation must be a weapon against AIDS. We cannot remain neutral against such appalling acts. We cannot merely pursue bland education and sanitized programs in public health.

Slavery of all kinds must end. Mass rape must end. Forced sex must end. Bad male behavior must end.

Tough love in stopping AIDS hasn't been tough enough. In Cuba, Nushawn Williams would have been executed. What if the government of Ethiopia hanged a man who infected his wife with HIV? It is time to take morally tough stands, or else another 10 to 15 million women and children will die.

Triage

In some parts of the world, bad behavior is entrenched. Doctors cannot bring peace to warring countries: this is not a medical problem but a political one. Similarly, physicians cannot end slavery or famine: these are larger problems than medicine can solve. Moreover, some countries have corrupt governments, corruption going back hundreds of years. It is naïve to think that do-gooder missionaries and physicians motivated by love and equipped with education can change much there.

We need to triage countries such as South Africa, where President Mbeki for a decade publicly resisted the fact that HIV causes AIDS and where he not only did not lead the fight against the spread of HIV, but helped to spread it by his poor example.

Pouring money and time into some countries is a waste. The point of triage is to intervene to leverage at-risk life into saved lives. We should ignore countries that don't need our help (North America, Europe, Thailand, Uganda) and ignore countries where nothing we do will make much difference (South Africa, Ethiopia, the Congo). Then we should focus on countries in the middle, perhaps India, where politicians lead and where people are changing their behavior.

And as for the sterling examples of Thailand, Brazil, and Cuba, well, no wonder! With their huge commercial sex industries, they combated HIV infections to avoid losing the hard currency flowing into their economies.

Similarly, if people don't care for their own safety, education and counseling will go only so far. After 25 years, most adults on the planet know that having unprotected sex, getting a transfusion of blood, or sharing needles can get you infected with HIV. If your own self-interest doesn't protect you now from HIV, more education certainly won't.

Besides, as one expert gripes, most AIDS education is bland and generic, and hence, of little value in teaching teenagers. It doesn't teach them how to negotiate usage of condoms during sex or how to safely use hard drugs. "We lack the political will to implement these things," he says.[30]

Among large portions of the world, primal drives for sexual pleasure, fueled by poor judgment under the influence of alcohol and other drugs, lead people to practice unprotected sex. In Russia, despair over the conversion to capitalism has fueled widespread prostitution and use of alcohol.

All these forces swamp educational efforts to stop AIDS. Wisdom lies in recognizing that we can't control the private actions of most people.

Survivors will be fastidiously aware of what behaviors can kill them, and they will teach their children to be similarly aware. Maybe a billion people may die from AIDS, but the other five billion will go on. Plagues, flu, and floods have wiped out similar millions before, but humanity has survived. Sadly, such deaths involve humanity's Darwinian evolution.

Structuralism

Activist groups such as Paul Farmer's Partners in Health emphasize that the cause of the spread of AIDS is not irresponsible personal behavior, but is a response toward evil *structures* of society. Education and prevention will never work until these structures change. Prevention is mere window dressing. Feminism focuses wrongly on individuals, and triage just breeds despair.

As some structuralists lament, "Obviously it is simpler to blame the victims for the rapid spread of AIDS in poor countries than to analyze the socioeconomic and political structures that underlie, frame, and often predetermine such personal 'choices.'"[31]

What evil structures? For starters, poverty, colonialism, apartheid and its legacy, racism, class injustice, and imperialism. Anthropologist Philippe Bourgois argues that in poor communities, lack of good jobs emasculates men who want to be good providers, who then turn to self-destructive behaviors out of frustration, using drugs, selling them, addicting women, and using violence to control others. Feminism for Bourgois ignores the "objective, structural desperation of a population without a viable economy."[32]

Poverty is a major cause of the spread of HIV infection. In the 1990s, thousands of poor farmers in China's Hena Province sold their plasma each week. They did so because they could not earn a good living by farming but could do so by selling plasma.

Plasma is collected by taking blood from the donor's body, separating the plasma, and returning the rest of the blood to the donor. In this way, donors can give weekly rather than donating once a month with whole blood.

Because the province's blood supply became infected with HIV, most of the donors became infected. Whole villages were wiped out. Moreover, because of the secrecy of the Chinese government, we have no idea how many Chinese patients received infected blood, plasma, or clotting factors. Millions of Chinese could be infected and not suspect it.

Too much of the world adopts the approach of "it won't happen here." As commentator Kent Sepkowitz bemoans, "For the past 25 years, the lessons learned about HIV prevention and control in one country have failed to inform decisions in others. As a result, the world has witnessed a slow-motion domino effect, as the disease overwhelms country after country."[33]

Leaders always deny that AIDS endangers the country (our blood is safe, we don't have prostitutes) and then, when cases of AIDS surface, those who are infected are blamed as deviant or foreign. As Sepkowitz says, "This sort of buck passing has delayed the control of AIDS in every country. By the time they finally appreciate the scale of the problem, they face a mature epidemic and the cost of lives and money has increased exponentially."

The connection between the spread of AIDS and structuralism may be put conceptually: *an unjust structure is an amplification system for HIV*. Women turn to prostitution to survive; male manual laborers use drugs to endure; poor hygiene and public health lead to diseases creating sores and infections, making HIV easier to transmit.

Feminism Replies

The key to stopping AIDS is to create social structures that empower women. Poor women around the world bear the brunt of AIDS. Such women know they are at-risk, but often can do little to protect themselves. Bearing the paycheck, and hence, food and clothing and other goods of life, men control these women. We will only stop AIDS when we give these women more say over voting, jobs, and sex.

Vaccines, vaginal gels, and female condoms need technological breakthroughs to be effective, and one day may be so. In the meantime, women must be allowed to say no to abusive infection by males and forced sexual slavery. Unless structures are created to help women, AIDS will grow and grow.

Maybe unfashionable, isn't old-fashioned feminism better than triaging 20 million people and forgetting about them? At least, feminism directed at people says that someone *cares* about them (versus the *indifference* of triage).

Structuralism is partly correct in that many of the evil structures of the world lead to the abuse, rape, killing, and HIV infection of women. We can help women without having a complete revolution in every society. Realistic change may need to be step by step rather than cataclysmic.

So basic rights for mothers, daughters, and wives can be implemented in small, faith-based communities, such as where clergy wield power in African villages. Money, food, and supplies, combined with faith and good will, can model sex only within marriage. Such an approach will also combat slavery, sexual exploitation of women and children, and be compatible with Islam.

Secular public health proposals that emphasize education may be inappropriate for faith-based, poor communities, where many people are illiterate and ignorant of the most basic scientific facts. Because AIDS is lethal and because a person has to get infected only once to get a lethal disease, such populations cannot wait to be taught to read or to be taught basic science. They need a solution now, and feminism is the answer.

Finally, we do not know that moral censure has not worked. Without it, who knows how many more millions might have died or have been infected? Fear of moral condemnation motivates many people, and maybe that is not a bad thing.

AIDS kills. AIDS is caused by HIV. It's immoral to infect someone with HIV. It's heinous to do so deliberately or with indifference. What other definition of an evil person do we need? Why not be a little moralistic here? After all, we're talking about *ethics*, not sanitation or legality.

Educational Prevention Responds

The champion of educational prevention rejects the moralism of feminism and structuralism. First, what's wrong with feminism in public health is that it really serves the emotions of the moralizer, not the one condemned. Moralizing did nothing to stop gay men from having sex after AIDS was discovered, but fear of death did. Moralizing only made matters worse.

The key claim is that feminism can change behavior. Is that true? One argument that it won't is that a lot of "tough love" has already been directed against using drugs, much less intravenous drugs. Similarly, a lot of moralism has been directed toward not having sex outside marriage, but has it worked?

If we execute men who infect their wives, who will bring home a paycheck to feed the wives? And feed the children? Execution sounds like a good idea, but if thought through, it's not. Seeing what would happen to them, wives would protect their husbands and not turn them in to authorities.

For workers in public health, triage is too pessimistic. Why not generalize that attitude and let everyone starve? Or go without penicillin? Why bother about the rest of the planet at all? Why not let the undeveloped world fight it out among itself and let the rich nations keep their distance?

But is this a *moral* point of view? Sipping wine leisurely while humanity dies? What does the Golden Rule enjoin us to do? Triage does not offer the world a moral solution; it gives up on finding one.

The essence of medical morality is to fight pragmatically for the good of the many, especially the tools of medicine. If we give up on that assumption, we might as well give up on medicine.

Triage Replies

The champion of triage replies, "You're right. If there are six billion people now on the planet and if a billion of them die of AIDS, mostly on the other side of the planet and unknown to me, I don't care. The planet already has too many people and it could easily lose a billion. When stories about AIDS appear on the news, I change the channel. In fact, to avoid such stories, I don't even watch the news anymore.

I may be morally deficient, but I have enough moral honesty to admit that I have no moral feelings of compassion, shame, or outrage about the mass of human deaths from AIDS. It's going to happen: it's a fact; it's accelerated Darwinian evolution; I don't think governments or missionaries can do anything about it; that's just the way it is. Give me my hot tub and another glass of wine."

Structuralists like economist Jeffrey Sachs argue that if Western nations transferred $150 billion a year to developing nations, by 2025 poverty could be wiped off the planet. Singer Bono has jumped on this approach. But will simply transferring money end poverty? And will ending poverty stop the spread of AIDS?

In *White Man's Burden,* World Bank senior research economist William Easterly criticizes humanitarian planners who impose their own solutions on developing countries, especially the idea that building infrastructure with foreign aid will end poverty.[34] Too many programs funded top-down, with no feedback from poor people.

With AIDS, Easterly argues that more life-years could be saved by not diverting money from antimalarial programs and childhood vaccinations and by fighting ordinary scourges such as tuberculosis. A million people still die each year from malaria in Africa.

Second, Easterly urges the West to focus on prevention rather than cure, especially by giving out condoms to the infected rather than expensive AIDS medicines.

Third, people's kids starve while they get antiretrovirals. HIV takes almost a decade to make people sick. One infected woman said she didn't need the medicines, but she did need a job for money to feed her family.

Finally, some countries may be hopeless. Twenty years ago, LiveAid concerts raised $100 million for Ethiopia, but little changed, and today, life in Ethiopia makes it among the lowest evolved countries on earth.

Educational Prevention Once Again

The champion of educational prevention also rejects the cynicism of triage. Both triage and feminism sound like solutions, but they are not. In fact, they serve the interests of those who espouse them, not the interests of the world's vulnerable women and children.

Triage would not have us offer expensive treatment to those infected but would concentrate on preventing new infections. In 2006, the standard of care for HIV infection is HAART, Highly Active AntiRetroviral Therapy, which costs $10,000 a person per year in developed countries and which 90 percent of HIV-infected people in the world do not get.

The key argument for offering HAART treatment at all in certain countries is that *it gives people a reason to get testing.* When Brazil offered HAART free to all its citizens, testing for HIV escalated and thousands came forth for treatment. Without free treatment, how many would have done so?

Triage is not an option. Let's call it what it is: global medical apartheid. The racial system of apartheid should not be replaced with a medical one.

Triage acquiesces to hopelessness, and hopelessness allows countries to spiral downward in war, rape, famine, and infection.

In 2001, breakthroughs occurred with the creation of the Global Fund to Fight AIDS, Tuberculosis, and Malaria and the Doha Agreement, allowing poor countries to buy or make generic anti-AIDS drugs. Powerful religious groups pushed the Bush administration to do more for victims of AIDS, which it did, and billions of U.S. aid poured forth. Seeing that otherwise, huge economies might be destroyed, the World Bank poured money into AIDS prevention. A similar threat to world security galvanized developed nations to respond. These efforts prevented millions of new infections and allowed two to three million people to live with HIV infection, people who in turn support millions of children.

CONCLUSION

Stopping the spread of AIDS is hard, and one reason is that dramatically different views exist about how to do it. One view's solution is a problem for another view.

Some of the proposed approaches are too drastic. Structuralism says we must change everything to fix AIDS: eliminate poverty, sexism, racism, and corruption. It asks too much.

Perhaps the only way to stop AIDS may be to experiment and adopt one view on a small scale, perhaps in a province, where the view can be fully implemented. Whether that approach is feminism, educational prevention, or structuralism, and given different religious backgrounds, provincial leaders, and scientific understanding, a particular approach might work better in one region rather than another. What worked in Brazil might not work in Biafra or Somalia.

And we must not ignore North America. The United States has 56,000 new HIV infections a year, 75 percent in men, especially among black men who are gay or bisexual or who have been in prison. One crusader says, "We must not make HIV infection a rite of passage" for such men.[35]

The problem discussed in this chapter is unprecedented in bioethics or modern medicine. It is unimaginable to contemplate a billion human HIV infections over the next five decades. The scale of death would dwarf the Black Plague, create hundreds of millions of orphans, bring down economies in developing nations, and create despair over continents.

Since the last edition of this text, the number of infections worldwide has stabilized or dropped, from 40 to 33 million people. Hopefully, and by the next edition, far fewer people will be infected because medicine and bioethics will have found ways to curb new infections.

FURTHER READING AND RESOURCES

Randy Shilts, *And the Band Played On*, New York, St. Martin's, 1987.

Alexander Irwin, Joyce Millen, and Dorothy Fallows, *Global AIDS: Myths and Facts*, Cambridge, MA, South End Press, 2003.

Anton A. Van Niekerk and Loretta M. Kopelman, *Ethics and AIDS in Africa*, Walnut Creek, CA, Left Coast Press, 2006.

DISCUSSION QUESTIONS

1. Explain how each of the views on stopping the spread of HIV tends to see the other four views as part of the problem of spreading HIV.
2. How could the blood have been screened in America and France, thus preventing thousands of deaths from AIDS?
3. How much can education do to prevent the spread of HIV? Are some people just evil and incapable of being educated to practice safe techniques?
4. How has there always been a trend to blame the victim, whether it's cholera, syphilis, or AIDS?
5. Is being gay, lesbian, or intersexual a choice or a matter of biology?
6. Do needle-exchange programs increase drug users or merely make using drugs safer?

CHAPTER 16

Medicine and Inequality

This chapter discusses finance of medical care in the United States. It discusses the history of medical finance in America and Canada. Its essential question for discussion is: should a just American society create a medical system to guarantee minimal care to all citizens?

MEDICAL FINANCE

Rosalyn Schwartz

Rosalyn Schwartz, age 47, white, lives in Ridgefield, New Jersey, and has a son, Andy. When she divorced in 1987, she lost the medical coverage from her husband's job.[1] The gift-wrap company where she works with five other employees (making around $19,000 a year) provides no medical coverage, though it might do so soon.

When Rosalyn tried to buy an individual policy, because she had an ulcer, a *preexisting condition*, insurance companies offered her only policies that excluded treatment for ulcers and that cost $4,000 a year.

In 1988, she found a small lump in her breast. Her physician said it might be cancerous and recommended removal, but Rosalyn postponed the lumpectomy, hoping that her employer would soon provide coverage.

In 1989, Rosalyn felt pain tear through her hip. By then her breast cancer had metastasized and had eaten into her hip, making her bones as fragile as glass. When she slipped and fell to the floor, her hip socket shattered. In the ambulance, she sobbed and could think only of costs. "Andy," she said. "I have no insurance. Tell them [at the hospital] I have no insurance. But you've just turned 18. Don't sign anything or you'll be responsible."

Some cancers are cells gone wild, so they must be excised and radiated as soon as possible. If such cancers reach the bone, it's bad.

Hospitalized for 23 days, Rosalyn underwent three surgeries. The total cost was $40,000, half paid by charity. Rosalyn owed the rest, which she paid off at $10 a month to each of 12 physicians and the hospital.

Unable to work after her surgery, Rosalyn received disability under Medicare amounting to $10,500 a year. Attempting now to purchase personal medical coverage, she discovered it would still cost her $4,000 a year, but it would not cover ulcers or cancer. Lacking such insurance, she forewent physical therapy, as well as bone scans every six months to check whether the cancer had returned.

A decade later, Rosalyn died.[2] Such is the life of one middle-aged working American woman who got sick and, after her divorce, had no medical coverage.[3]

In 2008, filmmaker Michael Moore made "Sicko," a devastating, funny critique of the various ways our patchwork system of insurance seeks to profit by denying coverage and by excluding benefits for sick people who need them (this film can be easily rented; parts of it are available on YouTube).

Medical Coverage in the United States

Universal medical coverage supports basic medical care for all citizens in a nation. One form is a *single-payer system* administered by one organization, usually a governmental agency, and funded by taxes. Most European countries provide single-payer, universal medical coverage, including Austria, Belgium, Denmark, Finland, France, Germany, the Netherlands, Norway, Portugal, Spain, Sweden, and the United Kingdom. So do Australia, Canada, Cuba, Japan, New Zealand, South Africa, and Taiwan.

America differs from other developed countries in having high expenditures per capita on medical care, yet not providing coverage for one-sixth of its citizens. The Institute of Medicine estimates that this gap leads to unnecessary deaths each year of 18,000 Americans.[4]

Another form of universal medical coverage is *mandated multi-plan coverage* where every citizen must purchase some form of medical coverage, either from a private or public plan, and all plans work under some governmental regulations. This is also called a *play-or-pay program;* its name comes from focusing on options for small employers, who must either play by offering medical insurance or pay a fine per employee for not doing so.

Massachusetts and Vermont recently led the way toward universal coverage. Their programs compromised between the right, which had pushed medical savings accounts, and the left, which had pushed a government-managed, single-payer system like Canada's. They required every citizen to have health insurance. Beginning in 2008, each citizen who filed a tax return had to indicate if he had health insurance; if he did not, he had to pay $129 extra in taxes. Insurers who did business in these states had to turn over lists of their clients to the state health department.[5]

American's Patchwork System of Medical Finance

Because America lacks one unified system of medical finance, explaining how the country's finance works is complex. America essentially has stumbled into a five-part patchwork system that covers most serious problems for most people most of the time, but which still allows some people to fall through the cracks. The section that follows describes these six parts.

1. Employment-Based Coverage and Private Medical Plans

About half of Americans get medical coverage though their employment.[6] This includes their spouses and children (including adult children up to their mid-20s). Coverage in retirement varies according to the largesse of the employee's former employer.

As a benefit to employees, employers provide medical coverage. Employers with many employees can negotiate lower rates than employers with few workers because larger numbers spread the costs of illness over more people. Because of their discounts, large employers usually offer the best medical plans.

Since World War II, private insurance plans have multiplied to over 300, each with its own rules, qualifications, reimbursement rates, and forms to be filled out by patients and physicians.[7] For the average physician, two full-time clerks deal exclusively with billing and insurance.

One disadvantage of employer-based coverage comes with small employers. As said, employers with fewer than 25 employees pay the highest rates. Small businesses trying to allocate capital for expansion, or struggling to make profits, or that cannot obtain inexpensive coverage, often cease to provide medical coverage to employees.

A second disadvantage of an employment-based plan is that when workers leave jobs, medical coverage eventually ceases. In 1985, Congress passed COBRA,[8] allowing employees to continue medical insurance at group rates for *18 months* by paying their share plus the employer's share of their former premiums. COBRA also covers spouses after divorce and also covers adult children.[9] Even with COBRA, many employees cannot afford to continue their coverage because (like Rosalyn Schwartz, who was eligible) they must now bear all this cost themselves, including the employer's former share, which may have been as high (for American auto workers) as 95 percent of the policy.

In 1996, the federal *Health Insurance Privacy and Portability Act (HIPPA)* required portability (i.e., transferability) for workers between similar plans and banned excluding preexisting conditions in such transfers (without this ban, workers with any medical problem would be trapped in their existing job).

A third disadvantage of employer plans is cost shifting. American hospitals are not reimbursed for providing medical care to the poor, but federal law forbids them from turning patients away in emergency rooms because of inability to pay. To compensate for losses from this care, hospitals shift costs and charge more for services for insured patients. Large employers resent such cost shifting, because it forces them, but not small employers, to subsidize the indigent. For this reason, large employers favored universal coverage in Oregon, Vermont, and Massachusetts.

A fourth disadvantage of employer-plans is that American employers claim the cost of insuring their employees is too high. In 1990, over $675 of the cost of each new Ford vehicle went to pay for medical coverage for employees.[10] Ford's retired employees had such generous coverage, with neither co-pays nor deductibles, that Ford and GM could not compete with foreign car companies.[11] In 2008, the huge financial burden of medical coverage for their employees and retirees helped cause the collapse of American automobile companies. Because of such high costs, some big employers (like many universities) created a two-class system with regular employees with salaries and good benefits versus part-time employees with no benefits.

A fifth disadvantage of the employment-based system occurs when illness or injury dislodges workers into chronic unemployment. Many people became poor because of medical conditions (cancer, schizophrenia, car accident) that then made them less desirable to employers who seek to reduce medical costs.

People who are unemployed or who work for a small company that offers no medical insurance may buy individual policies. About 7 percent of Americans do so, including the self-employed, seasonal workers, adult students, and people between jobs. However, as Rosalyn Schwartz discovered, individual policies usually are expensive and exclude just what is needed.

2. Medicare

When Americans reach age 65, Medicare covers about 80 percent of their expenses for hospitals and physicians. Medicare in 2005 covered 35 million Americans. Medicare is a single-payer system run by the federal government.

In creating it in 1965, Congress moved toward universal coverage. Lyndon Johnson wrangled it into law and aimed at helping poor, elderly people during illness, but Congress soon extended it to all Americans over 65.

The creation of Medicare stemmed from the evaluative premise that healthy, young citizens should pay for the medical care of sick, elderly citizens. A related idea lay behind Johnson's creation of the Great Society legislation of the 1960s, which created Head Start, food stamps, VISTA, and Aid to Families with Dependent Children (AFDC).

Medicare gave the elderly a medical security they had never previously known. Before, many elderly Americans worried whether they could afford physicians and hospitalization. Before, retired workers were on their own for medical coverage. Before, entering a hospital terrified the elderly for both medical and financial reasons.

Medicare also covers about four million people with disabilities under age 65, plus a hundred thousand people on dialysis under the End-Stage Renal Disease Act (ESRDA). The Medicare program in 2009 covered about 40 million Americans.[12]

Medicare is financed from mandatory payroll taxes—indicated on paycheck stubs as FICA (Federal Insurance Corporation of America). Medicare in 2005 cost $265 billion.[13]

In 2006, a Republican Congress under George W. Bush surprised its critics by expanding Medicare to cover costs of drugs for seniors in both sides of a "donut's hole," i.e., some initial costs, then a big gap, then all costs after the end of that gap.

3. Medicaid

A third arm of American health care is Medicaid, which also began in 1965 as part of Johnson's Great Society legislation. As a state program covering medical services, each state funds it differently, but federal matching funds guide each state's efforts and enforce national guidelines. All state Medicaid plans costs state taxpayers $35 billion in 1993, but these costs escalated over the next 20 years.[14]

"Entitlements" or "mandates" for medical services are the fastest growing part of state and federal budgets, and unless brought under control, they are predicted to wreak havoc on budgets, starting in 2010. Already in 2009, the recession forced state governments to choose between hospitals and prisons, schools and vaccinations.

Medicaid covers medical expenses only for poor people, especially those on public assistance, children of poor parents, poor seniors, people with disabilities, and adults with mental illness. So Medic*aid aids* the poor, whereas Medi*care cares* for the elderly.

Eligibility for Medicaid varies with each state. A citizen could qualify for Medicaid coverage with a much higher income in California than in Alabama. In New York in 2005, a single parent with two children could not have resources more than $6,000 or income more than $1,000 a month and qualify for Medicaid.

What Medicaid covers also varies from state to state. Over the last two decades, MediCal, MassHealth, and TennCare have covered the most services, and hence, had the most problems with their budgets.

Medicare does not cover nursing homes and long-term care. Only Medicaid does so. To qualify for Medicaid coverage for a nursing home, a senior citizen must exhaust all personal wealth, including sale of a personal home. To avoid sneaking around these rules and transferring assets to adult children, Medicaid now penalizes such transfers in the *five years* before application for a nursing home.

For people with mental illnesses such as schizophrenia, Medicaid pays for their drugs. Because most of these people take such drugs for life, state Medicaid plans pay a lot of money for their drugs. Like working, poor parents, people with schizophrenia face a dilemma between not working and getting their drugs free through Medicaid versus working a job with poor coverage for mental health and getting no drugs for their illness.

The bailout of 2008 by the federal government of American banks oddly included the Mental Health Parity Act, requiring insurers to cover by 2010 mental illnesses in the same way as physical illnesses.[15] This act was motivated partly to reverse incentives not to work.

An especially controversial aspect of American medical finance has been coverage for illegal immigrant workers. The Deficit Reduction Act of 2005 forbids Medicaid from covering services to noncitizens.

4. CHIP

Starting in 1997, the federal government began the State Children's Health Insurance Program (sCHIP, where the "s" is a placeholder for each state, e.g., UtahCHIP). Designed for those who earn too much to qualify for Medicaid yet are unable to cover their children through employment or private insurance, sCHIP works with each state's Medicaid program. Under it, children can obtain check-ups, prescriptions, dental work, and eye care, as well as services at hospitals and by physicians. The first act of Congress under President Barack Obama in January 2009 expanded sCHIP to cover 4 million additional children, up from 7 to 11 million, paid for by increasing federal taxes on cigarettes.

Before sCHIP, poor working parents faced the dilemma of going to work, losing eligibility for Medicaid, and then losing drugs and services of physicians for their children. If they became unemployed, they and their children became eligible for Medicaid. The sCHIP program thus reverses incentives for not working.

5. CHAMPUS/Tricare and the Veterans Administration Hospital System

A different medical system covers military personnel, their families, and veterans. While on active duty, members of the armed services see physicians through CHAMPUS/Tricare, which pays for them to see military or private physicians.

According to its website, "CHAMPUS is a health benefits program that covers medical necessities only. It provides authorized in-patient and outpatient care from civilian sources, on a cost-sharing basis. Retired military people are eligible, as well as dependents of active-duty, retired, and deceased military."[16]

Veterans may utilize a national system of hospitals and clinics run by the Veterans Health Administration (VHA). Founded after World War II in appreciation to America's veterans, the VHA is based on the moral premise that no one who served in the armed forces should later lack medical care.

The second-largest department of the federal government, with a budget of more than $60 billion, the VHA employs more physicians and nurses than any other institution in America. In recent decades, it has shed its reputation for shoddy care and has emerged as a national leader of good, efficient, electronic, medical care.[17]

The VHA covers veterans not only for surgery, drugs, and visits to physicians, but also for mental illness and long-term care in nursing homes. The Armed Services also run their own medical schools and pay for their members to attend nursing and medical schools in regular programs.

6. Health Care in Emergency Rooms

Part of America's medical system is the Emergency Medical Treatment and Active Labor Act (EMTALA) of 1986, which forbids emergency rooms from turning away patients who are medically unstable. All ER patients, regardless of coverage or ability to pay, must be stabilized before they are released.

This federal requirement means that emergency rooms serve as a national safety net for the uninsured and for illegal immigrants. States with large numbers of these kinds of patients face escalating costs for such coverage.

Medical Coverage in Canada

Canada has a fund for national medical coverage that functions much like Social Security in America. It covers every Canadian and all medically necessary services. It is also universal, portable, and publicly administered through a single payer.

High taxes on cigarettes, alcohol, and gasoline finance Canada's system. Each Canadian province sets its own policies by regulating the supply of services. For example, each province funds only a small number of hospitals with CT scanners and lithotripters (expensive machines that break up kidney stones with sound waves).

The Canadian system became national in 1962. Unlike America, private insurers do not restrain what tests Canadian physicians can order. Such physicians order whatever tests they want for patients and the tests are covered.

It is a myth that physicians in Canada work for the government. Like American physicians, they work for themselves and bill on a fee-for-service basis. Unlike American physicians, Canadian physicians cannot collude to raise fees.

The Canadian system for two decades has cost less than $2,000 American dollars per capita and covered all Canadians, whereas the American system has cost over $6,280 per capita and left 46 million Americans uncovered.[18]

Canadians boast about their medical system, especially when contrasted with the American system. Why? Here are some reasons.

First, Canadians live to about 80 years of life, Americans to about 77. Second, every pregnant Canadian woman gets free care, so Canada has one of the lowest infant morality rates of developed countries. In the United States, 17 percent of women experiencing childbirth undergo not only the natural fears of birth but also the anxiety of having no medical coverage to pay for their physicians or possible hospitalization.[19] Third, all Canadians can purchase affordable, long-term care in nursing homes. In the United States, virtually no one has this coverage.

In one poll in 1990, only 3 percent of Canadians considered the American medical system superior to their own. In the same poll and in contrast, nearly 30 percent thought Elvis Presley might still be alive.

The Canadian system doesn't cover everything. While paying most costs of hospitalization or physicians, it pays almost nothing for drugs or dentistry.

Canadians must wait for specialized care. In Nova Scotia, only one lithotripter exists, so patients there wait three months for an appointment. However, most stone busting is preventive and most kidney stones eventually drop and pass safely on their own. Surgery is available as an emergency alternative to lithotripsy. Furthermore, the only way to diminish the waiting list would be to buy more machines at enormous expense—each one costs millions of dollars.

Waits for specialized services are annoying. Because Canada limits the number of physicians in specialties, patients in Canada must wait longer than in America between initial referral and first appointment for oncologists and orthopedic surgeons—5.5 weeks to see an oncologist and 40 weeks to see an orthopedic surgeon.[20]

In 2005, Canada's Supreme Court struck down a crucial law that previously outlawed citizens from buying, or physicians or private insurers from selling, essential medical services.[21] That opened Pandora's box, and institutions such as Vancouver's Cambie Surgery Center began to perform knee surgeries for cash, without the usual two-year wait.[22] Rich Canadian patients then flocked to private clinics and hospitals.

Like America and Massachusetts (more later), Canada failed to recruit enough physicians in primary care. This will be a continuing problem for all countries with universal coverage.

Some critics also want a mixed health care system in Canada and America, like most European countries, where citizens could go to private clinics for some services. Canadian officials worry that such a system would drain specialists from its public system.

Clinton's Health Care Security Bill of 1993–1994

In 1993, President Bill Clinton proposed his Health Care Security Act to expand Medicare for all Americans. This act assumed two tenets: first, an *employer mandate:* all employers had to pay something toward medical insurance for their employees; second, formation of large *managed care plans.* The act assumed that such plans would compete against each other and that such competition would lower costs of health care.

Under managed care, a gatekeeper determines whether patients go forward to see a specialist or get admitted to a hospital. The gatekeeper is often a physician in primary care, but can also be a nurse or bureaucrat for the plan.

Both assumptions faced opposition. Small businesses fought the employer mandate because they feared being made to pay too much (at the time, thought to be between $1,600 and $1,900 per employee). Many said that, rather than provide such mandated medical coverage, they would not hire workers.

Second, many Americans dislike managed care. They dislike gatekeepers who may deny them the medical services to which they had become accustomed.

Elderly Americans especially feared being forced into managed care. They liked Medicare and wanted to keep it as it was. Because they voted in large numbers, politicians feared their power. Medicare has often been called by politicians the "third rail": touch it and you die (like the third rail of New York subways, which carries electricity).

The act's greatest financial problem was that it tried to simultaneously expand medical services and reduce costs. Not only did it hope to expand Medicare to cover 46 million uninsured Americans, it also planned to increase the number of services covered by Medicare. Moreover, the Americans with Disabilities Act mandated other kinds of expansion. All this contradicted the idea of lowering costs. Also, as said, owners of small businesses feared exorbitant taxes on them to pay for everything for everyone.

After a year of national discussion, the act failed to get to the floor of Congress for a vote. Perhaps the greatest reason for this failure is that President Clinton failed to clearly justify why a rich nation such as America should cover the medical needs of all its citizens. Instead of concentrating on this question, he got bogged down in details of how the plans would work, which soon bored most Americans.

Three States Fund Universal Coverage

In 1987, Oregon broadened its Medicaid plan to cover all Oregonians. Under its Oregon Health Plan (OHP), all employers, even small businesses, had to offer basic coverage by 1995 or pay a new payroll tax ("pay or play").

Oregon did not fund some expensive medical services such as in vitro fertilization, experimental therapies for people with AIDS, heart or liver transplants, or services in intensive care units for premature babies (later, to comply with the Americans with Disabilities Act, the OHP reversed this).

Although Oregon democratically developed OHP, when the parents of 7-year-old Coby Howard learned in 1988 that OHP would not pay for a bone-marrow transplant for his leukemia, they appealed to the news media for an exception. Surprisingly, Coby died a few months later, a rare failure of the rule of rescue.

In 1993, OHP had spent $84 million, but only $34 million had been allocated for it; overall, it faced a predicted $1.2 billion shortfall.[23] To save money, OHP in 2003 reduced benefits and required higher deductibles and co-payments.[24] Between 2003 and 2005, two-thirds of its members lost their insurance coverage, and over three-fourths went uninsured for more than six months. Despite a restoration of some coverage in 2004, many of those dropped continued to experience problems obtaining medical care. In short, OHP proved more expensive than Oregonians could afford.

Twenty years after Oregon did so, Massachusetts and Vermont cranked up their own systems of universal medical coverage. Beginning in 2008, each citizen of these states who filed a tax return had to indicate if he had health insurance.[25] In Massachusetts, the poorest residents (making under $10,000) got access to medical coverage with no premiums and no deductibles.

Where Massachusetts penalized noncompliance, Vermont encouraged its uninsured residents to enroll in its Catamount Health. Under it, and for about $500 a month, families got the same coverage as Blue Cross/Blue Shield (BCBS), with tiered co-pays for drugs and the same deductibles.[26] On a sliding scale, Vermont subsidized families making up to 300 percent of the poverty level (about $30,000 for one parent and $60,000 for a family of four).[27]

Vermont's plan recognized that people with chronic conditions (diabetes, heart disease, obesity, high blood pressure) consumed 80 percent of the medical dollar. It covered screening, counseling, and prevention for people with these conditions to try to reduce more expensive interventions later.

Employers with more than ten employees who do not provide medical coverage must pay the state medical fund $295 per employee. Massachusetts/CHIP expanded to cover all expenses of children in families up to 300 percent of the poverty level.[28]

Both plans are costly. In Massachusetts, Medicaid payments for medical care went up to $90 million by 2009, about what private insurers formerly paid. One scholar predicted that working families (who will pay $14,000 a year) won't be able to afford it and will go bankrupt because physicians and patients in the plan have no incentives to cut costs.[29]

Both plans put the lie to the idea that universal coverage must be a government-run single-payer system. By cobbling together several plans, these states managed to provide coverage for their citizens.

In 2007, California, Illinois, and Pennsylvania planned sweeping reforms designed to offer all their citizens medical coverage, but the recession of 2008 killed those plans. By November 2007, after Massachusetts required everyone in the state to purchase medical coverage or lose a $219 personal tax exemption, 200,000 of 600,000 eligible people enrolled. Those who didn't enroll lost their $219 credit and chanced going without coverage.

By April 2008, the number of people enrolled in the Massachusetts plan swelled to 340,000, some of whom had long postponed care, generating a crisis in finding a primary care physician willing to treat new patients.[30] By March 2009, 432,000 people were covered, leaving only 2.6 percent of the state's residents lacking coverage.[31] Already being the state that spent the most on medical care per resident, in 2009 Massachusetts experienced a budget deficit of $4 billion and sought ways to rein in medical costs that had been growing faster than the national average over the previous decade. The state also experienced a problem finding enough physicians in primary care to see the new influx of patients, making worse the national crisis of too few physicians entering primary care.

Expanding Medicare? For and Against AmeriCare

Why not expand Medicare to cover all Americans regardless of age and call such an expanded Medicare system "AmeriCare?" AmeriCare could absorb other systems of medical coverage, including Medicaid, insurance for federal employees, CHAMPUS, all government disability funds, and medical payments covered under automobile insurance.

Favoring AmeriCare #1: Greater Efficiency

AmeriCare could eliminate the overhead, profit, and waste of multiple private insurers. About 4 to 12 percent of health care costs represent fees and profits of private insurance plans, $100 billion in 2005.[32] By comparison, Medicare has maintained reasonable administrative expenses, about 2.5 percent of total expenditures.[33] The crucial concept behind AmeriCare is to transfer that $100 billion to AmeriCare to cover services for the uninsured.

Medicare has been successful. Elderly Americans enjoy a technologically advanced system. It is not the fault of Medicare that the elderly still spend 15 percent of their income on medical services; this is attributable simply to increases, first in the cost of normal services, and second in the vast increase in the number and variety of services covered.

From a physician's viewpoint, AmeriCare would eliminate hiring personnel to deal with many private insurers. AmeriCare would also reduce the delay of payments from many private insurers to physicians.[34]

Hospitals presently get about half their revenues from Medicare. Expanding it will simply broaden it, rather than creating an untried system. Medicare could be gradually expanded either in the way Congress added a drug benefit in 2006, or by age groups, first dropping eligibility from age 65 to age 55. This would allow for periodic assessment and modifications.

Opposing AmeriCare #1: Not Another Federal Bureaucracy

AmeriCare would create a bloated, unresponsive federal bureaucracy. During the 1960s and 1970s, the Veterans Administration became such a bureaucracy. The federal government cannot do certain things well, and one of them is health care.

An expanded Medicare system would become another End-Stage Renal Disease Program, with runaway costs. What everyone pays for, nobody pays for. In public systems, everyone will seek his own advantage to the detriment of the overall good. This is the age-old story, played out long ago in England in the *tragedy of the commons:* the owner of each flock increased the number of sheep he grazed on town land—the commons—until it was so overgrazed that the grass disappeared and the commons was destroyed.[35]

What is the proper role of the federal government in medical care? Consider federal funding for end-stage renal disease, artificial hearts, and AIDS, which is too politicized and occurs at the expense of other diseases, such as cancer. American government is being asked to do too many things for too many people.

With one-seventh of the American economy, and one-sixth of new jobs at stake in health care, do we want to take the chance of a federally administered system?

Favoring Medicare #2: Eliminating Experience Rating

Private insurers issue policies using either community or experience rating. In *community rating,* they evaluate risk for a large employer, state, or area and charge the same to every policyholder in that group. Community rating favors ill people because they cannot be excluded and healthy people subsidize them. National, universal medical coverage spreads community rating over an entire country.

Experience rating charges an individual or small business based on the characteristics of the person or employees, and previous illnesses or small numbers dramatically increase costs. In extreme cases, insurers maximize profits by selling policies to healthy young people who are unlikely to make claims and by avoiding people who are sick, old, disabled, or at high risk of accidents—that is, people likely to make expensive claims. Insurers seeking to maximize profits thus exclude the sickest people from coverage.

Some history about medical insurance in America may enlighten the situation. During the 1930s, surgeons and physicians founded BCBS to ensure that patients could pay them after hospitalization for catastrophic conditions. By state law, the "Blues" were nonprofit organizations; as such, in most states, they paid no state or federal taxes and no taxes on the premiums they collected.

In return for their nonprofit status, BCBS companies had to insure everyone who wanted to be insured, i.e., had to adopt community rating. Because BCBS had a state-permitted monopoly on medical coverage between the 1930s and the 1960s, this program worked for everyone: BCBS insured everyone who wanted insurance, and rates remained reasonable.

In the early 1970s, changes in federal regulations allowed commercial insurance companies of a new kind to emerge. These companies used experience rating, and they cherry picked the healthiest customers, leaving BCBS as the insurer of last resort for the unhealthiest and neediest customers.[36]

These factors help us understand what eventually happened to Empire BCBS in New York: new commercial companies took its best customers and left it with only the sickest customers, such as those with AIDS. As a result, Empire BCBS raised premiums for its remaining customers by 100 percent, but still nearly went bankrupt.

Another target of cherry picking, Kentucky BCBS, between the early 1960s and the late 1970s, saw its share of policies statewide drop from 90 to 30 percent. Some states later made cherry picking illegal.

If you wanted to make the most money by selling medical coverage to people, you would cherry pick and cover only companies with healthy young people, e.g., those working for Google, who were unlikely to make claims and who had employer-paid premiums. You would decline to cover employees and their families at pest-control companies.

People misunderstand "medical insurance" a misleading phrase. Thirty years ago, it meant simply insurance—a hedge against a dreaded but remote possibility. People then bought medical insurance hoping they'd never have to use it. As such, policies covered catastrophes like automobile accidents or diagnoses of cancer.

Gradually, medical policies evolved into prepaid group medical coverage. They expanded to cover not just catastrophic but all "major medical" expenses. This was logical: if people would pay small premiums to protect themselves against catastrophic risks, why not pay somewhat more to protect against common risks? Thus "insurance" grew until it included every medical service, and today, people complain when their insurance doesn't cover everything, as if that is what the term means.

Many people mistakenly believe that most Americans without medical coverage are *unemployed*. In fact, most Americans without medical coverage *work*.[37] Most waiters and waitresses lack employer-sponsored medical insurance, as do most workers in small businesses. Only the rare business that employs fewer than ten people, one in ten, provides medical coverage.[38]

AmeriCare would ban experience rating and for-profit medical insurance. Systems of universal coverage assume that insurance is a moral enterprise of sharing risk to help those with bad genes or those who are victims of accidents. It rejects the idea that selling medical insurance should be a way to make profits.

One other point: because BCBS was created by physicians and surgeons, it reimburses *procedures* well, but not *preventive services*. Specialists who do procedures receive far more than physicians in primary care who talk to patients: an ophthalmologist gets $2,000 for removing a cataract in an hour but a geriatric psychiatrist only gets $80 for talking to the same patient afterward. No wonder that few young physicians go into low-paying geriatrics, pediatrics, internal medicine, and family medicine. Given that, isn't the American system broken, spending more and more on fewer and fewer people for less and less care?

Opposing AmeriCare #2: Health Care Is Not a Right

AmeriCare would make access to health care a *right* of all American citizens. Elderly Americans now think of Medicare as a right, and most Americans would come to think of AmeriCare as a right. Is that what we want?

Problems at the margins would be difficult: who is a citizen and entitled to national care? A baby born here? An immigrant? How long must one live here before becoming eligible? Would it be right to let some move here and, say, after 7 years, have the same medical benefits as someone who has paid into the system for 30 years?

Supporters of AmeriCare claim that citizens have a right to *basic* health care. The problem here is conceptual: no one can agree on what is basic. Basic care such as dialysis in America is luxurious in Mexico or Kenya. When American physicians visit developing countries, they despair that they cannot provide the basic care of American medicine.

As medicine improves, what is minimal becomes normal, what is extraordinary becomes ordinary. So in 1962 kidney dialysis was extraordinary; now it is ordinary. In the 1970s, kidney transplants were extraordinary; now they are ordinary. And so on.

What this means is that there is no logical point after which we must stop providing health care, and before which coverage is a right, and after which, it is not. It all blends together, and once you make one part of the continuum a right, soon the whole thing will be.

Favoring AmeriCare #3: Justice and Fairness

Universal medical coverage may be required as a matter of *justice*. Philosopher John Rawls believed that the term *justice* applies to the design of a society's structure, and health care is part of that structure. According to Rawls, principles of justice stem from a hypothetical social contract where citizens come together to choose under *a veil of ignorance* about their own age, race, religion, sex, health, wealth, abilities, and talents. In other words, they cannot bias their choices by considering arbitrary personal characteristics.

Under these conditions, Rawls believes that rational people would not gamble with the structure of their society but would choose those structures that gave people maximal equal liberty. But some liberty could be sacrificed to achieve greater equality. To Rawls, inequality is justifiable when it works to the advantage of those who are the worst off. This is Rawls's *difference principle.*

An essential part of Rawls's concept of justice is the recognition that the world is naturally unfair: some people are born into rich families, some into poor ones; some people are born healthy, others with spina bifida. For Rawls, government can either worsen such inequalities or lessen them. For Rawls, governments that sharpen inequality are unjust; governments that reduce it are just.

Rawls's veil of ignorance can be seen as a device for ensuring that the golden rule informs our decisions about the structure of a just society. Underlying this approach is the ability to imagine ourselves as the worst off—to see ourselves as sick, hurt, poor, and uninsured; to imagine how bad it would be to have a serious accident, and how much worse it would be to have no way to pay for the care we need.

How might Rawls's approach be applied to our own system? The last 35 years, 1975–2010, have not been good for the poor in America. Between 1970 and 2001, the gap between the richest 5 percent of Americans and average Americans widened, as the former's wealth jumped from $33,000 to $265,000 while the latter's inched only from $2,000 to $10,100.[39]

Over these years, more and more workers had to work longer and longer just to keep what they had. Some jobs that once paid $20 an hour now paid $7. If, as Rawls assumes, a just society is egalitarian, then American society became more unjust.

Our existing medical system, in which more than 46,000,000 Americans lack coverage, is an unjust, structural inequality at a level where life-and-death decisions are made. We know that inherited genes cause many diseases and no one is responsible for the genes he or she inherits. Why allow the structure of medical finance to intensify the injustices of fate?

According to Rawls's difference principle, an unequal medical structure would be just only if the poor were better off under it than under an egalitarian system. In the present, unequal American medical system, that is obviously false.

Opposing AmeriCare #3: Out-of-Control Costs

The more health care is seen as a right, the more life becomes medicalized, that is, people tend to seek medical care in more and more circumstances. That happened in Australia, whose system once covered payments for in vitro fertilization. Furthermore, people now live much longer—partly because of the care Medicare provides—and people who live to be old cost the most.

A major issue about health care is that increasing access and services entails increases in costs. Fiscal conservatives say that our experience with Medicare has taught us an important lesson: the system cannot expand the number of patients covered or the range of services offered and simultaneously decrease costs.

In 2006, the trustees of Medicare and Social Security announced that, without higher taxes, Medicare will go bankrupt in 2018, 12 years sooner than predicted when George W. Bush took office in 2001.[40] Despite this announcement, Congress passed a new benefit in 2006 for Medicare recipients, covering their drugs up to $2,250 and then (after the "donut's hole") after they spend $5,100.[41]

As libertarian University of Chicago law professor Richard Epstein emphasizes, the cost of universalizing Medicare dramatically increases as the system moves from insuring each smaller segment of the 46,000,000 uninsured Americans.[42] Covering most children is relatively cheap. Covering most of the adult, working poor is not exorbitant. But covering the last 10 percent is expensive, because such percentages represent the real cost-busters that all private systems avoid. These patients suffer diabetes, schizophrenia, or congestive heart failure. If a national system entitles them to the best care, it will be difficult for it to say when a just limit of care has been reached.

Furthermore, reformers often want to increase services. Each increase in service provided to all Americans costs more money. The increases in services that are most commonly mentioned are: long-term care in nursing homes, home health care, hospice care, transportation to medical facilities, and dental services.

Libertarians such as Epstein believe Clinton's Health Security Act previewed exactly what would go wrong when the government mandated medical coverage. Clinton's act first ran into trouble with libertarians over its vague estimates of cost. Even the act's advocates said it might entail an extra tax on income of 10 percent. President Obama wanted to tax those making over $250,000 more to pay for his plans.

Another problem was making it illegal, as Canada did, to purchase extra health care outside a national system. It is one thing to guarantee everyone a basic minimum of health care, but quite another to force everyone into the same system and to deny them opportunities to pay for extra care. The latter seemed un-American.

Surprisingly, many recipients of Medicare opposed Clinton's Act, perceiving that the cost-containment goals could be obtained only by limiting funds. Put differently, and as Richard Lamm says (below), the costs of giving care to the most expensive uninsured patients can conflict with the goal of giving maximal benefits to Americans over age 65.

In general, libertarians just do not believe that the American government can control costs and provide universal access, as happened in Canada, Germany, and Australia. They fear that government will limit freedoms of physicians, businesses, and mandate expensive services requiring higher taxes.

Favoring AmeriCare #4: Market Solutions Won't Work

It is sometimes argued that health care could be controlled by letting medicine operate as a true market, subject to the laws of supply and demand. Markets regulate other goods and services without bloated bureaucracies and wasteful costs. Why not medicine, too?

In a true market, people would buy health care, such as a knee operation, with their own money. There would be no medical insurance and thus no reimbursement from insurers. Because people would have to pay for their care themselves, prices would tumble.

For a routine eye examination, patients might choose a nurse practitioner charging $10, a primary care physician charging $30, or an ophthalmologist charging $300. Given these alternatives, most would not choose the ophthalmologist, and so ophthalmologists would lower their fees to compete, unless they could somehow demonstrate that their services were worth more. On the other hand, if covered by their medical plan, most Americans would go to an ophthalmologist.

Such a true market would lower costs, but a market in medicine also has burdens, especially for sick and elderly patients. When people have just discovered they have cancer or multiple sclerosis, they do not always make good decisions. As one expert group concluded:

> The special nature of older persons and their health problems argues for caution in relying primarily on private solutions to providing health care for them. . . . In particular, the elderly are less equipped to deal with a marketplace of health care than younger, working persons. Partly because elderly persons are more likely to suffer from physical and mental impairments (including eyesight, hearing, and memory), they have more trouble than younger persons in comprehending the increasingly complex insurance arrangements now available. The elderly also usually lack the counsel of the purchasing agents and benefits representatives who serve younger, employed populations. Although some retired persons may be able to navigate our health care system, many others will not fare well in the rough and tumble of a health care marketplace.[43]

In a true market, medical professions would become hardboiled, doing wallet biopsies before helping anyone (read A. J. Cronin's autobiographical *The Citadel* to see how physicians once practiced this way). A real market in medicine would be a harsh, cruel system where patients and professionals no longer worked together to overcome illness, but where each bargained with the other for financial gain.

It is also true that if health care were like other commodities—rather than being subsidized as it now is—many people who could afford care would make foolish decisions. If they had to choose between a new car and a hip replacement, some would choose the car. Moreover, some people might be tempted or pressured to sacrifice health care for the sake of their families, or a parent might give up a hip replacement and put the money toward a house for her family. In this regard, a true market is exactly what people who lack insurance face today.

Opposing AmeriCare #4: Intergenerational Injustice

Many elderly citizens mistakenly believe that Medicare recipients have already paid for their benefits through FICA taxes. One popular book about Medicare benefits states, "The most fundamental point is that Medicare is not a gift. You paid for it while you were working. Medicare owes you services in just the same way that a health insurer to whom you have paid premiums owes them to you."[44]

In fact, today's workers by their FICA taxes pay for the Medicare benefits going to today's elderly.[45] After the first few years on Medicare, most beneficiaries receive benefits amounting to far more than they paid in.

Richard Lamm, governor of Colorado from 1978 to 1987, once set off a national debate about exorbitant medical costs when he attacked the high costs of organ transplants and the amount spent on the last years of Americans' lives. He wrote:

> Once we accept the fact that there are limits to what the nation can afford (and increasingly, people are recognizing this truth), then we will begin a process of asking how to get the most health benefits for the most Americans for our money. We should have asked this question years ago. It is outrageous that this country spends five to eight times what other countries spend, and yet has no better health outcome. America is going to demand more accountability for the more than one billion dollars a day it now spends on health care. Many countries give a high level of health care to all their citizens for a fraction of what we spend, and yet keep them healthier. We are no longer rich enough to give a blank check to an inefficient health care industry.
>
> Once we start to apply even minimum management standards to the health care industry, we will see some substantial changes. If we ask how to get the most health benefits for the greatest number of Americans for our tax dollars, many of today's practices will not meet the test. If we zero-budget all that we now do in health care, we shall inevitably close unnecessary hospitals, close excess ICU units, and look much more closely at utilization factors and outcomes.
>
> We shall have to develop a concept of cost-effective medicine. Virtually every health care provider will agree that much of what we do today in medicine has "marginal utility." When a society faces fiscal reality and seeks to optimize its dollars, it not only starts on the road to financial sanity, but it also brings dramatic change to existing medical practices. Dialysis and transplantation will undoubtedly undergo major change. The "opportunity costs" in other areas of medicine are clearly greater than much of what is being done today. The bottom line is that we can save more lives and bring better health care to more Americans for many of the dollars we are spending today.

> Economist Lester Thurow suggests that, to impress upon health providers what they are doing when they order marginal services, we should require them to imagine an American worker sentenced to a period of slavery long enough to pay the medical bill for that procedure. Dr. Thomas Starzl recently gave a liver transplant to a 76-year-old woman. It cost $240,000. Dr. Starzl should understand that with the average U.S. family making $24,000 a year, he has sentenced 10 U.S. families to work all year so that he could transplant a 76-year-old woman.[46]

If Governor Lamm is correct, then expansion of Medicare must be done by increasing taxation on present Americans. If that is politically impossible, and if financing is done only by long-term borrowing that future Americans must pay off, it would be unjust to young Americans to create AmeriCare.

Existing Medicare will no doubt be saved. What will likely happen is that the age of eligibility will be raised, say to 67, and later, perhaps 70. The Medicare payroll tax will increase, say from 2.9 to 3.5 percent, and then later, perhaps to 4 or 5 percent. The top amount taxed by Medicare will also keep rising. If AmeriCare were created, this tax would almost immediately jump to 10 percent. All this will be the yoke of taxation on the backs of America's workers, who have no choice but to have new taxes taken out of their paychecks.

Opposing AmeriCare #5: Socialized Medicine Reduces Liberties

Democracies try to balance two competing values: equality and liberty. A system once in equilibrium with perfect financial equality must forbid inheritance of money, unequal trades, or unequal pay, or else the system will soon create citizens of unequal wealth.

We might conceive of equality and individual liberty as the X and Y axes of Cartesian coordinates. The more we move to perfect equality, the more individual liberty vanishes. For example, for many decades America had no income tax: citizens kept all the money they made. The programs of the Great Society transferred money from the working to the needy. The liberty of some to keep all their money was reduced to increase financial and medical equality for all.

Transfers of income mean taxation, and all taxation is involuntary. Involuntary taxation to some is a kind of working slavery, where a certain portion of the year is required just to pay one's taxes, say, the first six months. Critics say the cost of AmeriCare is too high if everyone must work another month against their will to pay for it.

For universal coverage to work, patients also cannot be allowed to opt out of the system. This is like having a situation of perfect equality and then allowing unequal trades. This problem undermined the Canadian system. Similarly, physicians would not be allowed to sell their services privately or avoid being in AmeriCare.

Favoring AmeriCare #5: AmeriCare Is Not Socialized Medicine?

Some people would call AmeriCare "socialized medicine." Lest that emotional phrase freeze our thought consider exactly what "socialized" means. "Socialized" could mean simply "publicly owned." If so, that is not necessarily a bad thing, or even unusual. In America, highways and waterways, public schools, state colleges and universities, the armed forces, airwaves, the air, the skies, and national parks are publicly owned. When America was founded, private toll-roads were common and some people tried to own rivers and ports, charging tolls on ships that came and went, until the U.S. Supreme Court decided that American waterways were public goods.

When Congress debated Medicare in 1965, the American Medical Association (AMA) opposed it as socialized medicine. In 2009, the AMA opposed President Obama's plans for universal coverage (although only one-third of American physicians joined the AMA). American physicians feared that government-administered care financed by taxes would mean government-controlled care,[47] and that all physicians would soon be employees of the federal government.

To placate these physicians, a crucial decision was then made: under Medicare, physicians would be reimbursed on a fee-for-service basis. Eventually, this arrangement would make physicians rich and would give them the best of both worlds: freedom to work independently rather than as government employees and freedom to order infinite services for their patients—services that would be taken care of by government-enforced payments in the form of higher and higher FICA taxes.

So if universal coverage is not necessarily socialized medicine, what could it be? Four answers are most often discussed: First, it could be a single-payer system, such as AmeriCare, in which the federal government would tax all Americans and reimburse physicians on a fee-for-service basis. Second, it could be an *American medical service*—a system in which all medical professionals work for the federal government. Third, it could be an *employer-mandated system* like Oregon and Massachusetts where federal law requires every employer to buy basic medical coverage for every employee and establishes a separate government-financed system for unemployed people. Fourth, it could be a *voucher system,* where all Americans receive government-funded vouchers to buy health care directly from hospitals or insurers.

Opposing AmeriCare #6: Illegal Immigrants

The elephant in the room of universal medical coverage is illegal immigrants. In the fall of 2006, America's population reached 300 million people, a growth of 100 million people since 1967. About 53 percent of the new Americans were recent immigrants, both legal and illegal, and their children.

The majority of these immigrants are illegal workers. Covering them for medical care will break the bank. Moreover, if they are covered, workers with expensive diseases and disabilities will flock to America to get coverage for their conditions. This is what is known in the insurance industry as *adverse selection.*

Whether hospitals admit illegal immigrants varies from hospital to hospital, state to state. Reimbursement figures show that the largest group of illegal immigrant patients is pregnant women.[48]

Consider two hospitals in the Dallas-Ft. Worth area: Parkland Hospital in Dallas does not ask immigrants about their national status and pregnant mothers from Mexico flock to it to give birth, whereas for treatment, JPS Health Network requires proof of American citizenship, and hence, sees few illegal pregnant women.[49]

In 2005, California spent over $1 billion on medical care for illegal immigrants. The other top states giving such care were Arizona, Texas, New York, and Illinois.

If children are born in America, their births are reimbursed by Medicaid and then the child is an American citizen, with K-12 public schooling available to him.

Critics claim that America cannot afford to open its borders and to give away medical coverage and jobs to everyone who wants to enter.

Also vexing is whether to start illegal immigrants on chemotherapy for cancer or hemodialysis for kidney failure. Once such therapies begin, they are difficult to stop. Once they are started for some immigrants, it is difficult not to do them for other immigrants. But the more readily such expensive medical services are given, the greater the incentives for people to slip into America illegally to get them, and to avoid returning to their own countries, where treatment is unavailable.

As for Vermont and Massachusetts, how many illegal workers do they have? Vermont is one of the whitest states in the country with few jobs in meat processing, janitoring, and other low-skilled positions that attract immigrants.

Favoring AmeriCare #6: Illegal Immigrants

Some myths abound about illegal workers. Most Americans do not believe that such workers pay FICA and income taxes, but taxes are deducted from their paychecks.[50] So workers from Central and South America who work as janitors or cut up meat in factories subsidize Social Security checks and hospital care for senior Americans.

Anti-immigration advocates claim that illegal workers burden American's hospitals and drain resources from traditional Americans. Starting in 1996, reforms to welfare disqualified illegal immigrants from receiving welfare, food stamps, subsidized housing, Medicaid, and Medicare. However, if injured, immigrants must be treated and stabilized in emergency rooms.

In 1996, the Internal Revenue Service (IRS) began issuing identification numbers to illegal workers to take their taxes. You can be a gangster or an illegal worker in this country, and other authorities may take their time dealing with you, but in the meantime, the IRS demands your taxes. Each year, half of the seven million illegal workers use such ID numbers to file federal and state returns and pay the same taxes as traditional Americans.[51]

Obama's Push for Universal Coverage

President Barack Obama in 2009 tried to create universal coverage for all Americans. Given debts created to overcome the recession then, critics and supporters agreed that long-term success of such expansion hinged on controlling costs. On the other hand, entrenched interests historically resisted such controls. So Congress needed to find a way to console specialists, drug companies, private insurers, and small businesses, so they would not fight universal coverage, while still expanding coverage to all and controlling costs.

One option being discussed was expanding the present system covering federal employees to be a public program that uninsured Americans could join. Another was a national insurance "exchange," setting federal standards for all private insurers. Finally, the "play or pay" strategy of some states for small businesses was also being discussed, as well as removing the exemption on taxes on health premiums paid by employees and employees.

As this book went to press, hopes for expanded coverage were in doubt. Critics feared the lower costs and premiums of expanded coverage would kill off expensive, for-profit insurance companies—a result the Obama administration approved. Small businesses, for whom nearly half of Americans work, feared a mandate to provide coverage or be taxed the same as larger businesses, as this might bankrupt some small companies.

Finally, ethics became a big issue as suggestions about voluntary counseling at the end of life appeared to some to be discrimination against people with disabilities needing expensive care and seemed to smack of cost control by encouraging people to accept medical realities.

FURTHER READING AND RESOURCES

Ezekiel Emanuel, *The Ends of Human Life: Medical Ethics in a Liberal Polity*, Cambridge, MA, Harvard University Press, 1992.

Richard Epstein, *Mortal Peril? Our Inalienable Right to Health Care?* New York, Basic Books, 1997,

Thomas Bodenheimer and Kevin Grumbac, *Understanding Health Policy*, 5th ed., New York, McGraw-Hill, 2008.

DISCUSSION QUESTIONS

1. How is community rating generally Rawlsian in nature and how is experience rating more libertarian?
2. How did Canada's system work for many years by forbidding physicians and patients from contracting with each other for money outside the national system? Why was this necessary?
3. Does a just society offer its citizens some minimal level of medical care? How would that minimal level be defined?
4. Should illegal immigrants be entitled to medical care? If not, should physicians work for the Immigration and Naturalization Service and report illegal immigrants in the emergency room?
5. What are some of the common misconceptions about medical coverage in America?

CHAPTER 17

David Reimer: The "John/Joan Case"[1]

Throughout history, some babies have had ambiguous genitalia at birth, partially formed sex organs, microorgans, or organs of both sexes. Historically, the latter were called "hermaphrodites" from the combination of the Greek gods Hermes and Aphrodite. Later, sexologists used the more neutral phrase *intersex* children or children with developmental sex disorders. Exactly which phrase is best to use to refer to such people is an ongoing controversy, some advocates preferring the phrase "people with developmental sex disorders" and physicians, "intersex people." This chapter uses "intersex people."

The first case of attempted surgical sex reassignment was that of Lili Elbe in Berlin around 1931, performed by Mangus Hirschfield through five operations, resulting in death.

Intersex people may be more common than is often assumed and have an incidence as high as 1 per 5,000. They create problems in sports where people must be classified either as female or as male. In 2009, 18-year-old South African runner Caster Semenya had been running as a girl, but gender tests showed she had no ovaries or uterus and she did have internal testes that produced testosterone.[2]

The most common causes of intersexuality are congenital adrenal hyperplasia (CAH) and complete androgen insensitivity syndrome (CAIS). Intersex includes anomalies of sex chromosomes, the gonads, the reproductive ducts, and genitals, including congenitally ambiguous genitals, contrasting internal and external sex anatomy, incomplete development of sex anatomy, sex chromosome anomalies, and disorders of gonadal development.[3] The definitions of "intersex" and "developmental sex disorders" (DSD) are contested. Advocates push a broader definition of these terms to include more people. Because of shame and secrecy surrounding people with intersex, this condition may be underreported.[4]

Within the last half-century, surgeons and endocrinologists tried to normalize such children. This chapter focuses on these efforts and the famous "John/Joan" case of David Reimer, who was born a boy and raised as a girl. In the last 20 years, advocates for intersex people have argued that physicians and psychologists intervene mistakenly so often that such children would be better off being raised as they were born. Ideally, supportive parents would accept them as they are and not make them live in shame after surgical-hormonal sex assignment. The other side argues that a child, for happy adjustment in school and in a family, *must* leave the hospital as a boy or a girl. Whether this is true is the essential question of this chapter.

DAVID REIMER'S CASE

When Ron and Janet Reimer had twin boys in 1966 in Winnipeg, Canada, the Menonite-raised couple felt joy. Eight months later, Bruce and Brian developed problems urinating from phimosis (a minor problem where the foreskin cannot be fully retracted from the head of the penis) and their pediatrician recommended circumcision. Bruce went first and the physician botched the operation, leaving him without a penis.

Devastated by this malpractice, Ron and Janet forewent surgery on the other twin, Brian, and took Bruce home, saddened that he would never be able to reproduce or have sex. Ten months later in 1967, they heard John Money on television discussing gender surgery at Johns Hopkins Hospital.

Money, a brilliant, iconoclastic psychologist, pioneered the field of sexology and originated the distinction between biological sex and gender identity, e.g., you can have the chromosomes of a female but think of yourself as a male. At the time, behaviorism ruled in psychology and Money strongly believed that gender identity was constructed from the experiences of the child—experiences that could be shaped to control the eventual gender of the adult.

Money described how Hopkins had just performed two male-to-female sex-change surgeries and had opened a clinic for further operations. Money claimed that biology did not determine sexual orientation but early childhood experiences and hormones did, and that both could be manipulated to create wanted genders. Based on his studies of 151 pairs of hermaphrodites who had been raised male or female, Money concluded that, "The psychological sex in these circumstances does not always agree with the genetic sex or with whether the sex glands are male or female."[5] Money claimed that whether an adult lived as a female or male depended on how each was raised, not on their underlying biological sex.

Money cofounded the field of sexology, taught at Johns Hopkins Medical School for 55 years, and cofounded its famous clinic of sex reassignment surgery. He created important concepts, such as the distinction between gender identity and the traditional idea of a biological sex. *Gender identity* refers to how one sees oneself and behaves as male, female, or in-between. *Gender role* refers to how one acts in public, or how the public expects one to act, as a male, female, or in-between. Both differ from the idea of a *biological sex*, which is determined by one's chromosomes.

Money believed that intersex children were "experiments in nature" in understanding whether biology or upbringing determined an adult's gender role and sexual attraction. This *nature-nurture debate* has been ongoing in the science of human development for centuries.

Money strongly believed that biology was not destiny and that what really mattered was conditioning, early rehearsal, and socialization. Contacted by the Reimers, he welcomed the chance to see their son and promised his help.

In this embrace, Money had another motive. New evidence had appeared that exposure of the fetus to hormones during gestation organized sexual differentiation. If this were true, then people were born male and could not escape their sexual orientation. What Money needed, his critics said, was a human who was born male, made into a female, and then happily lived as a female.

Ideally, there would also need to be a control, for otherwise too many factors might influence the outcomes. So for Money, the Reimers's call was a gift from Heaven, because Bruce had an identical twin brother who was being raised as a boy.

Money convinced the Reimers to raise Bruce as a girl, calling him "Brenda," and they agreed to surgical removal of Bruce's testes. They also agreed to later create a vagina for Bruce through surgery.

But first, according to Money, it was important to create a gender identity for Bruce as "Brenda." Money believed that a *gender identity gate* was open only between two and three years of age, after which the gate closed and locked the child into a gender.

At home in Canada, Brenda resisted being a girl and wanted to do the same things as her twin brother, Brian, such as climb trees, play with soldiers, and urinate standing up. She disliked wearing dresses, sitting with girls, playing with dolls, and going to Girl Scout meetings. The Reimers hid Brenda's true identity from neighbors, teachers, and relatives, who thought of Brenda only as a disruptive tomboy and who didn't suspect what was really occurring.

Money stipulated that he had to see both twins twice a year in therapy sessions, which the parents were barred from attending. He believed it important for Brenda to self-identify as a female, especially by "owning" her identity, and he tried to push her into femininity.

Quite ahead of any true results, in 1972 Money caused a sensation at a meeting of the American Association for the Advancement of Science (AAAS) and make stupendous claims about his research. Eerily, this foreshadowed a similarly sensational announcement in of the 2004 AAAS meeting by South Korean researcher Hwang Woo Suk that he had cloned viable human embryos and derived viable stem cells from them.[6] Unfortunately, both claims were fraudulent.

Whether Money knew or admitted that he committed fraud is unclear. He appears to have been a "true believer" and totally committed to his view about the primacy of nurture and early rehearsal in childhood. Those who knew him at Hopkins suggest that some of his intensity about this issue stemmed from his own troubled early childhood in a repressive Christian sect in Australia.

Money claimed that Brenda was happy as a girl and that his research had been validated. He claimed that anyone could be raised male or female and be happy as an adult. Feminists and psychologists loved his results, for they destroyed sex-role stereotypes and raised the importance of psychology in the eyes of the world. Unfortunately, like other later frauds, this fraud had major consequences on how others acted: "Money's case was decisive in the universal acceptance not only of the theory that human beings are psychosexually malleable at birth, but also of sex reassignment surgery as treatment of infants with ambiguous or injured genitalia."[7]

Back home, Brenda increasingly resisted being treated as a female and refused to consent to her upcoming vaginal surgery. When the twins saw Money, the psychologist made them strip and—in what now would be regarded as child abuse—made Brian mimic sexual copulation with Brenda as s/he was made to lie on her back with her legs spread. Nude, Brian was also forced to mount nude Brenda from behind. Years later, both twins felt deeply traumatized by these forced-sex-play sessions. For his part, Money believed that later sexual orientation stemmed from childhood sex-play and rehearsal of sexual behavior.

The twins understandably resisted visiting Money. The parents did not know what Money was doing with their children, impressed as they were by Money's credentials, his appointment at Hopkins, and the reputation of that institution. The twins thought wrongly that their parents knew and had consented to what Money was doing with them.

The parents moved to another city to see if a change in school or neighbors would help, but the move proved disastrous. As Brenda approached her 11th birthday and fought off surgery, things worsened for the couple: Ron drank and Janet attempted suicide. Amazingly, and in published accounts, Money portrayed the parents as happy with their decisions about Brenda. He wrote about the case often, calling it the "John/Joan" case.

Like many intersex children sexed surgically one way or the other at birth, Brenda was never told what had been done to her. Today, people are living as adults and do not know they were born with ambiguous genitalia and assigned a sex at birth.

Increasingly suffering feelings that, "I'm a boy in girl's clothes," Brenda resisted starting hormone shots to feminize her appearance. For six months, Money convinced pediatricians in Winnipeg to give Brenda estrogen shots. On a visit to Baltimore and alone with Brenda, Money introduced her to an adult male patient who had undergone a sex change. Brenda/David ran from the room, pursued by Money and staff, down a flight of stairs, and out of the hospital, finally helped by a sympathetic employee to get back to her parents in their hotel room. There, she threatened to kill herself if ever forced to see Money alone again.

After a team of reporters from the British Broadcasting Corporation (BBC) unearthed problems with Money's optimistic reports about Brenda, doctors in Winnipeg and Baltimore grew increasingly anxious about the case. After a crisis, Brenda's father told her the truth about her origin. Rather than being shocked, the child said, "I was *relieved*. Suddenly it all made sense why I felt the way I did. I wasn't some sort of weirdo. I wasn't crazy."[8]

Brenda almost instantly decided to live as a boy. Almost 15 years old, he started dressing as a boy and took the name "David." He switched from getting injections of estrogen to getting injections of testosterone.

As a boy, David soon started hanging out with girls and starting dating. He found a girl he liked and told her the truth about his life. She already had figured it out. She was unmarried with kids from two different men, and wanted to marry David. They were married in 1990.

Meanwhile in the medical literature, a graduate student in science, Milton Diamond, became interested in David's case. Money attacked Diamond. David learned that false reports about his happiness were letting Money and surgeons change other children.

David eventually went public and, deeply wounded, attempted to refute Money's claims. His twin brother, who had been neglected during his childhood as "the normal one" while his parents focused on David, died of a drug overdose in 2002. David made good money from a book about himself, *As Nature Made Him*, and a movie based on him, but he squandered it in bad investments. His wife left him, and all these losses—twin, wife, money—drove him to kill himself in 2004.

David Reimer's case was atypical of intersex people because it was entirely caused by humans: first by human error, then by human decisions. Most intersex babies come out because of the deviations in anatomical development of the fetus and because—we believe—of exposure during fetal gestation to hormones and unknown chemicals.

ETHICAL ISSUES

What Is Normal and Who Defines It?

Eng and Chang Bunker (1811–1874), Chinese conjoined twins born in Siam (now called Thailand), traveled with P. T. Barnum's circus as "The Siamese Twins" Because they were treated with dignity and paid well for exhibiting themselves, they earned enough to buy a farm, marry two women, and have many normal children.

Conjoined twins Abigail and Brittany Hensel were born in 1990 in Minnesota and are now happily adjusted young adults. The Hansel twins had parents who taught them that the world was abnormal for rejecting them as they were and that they were normal as they were born. Attitudes of parents and medical staff are also important in determining the developing self-esteem of children with intersex.

In ordinary life, anatomy matters a lot. Our anatomy limits what we can do and how we experience the world. Socially, we *expect behavior* based on other people's anatomy. We *normalize ourselves* each day by combing our hair, dressing, etc. Our chaotic social world is also *more predictable* because of gender normalization.

Therefore, people of ambiguous anatomy frustrate us: we don't know what to expect from them or where they fit in. They create a problem for us, for society, so we seek to normalize them or regard them as "freaks" with stigma.

Secrecy in the Child's Best Interest

Most families cannot accept a child with ambiguous genitalia or mixed organs. In elementary school, bathrooms do not exist for "others." For normal development, a child must have a gender identity. Therefore, it is best for the child to have a clear gender assigned, one way or the other, than to have a mixed one or none at all.

Everyone who knows that a woman who's pregnant wants to know the gender of the baby at birth. Most people learn the gender of the fetus before birth, setting up a definite expectation. Families express disgust at going home with, not a boy or girl, but an "it." There are pink baby clothes and blue baby clothes, but no purple baby clothes.

Androgeny, having the appearance and affect of neither gender, is not a good option. If the person's sexual orientation is heterosexual, others will mistakenly interpret the lack of a clear gender as evidence of homosexual orientation.

Furthermore, most children do not need to know about their problems at birth with ambiguous genitalia. If such problems can be corrected, or given a better appearance, then the adult can live and function normally. In fact, many people may never know they were "sexed" at birth and they will live happy lives regardless.

Finally, surgeons and parents at birth do the best they can. They believed that lack of gender at birth was a social emergency and that a decision had to be made. It is wrong to second-guess them years later.

Ending the Shame and Secrecy

In his 20s David Reimer met Cheryl Chase, who soon became the leading advocate for intersex people to know their true origins and to make their own decisions about gender and sexuality.

At birth, Chase had ambiguous genitalia and was first sexed as a boy, but after 18 months and an unusual appearance, doctors decided to make her a girl. Chase's life refuted Money's claim that nurture can make an intersex child into one gender or the other with happy adults. Cheryl never felt completely male or female and lived between genders.

Cheryl Chase argues that, "What most harms the intersex child is the attitude that the child suffers from something shameful that must be concealed and never publicly acknowledged."[9] She argues that such children would be better off being told the truth and being allowed to choose, in early adolescence, which gender they want to be. Ideally, the parents would embrace the child as he/she is and not be ashamed.

In the late 1990s, Chase and other intersex people challenged the view of Hopkins/Money that early surgery and hormones were good for children with intersex. They picketed a meeting in 1996 of the American Academy of Pediatrics. With David Reimer's public testimony falsifying Money's claims that biology doesn't matter to gender, other intersex people emerged and claimed they were wrongly assigned a gender by surgery at birth and irreversibly harmed. Some committed suicide. At the same time, a more sophisticated view emerged in endocrinology, genetics, and medicine about normal sexual development and intersex.

This situation parallels that of parents of conjoined twins. As Alice Dregger argues, most parents consider this an emergency and desire for surgeons to normalize the twins into singletons, even at the tragic cost of killing or maiming one or both children.[10] With Abigail and Brittany Henson, their parents did not make the girls ashamed of their unique anatomy and the girls as adults seem remarkably well-adjusted.

Alice Dregger and Cheryl Chase argue that first, physicians and families should wait until the child/adolescent can decide for itself what gender it is; second, that physicians should help families understand that an intersex child can be happy with an ambiguous gender; third, that if physicians and families guess wrong about gender, that intersex children can be irreversibly harmed, and finally, that the crisis at birth about gender is socially constructed and mediated by ignorance and fear.

The American Academy of Pediatrics disagreed. In its famous 2000 guidelines on how to deal with intersex children, it wrote, "The birth of a child with ambiguous genitalia constitutes a social emergency."[11] By sexing a child immediately at birth, it hopes to prevent later harms, such as uterine infections, cancer, and infertility. It also hopes to provide the child with working genitalia for first, sexual satisfaction in the future, and second, a stable gender identity. It wants to foster parental bonding with a gender-defined child and help the child to avoid being different.

Nature or Nurture, or Both?

When it comes to feeling attracted to members of the opposite sex, or one's gender identity, things may be more complex than either having certain chromosomes or being raised as a boy or girl. Milton Diamond of the University of Hawaii was a graduate student in the 1970s when his lab discovered that exposure to hormones of a region of the Y chromosome (the SRY gene) organizes pluripotent anatomical tissue into male or female sex organs. Testosterone organizes formation of Wolffian ducts, which then become the internal, male reproductive system. Mullerian Inhibiting Hormone (MIH) simultaneously tells the precursor to Mullerian ducts, out of which the internal, female reproductive system is formed, to disintegrate, allowing the fetus to develop the male sex organs.

As a graduate student, Diamond came to believe that biology and hormones made gender identity, not childhood socialization, and hence, became a lifelong critic of John Money's views and specifically, Money's attempt to reassign David's gender and Money's attempts with several other cases of intersex babies.[12] Money attempted to suppress Diamond's work and at one conference, actually hit Diamond.

The work of Diamond and others partially explains how intersex children come to exist. A biologically female fetus may be exposed to testosterone from a mother's unknown tumor, from her taking steroids, or from idiosyncratic sources. This will give the child and adult a masculine or androgenous, unfeminine appearance.

So "biology may be destiny," but it's a biology that's part genes and part what happens to the fetus in utero. But Money's work seems wrong: by the time the child emerges in birth, how it's raised won't affect its later gender orientation.

Ken Kipnis's Proposals

Professor Kenneth Kipnis, a prominent bioethicist who has studied these issues, made three recommendations (with his colleague, Milton Diamond) in 1998 about sex reassignment surgery.[13] First, impose a moratorium on surgical assignment of gender: (a) without the consent of the patient and (b) until evidence-based medicine proves that such surgery helps more than it harms. Second, do not restart such surgery until comprehensive look-back studies show how and when benefits of such surgery can be obtained. Finally, undo the deceptions by past physicians to living patients about such surgeries imposed on them as infants.

Before agreeing to surgery on their children, Kipnis proposes that parents give "bullet-proof" informed consent and understand that surgery may compromise sexual sensation; end ability to have children; may conflict with the later adult's feeling of true gender identity; has not been proven to be beneficial, and has been opposed by some experts.

Kipnis also argues that because so few intersex children were told the truth, many as adults don't know what happened to them. Moreover, because of secrecy, no long-term outcome studies have been done. Like the juggernaut to normalize conjoined twins without good, long-term data to support it, what has been done to intersex babies is done in (what Kipnis calls) "an epistemic black hole." That is a bad way to operate.

As such, assignment of gender at birth is chancy and some adults later will feel that the wrong choice was made. How many adults seeking sex reassignment surgery were sexed at birth and never told by their parents? We do not know.

Medical Exceptions

Where not intervening with intersex children will be medically harmful to the children, it is morally imperative to do so. But the definition of "medically harmful" must be very tight and not stretched to considerations of appearance or social norms.

CAH is one such condition, where the child lacks a key enzyme and experiences vomiting due to "salt wasting," resulting in severe dehydration and, if untreated, death. It results from excess or deficient production of sex steroids. Almost all (95 percent) cases of CAH are from an autosomal recessive genetic condition called 21-hydroxylase deficiency. Newborn screening in many states picks up this condition and it can be corrected at birth by adding or subtracting hormones or giving salt.

Although not medically threatening, everyone seems comfortable reducing the size of a very large clitoris (clitoromegaly) to give the girl a more normal appearance later as an adult.

The Dutch Approach

In contemporary Holland, long considered an enlightened country about sex, intersex children attend a special clinic where they are given hormones to delay the appearance of their sexual organs.[14] Such children suffer high rates of attempts at suicide, self-mutilation (they hate their bodies and cut their bodies), and loathing of their gender. They frequently report feeling trapped in the body of the wrong gender, or having feelings of no clear gender.

Dutch professionals seek delays to enable such children to explore their sexuality and choices about gender in a supportive atmosphere, in contrast to the one most were raised in. In such a context, some may choose surgical assignment but some may choose to live as they are, like adult conjoined twins.

CONCLUSION

No parent expects an intersex child, but then again, no parent expects a child with any disability, noticeable difference, or aberration. From this fact, it doesn't follow that physicians must take a chance and try to normalize each child, guessing which way is right.

Between 2000 and 2006, the American Academy of Pediatrics drastically altered its views on intersex babies. Its 2006 Consensus Statement no longer considers the birth of an intersex baby to be a surgical emergency.[15] Few pediatric surgeons or pediatric endocrinologists today take decisions to sex a child at birth lightly, and even fewer would follow Money's lead and sex a child against its biological gender.

It is often understandable that many parents will have trouble accepting that they have an intersex child and will be uncomfortable with a child's ambiguous gender or ambiguous sexuality. Sex assignment before leaving the hospital may seem like a magic wand, making the problem go away—at least for a while. It is also possible that most people so sexed are happy and that only unhappy ones speak out as advocates.

FURTHER READING AND RESOURCES

Consortium on the Management of Disorders of Sex Development, *Clinical Guidelines of the Management of Disorders of Sex Development in Childhood*, 2006, Intersex Society of North America.

Alice Dregger, *One of Us: Conjoined Twins and the Future of the Normal*, Cambridge, MA, Harvard University Press, 2005.

David Benatar, ed., *Cutting to the Core: Exploring the Ethics of Contested Surgeries*, Lanham, MD, Rowman & Littlefield, 2006.

Linda Geddes, "Puberty Blockers Recommended for Transsexual Teens," *New Scientist*, December 10, 2008.

Merle Spriggs and Julian Savulescu, "The Ethics of Surgically Assigning Sex for Intersex Children," in Benatar (ed.), *Cutting to the Core*.

Leslie Feinberg, *TransGender Warriors: Making History from Joan of Arc to Dennis Rodman*, Boston, MA, Beacon Press, 1996.

L. Sax, "How Common Is Intersex? A Response to Ann Fausto-Sterling, *Journal of Sex Research* 39, no. 3, 1747–8.

Ken Kipnis and Milton Diamond, "Pediatric Ethics and the Surgical Assignment of Sex," *Journal of Clinical Ethics* 9, no. 3, 1998.

Heather Draper and Neil Evans, "Transexualism and Gender Reassignment Surgery," in Benatar (ed.) *Cutting to the Core*.

Jeffrey Eugenides, *Middlesex*, New York, Picador, 2003.

DISCUSSION QUESTIONS

1. Could most families handle raising an intersex child of ambiguous gender? Most schools?
2. Would an intersex child with ambiguous gender be subjected to ridicule and abuse by other children?
3. One family reportedly was wrongly told their fetus was male and planned the nursery in blue. When told at birth that the child was female, the parents demanded the child be sexed as a male. When surgeons there refused and at another hospital, they went to another hospital in another state, where the operation was done. Was this wrong?
4. Is sex reassignment surgery a good thing for adults not told of their unique origins? If told, might some adults decide not to seek such surgery?

CHAPTER 18

Ethical Theories and Bioethics

Bioethicists dispute exactly how ethical theory informs correct decisions in medicine. This chapter surveys major ethical theories that figure in bioethics, emphasizing their historical origins. The discussion illustrates how conflicts between theories, or the values underlying them, generate one ongoing controversy in bioethics. The chapter ends by discussing principlism and case-based approaches. Its essential question concerns what, if any one thing, makes an act right, and hence, given various answers to that question, which theoretical approach is best for bioethics.

THE QUESTIONS OF ETHICAL THEORY

One approach to ethical theory asks, "What makes an act right?" This approach underlies the answers of utilitarianism (utility), theology (the will of God), Kantianism (universalizability), social contracts (rules chosen under fair conditions), cultural relativism (the norms of one's culture), emotivism (feelings), subjectivism and egoism (my interests), and nihilism (nothing). This approach assumes that ethicists can discover one unchanging, monistic thing that "makes" an act right, in the same way that scientists discover natural laws of the universe.

This question shall guide our journey through philosophical thinking about ethical theories over two thousand years. Obviously, no short chapter can do justice to such a topic, which itself is the subject of many advanced courses for majors and graduate students in philosophy.

Virtue Ethics: The Greeks

Virtue ethics emphasizes the central role of formed character in the life of ethics. Virtue ethics rejects a content-based answer to the question, "What makes an act right?" substituting the judgment of the good person in a specific situation.

Virtue ethics is a big tent and includes ancient Greek ethics, theistic ethics, and to some extent, Kantian ethics.[1] Ancient Greek philosophers (fifth century BCE and before) advocated virtue ethics. Indeed, "ethics" derives from the Greek *ethos*, meaning "disposition" or "trait." In turn, *ethos* constituted part of the *ethike aretai*, where *arete* connotes excellence, good, and skill. So *ethike aretai* are good traits, excellent habits, or skills of living well.

Pre-Socratic ethics concerned *ethike arete* in performing a role. Take the role of being a soldier. If one asked, "What is the goal of being a soldier?" others answered: "to defend one's country." And again, "What excellences are needed to defend one's country?" The answers: physical strength, courage, skill in using weapons, organization in fighting in groups, temperance, and cunning—the *aretai* or virtues of a good soldier.

In Greek medicine, if we want to know what makes a good physician, we need to know the role of the physician. If that role is to heal the sick, then the physician needs virtues of compassion, knowledge of healing, and skill in human relations.

In a move of ethical genius, Socrates transcended role-defined ethics and asked about the *ethika aretai* not just of a particular role but more generally of a good person. His partial answers were supplemented by his student, Plato, and even more concretely by Plato's student, Aristotle.

The distillation of these three great thinkers for virtue ethics is that the human *ethika aretai* are courage, temperance, wisdom, and justice—the excellences necessary to function well as a good human. Today we know them as *the cardinal virtues.*

So we should ask not only, "What virtues should a good physician possess?" but also, "What virtues should a good person possess who happens to be a physician?" The narrow question is, "What should a good physician do?" The broader question is, "What should a *good person* do?"

This conflict matters when physicians perform conflicting roles of healer, experimenter, or triage officer. As defined by Kant or theism, a good person may not do some things that a good physician-researcher would so, such as pushing a human subject hard in an experiment that has little chance of helping that patient but which might help future patients.

Even in ancient Greece, physicians had conflicting roles. Most were naturalists, but one branch followed Hippocrates, adopting a sanctity-of-life ethics that banned abortion, surgery, and helping patients die. In contrast, most Greek physicians adopted a quality-of-life view, believing that it was futile to maintain lives of suffering, so they often helped terminal patients to die.

Role-based ethics suffer problems when role conflict or when the wider society calls into question whether the role has been properly defined. Greek virtues celebrated Hellenistic culture and despised the cultures of the peoples they conquered. Indeed, Aristotle's student, Alexander the Great, attempted to impose by force Greek values, culture, and language on the people of the empire he created. So the quality-of-life attitude of Greek physicians extolled courage, nobility, and honor in facing life's end, whereas the sanctity-of-life ethic of Hippocratic physicians opposed these attitudes, and hence, that role for physicians.

Virtue Ethics: Christianity In the fourth century CE, Christianity added its theological virtues of faith, hope, and charity to the cardinal virtues, bringing the total to seven. Christianity had its contrasting seven deadly sins—sloth, lust, envy, greed, anger, gluttony, and the master vice, pride.

Good physicians always exhibit compassion. This virtue comes from Christianity and its monastic tradition, where lives focus on helping others. Etymologically, "compassion" means "to suffer with," as Christians believe that Jesus suffered with, and for, humans on the Cross.

Where naturalistic physicians emphasized technical competence, religious physicians emphasized compassion. When death ends the value of technical competence, physicians need compassion. Because death always wins over competence, physicians always need compassion.

Role-defined ethics underlie the apprentice system in medical education, where medical students gradually assume more responsibility in assisting older physicians. The attending physician teaches the resident, who teaches the intern, who teaches the third-year student.

In contrast, the three great religions of the West emphasize duties to the poor and sick: the rabbinic ethics of Bar Hillel stress acts that help one's fellow man; Jesus says that as you treat the poor, so you treat Him; and Mohammed made the *zakat*, the tax on property for the poor, one of the pillars of Islam. So for a Jew, a Christian, or a Muslim, a good physician is first a Jew, a Christian, or a Muslim, and second a physician.

As such, care for the poor is part of being *a Christian physician*. This physician's license, knowledge, and wisdom are not just rights to maximal income, but a calling. In the movie *Chariots of Fire*, the Presbyterian Olympic runner says, "I run not for me but to glorify the Lord" and will not compete in races on the Sabbath. Similarly, to use a medical degree only to make money or to pursue fame is to abuse a degree given in trust from God.

Virtue theory in bioethics has other limitations. It admits that it has little to say in advance about particular issues because practical judgment or *phronesis* will balance many interests in finding the best outcome in each case. What is important, it asserts, is that the person making the decision is informed, smart, decisive, skilled with people, and temperate. So it implies that some physicians will be much better than others in making good ethical decisions.

Natural Law

When Rome conquered Greece, Greek culture in turn captured Rome. Rome's stoic philosophers elevated one aspect of the Greek worldview to a higher level. Rules for human beings, they argued, were so embedded in the texture of the world that they were *law* for humans. These laws came to be known as "natural laws." They were apprehended by unaided reason, without Scripture or divine revelation.

The notion of a lawgiver lies behind natural law. In the eleventh century, Thomas Aquinas synthesized Aristotelianism with Christian ideas to create his *Thomistic* worldview.

Aquinas made explicit the connection between God and natural laws: a rational God made the world work rationally and gave humans reason to discover these laws. So studying Thomistic ethics is a rational process of discovery of those rules. Correct *descriptions* of the world would yield correct *prescriptions* about how to act. To act rationally is to act morally, which in turn is to act in accordance with natural law.

These rules commanded humans to resist their feelings. St. Augustine taught in the fourth century CE that sin contaminated human feeling and, as such, lust, sloth, avarice, and pride infected humans. In stunning contrast to modern times, for Aquinas, ethics was *not* about examining one's feelings but about following the natural rules laid down by God.

So natural law condemned homosexuality. Aquinas believed that God made two sexes for procreation and that it was natural and rational for a man and woman to mate to have children. On the other hand, for two people of the same gender to have sex was contrary to natural law, and hence, immoral.

One problem with natural law theory is that what is considered against natural law may vary over the centuries. Many today do not consider homosexuality to be unnatural, especially because it has been practiced since the beginning of human history and because some great cultures, such as the ancient Greeks, celebrated it as ideal.

For natural law theory, consider marriage and children. Natural law regards loving sexual relations between a married man and woman as natural and good, and the natural product of such sex is children. But many forms of assisted reproduction today—in vitro fertilization, egg transfer, surrogate mothers, and artificial insemination of donor sperm—violate natural law because they don't involve sex between married men and women.

Natural law applied to bioethics suffers two main problems: it tends to conflate "natural" with "primitive" or "traditional," and hence, it has no way to accommodate change or progress in medicine, e.g., in helping married couples produce wanted children.

Natural law theory bequeathed to bioethics the famous *doctrine of double effect*. This doctrine holds that if an action had two effects, one good and the other evil, the evil effect was morally permitted: (1) if the action was good in itself or not evil, (2) if the good followed as immediately from the cause as did the evil effect, (3) if only the good effect was intended, and (4) if there was as important a reason for performing the action as for allowing the evil effect.

This doctrine justifies an exception to abortions with an ectopic pregnancy (an embryo growing in a fallopian tube) or a cancerous uterus (where uterus and fetus had to be removed together). In both cases, this doctrine allowed abortions only if the direct intention was to save the life of the mother and other conditions above were followed.

This doctrine forbids physicians from assisting in executions, since it forbids an intention to kill. On the other hand, it allows increasing dosages of morphine for terminal patients, so long as the intention is to relieve suffering, not to kill the patient. (This idea entered the case of Ana Pou, the New Orleans physician caught by Hurricane Katrina—see Chapter 3).

The *principle of totality* also derives from natural law. It says that the human body may be changed only to ensure the proper functioning of that body. The underlying idea is that one's body is not something that one owns, but that one holds in trust for God: "The body is the temple of the Lord." So a gangrenous leg may be amputated or a cancerous breast removed, because these diseases threaten the body's overall health.

According to this principle, we are given our bodies as they are for a reason and we should not change our bodies for frivolous reasons. Thus the principle of totality rules out all forms of sterilization to prevent pregnancy—vasectomy, tubal ligation, and hysterectomy—because to be able to create babies is a natural function of the bodies of men and women. The principle also forbids cosmetic surgery solely to change one's appearance, such as breast reduction or augmentation, rhinoplasty, and liposuction. The principle also forbids physicians from assisting athletes to increase muscle strength by using anabolic steroids, or by using germ-line enhancement to create more ideal bodies.

This principle is deeply embedded in our feelings. When people in 1996 saw a genetically altered mouse with a human ear growing out of its back, they were disgusted. The mouse's creators had violated the bodily integrity of both humans and mice. Similar feelings arise about other chimeras, even with such procedures as putting genes from salmon into genetically modified tomatoes.

So the principle of totality says that God, or evolutionary wisdom, wisely created human bodies, or different species as they are, and that humans shouldn't meddle with these results. To meddle courts retribution, either by God or Nature.

Kantian Ethics

Immanuel Kant (1724–1804) lived during the Enlightenment and believed in the power of reason to solve human problems. Raised by religiously conservative Protestant parents, Kant accepted conservative religious ethics at his university until he studied science, whereupon he doubted some of his former beliefs.[2] While continuing to accept basic Christian values, he ached to justify those values in some rational way. Rather than basing them on beliefs about God or an afterlife, he based these values on "pure reason."

The distinctive elements of Kantian ethics are these:

Ethics is not a matter of consequences but of duty. Why an act is done is more important than its results. Specifically, an act must be done from the right motive, and the right motive is the desire to do one's duty. Indeed, there is only one correct motive in Kantian ethics and that is the desire to be a good person, to do what is right, to have a "pure will."

Kant's ethics celebrate duty (and are therefore called *deontological*, from *deontos*, duty) because they emphasize acting from obligation, not from desire or feeling. We should praise only medical acts done because of duty, not from compassion. For Kant, the correct motive for treating a patient well is not because a physician feels like doing so, but because it is the right thing to do. When we act morally, Kant says, reason tells feelings what to do, not the other way around, as in popular culture.

Kant says the only thing valuable in the world is a good will, the trait of character indicating a willingness to choose the right act simply because it's right. But how do we know what is right? What is our duty? Kant gives two formulations.

1. A right act has a maxim that is *universal*. An act is right if one can will its maxim or rule to be acted on by all others. "Lie to get out of keeping a promise" cannot be so willed because if everyone acted this way, promise keeping would mean nothing.
2. A right act always treats other humans as "ends-in-themselves," never as a "mere means." To treat another person as an "end in himself" is to treat him as having absolute, infinite moral worth, not relative worth. His welfare cannot be

sacrificed to the good of others or to one's own desires. So parents cannot create one child to help another, as with *savior siblings*.

Consider the nurse who discovers a physician failed to tell a patient an important piece of information years ago. Now it is too late for the information to do the patient any good. A consequentialist might argue that she should not tell because the patient won't benefit. But for Kant, the patient must be told the truth. The only universal rule is "Always tell patients the truth." Such a rule is the basis of trust and of treating patients as "ends in themselves." If the nurse were the patient, she would want to know the truth. The nurse may *feel* that she shouldn't reveal the truth but only her reason will tell her what her real duty is.

Also for Kant, people are free only when they act rationally. Kant would agree that much of how we act is governed by our emotions, as well as our biology. But controversially, Kant denies that we act morally when we do the right thing because we are accustomed to it, because it feels right, or because our society favors the act. We act morally only when we exercise our understanding of why certain rules are right and then freely choose to bind our actions to those rules. Kant calls the capacity to act this way *autonomy*. For him, it gives humans higher worth and dignity than animals.

Kantian ethics has several problems. First, Kant is regarded as the supreme rationalist in ethics because he claimed that anyone who disagreed with him was guilty of a contradiction. But as John Stuart Mill famously argued against Kant, elitist Greek ethics or pursuing the greatest good for the greatest number is not self-contradictory.

In his Enlightenment project, most scholars believe that Kant failed. The Scottish skeptic David Hume argued against Kant that ethics is mostly socially valuable feelings. This view in ethics is called *emotivism*. Charles Darwin and the father of psychiatry, Sigmund Freud, later agreed with Hume that reason is the tip of the moral iceberg. Because so much of ethical life is emotional, little is changeable by reason.

Regarding the place of reason in ethics, emotivism and Kantian ethics face each other as poles, while other views lie between, such as those of Aristotle and his modern follower, Martha Nussbaum, that feelings can be educated by culture, therapy, and schooling.

Kantian ethics also fails to tell us how to resolve conflicts between competing maxims. Worse, critics such as John Stuart Mill believe that Kantians indirectly appeal to consequences in thinking about what to universalize. Finally, the ideal of treating each person as if he had infinite value is not always practical: it does not tell us how to deliberate about tradeoffs when some humans die in triage situations.

Nevertheless, Kant provides useful insights to medical ethics. He would favor using a lottery to distribute a lifesaving, but scarce new drug. His emphasis on people as "ends in themselves" explains the outrage that people have felt when learning of research done by Nazi physicians. Finally, Kantian autonomy explains why informed consent grounds participation in medical experiments. Also, when combined with the political autonomy of citizens of democracies, Kantian autonomy sets the stage for modern medical ethics.

Utilitarianism and Consequentialism

Utilitarianism originated in late eighteenth- and early nineteenth-century England as a secular replacement for Christian ethics. Its essential idea is that right acts produce the greatest amount of good for the greatest number of beings, which it called "utility."

Like the Taliban today, the Puritans then wanted everyone to obey their religious rules. In contrast, utilitarians thought morality should minimize harm to people and maximize group welfare. For Christians, Jews, or Muslims, morality is inconceivable without God's existence, but not so for utilitarians.

Utilitarianism aimed to humanize outmoded institutions. Developed by reformers Jeremy Bentham (1748–1832) and John Stuart Mill (1806–1873), it focused on changes that could benefit the majority of people.

Utilitarianism did not urge people to turn the other cheek and hope for justice in another life, nor did it exalt those virtues so cherished by England's aristocracy: stylish dress and manners, personal honor, literacy, scientific and artistic accomplishment, and appreciation of the arts. Hence, to aristocrats, being "utilitarian" is to be crass by being too practical.

The foundation for reform by Utilitarians came in 1832 in eliminating boroughs controlled by one landlord and in extending the vote to all citizens with property. At midcentury, utilitarians campaigned against slavery and the harsh factory conditions made famous by Charles Dickens in novels such as *Hard Times*. They attacked the harsh penal system, passed the Corn Laws, ended debtor's prison, opposed capital punishment for petty thefts, and advocated the vote for women. They urged public hospitals for the poor, the penny post, and facilities for clean water, waste disposal, and sewers.

Utilitarianism's teaching can be summed up in four basic tenets:

1. *Consequentialism*: Consequences count, not motives or intentions.
2. *Maximization*: The number of beings affected by a consequences matters; the more beings affected, the more important the result.
3. *A theory of value* (or of "good"): Good consequences are defined by pleasure *(hedonic utilitarianism)* or what people prefer *(preference utilitarianism)* or by some other good thing.
4. *A scope-of-morality premise*: Each being's happiness is to count as one and no more and beings who count are to be made explicit, whether these are only humans or all sentient creatures.

For utilitarians, right acts then produce the greatest amount of good consequences (versus motives) for the greatest number of beings.

Each of these tenets can be controversial. Bentham emphasized that the meaning of (4) was whether a being could suffer, not whether it was human or animal. As such, utilitarianism includes animals in its calculations of the "greatest number."

To modern ethicist Peter Singer, utilitarianism rightly included the sufferings of animals with those of humans. Utilitarianism also takes a larger view than most moral viewpoints and implies that every being's happiness on the planet matters, not just citizens of my society.

Virtue ethicists and Kantians regard a person's motives as a sign of his character. John Stuart Mill says that the drowning man doesn't care why the lifeguard is swimming out to sea to rescue him, just that the lifeguard is coming. Utilitarians think motives count only insofar as they tend to produce the greatest good.

In medicine, does it matter whether a physician listens because she really cares about patients or because she's found that having satisfied patients is an effective way to maximize income? A utilitarian might argue that if she is talented, whether she really cares about her patients matters little; in either case, her behavior produces good consequences to real people. For a larger view, she may do more good bringing clean water to a village than by being a medical missionary.

Utilitarianism also contains a theory of value, that is, a theory about what is a harmful consequence and about what is a good one. The simplest theory of value is *hedonic utilitarianism,* which equates a good consequence with pleasure, and harm, with pain. *Negative utilitarianism* focuses on relieving the greatest misery for the greatest number, as in famine relief; *positive utilitarianism* focuses on benefiting humanity. Utilitarian theorists debate whether some things are intrinsically valuable, such as pride and honor, or whether they are good only because they create good feelings in people over the longrun.

A compromise view is called *preference utilitarianism,* and its adherents believe that utility is maximized by furthering the preferences that people have. Preference utilitarianism is compatible with a base of subjective feelings in ethics, whereas intrinsic value utilitarianism is not.

The maximization tenet can get utilitarians into trouble. Wouldn't utilitarianism be willing to violate the traditional sanctity-of-life principle to save many people? Here, utilitarians bite the bullet: they think that the Nazi generals who tried to kill Hitler in 1944 at Wolf's Lair were justified; they think that on the expedition to the South Pole, commander Robert Scott should have allowed his crew member with the gangrenous leg to die, rather than slowing down the whole party by carrying the injured man, which resulted in the death of all. They think that if an FBI sniper sees a terrorist about to detonate a bomb in a skyscraper full of innocent people, the sniper should shoot the terrorist.

These are the easy cases. The hard ones come in population policy. If more happiness is better than less, why shouldn't we create the maximal number of people on the planet? So long as each new life has more happiness than misery, and so long as everyone else's life has at least the same amount of happiness as someone else's, shouldn't we produce more? This "total view" of utilitarianism is universally seen as what philosopher Derek Parfit calls "The Repugnant Conclusion," because we think the average happiness is more important. But it is difficult to see why utilitarianism entails maximizing average happiness and not the total good, so it may be stuck with this counterintuitive implication.

More specifically to medical ethics, wouldn't utilitarianism permit the sacrifice of an innocent, healthy person to transfer his organs to four patients who needed them to live?[3] Aren't four people alive better than one? If consequences and numbers define morality, what's wrong with doing so? Yet we know it's wrong to sacrifice a person like this.

One traditional reply among utilitarians is to distinguish between *act* and *rule utilitarianism*. Rule utilitarians believe that normal moral rules, such as "First, do no harm" in medicine, maximize utility over decades. *Act utilitarians* advocate judging each act's utility. Some act utilitarians think *rule utilitarianism* has a dilemma: if there are exceptions, then you ultimately have act utilitarianism (since you never know in advance whether a particular situation needs to be judged as an exception); if there are no exceptions, then you are close to a Kantian and only a nominal utilitarian. If the rule, "First, do no harm" has no exceptions in medical ethics, it may explain why it is wrong to destroy an innocent person to transplant his organs to four others.

In medicine, utilitarianism rules public health and triage. The goals of public health fit with this theory. Improvements in public health have helped more people live longer (created more "utility") than all the drugs and surgeries ever invented. When English physician John Snow in 1849 advocated clean water to prevent cholera epidemics (spread by dirty water), he acted like a good utilitarian. Unfortunately, it took 40 years and many cholera epidemics for Snow's ideas to prevail.

Triage allocates scarce resources during emergencies when not all will live. Because consequences count, utilitarian physicians should *not* treat each patient equally, but should focus on those who can be benefited. Rigorous application of this principle gives utilitarianism its famous hard edge: physicians should abandon those who will *die* anyway and, just as ruthlessly, abandon those who will *live* anyway. Physicians at the scene should help only those who waver between life and death and for whom intervention can tilt the balance toward life. The goal is to save the maximal number of lives.

This point illustrates an ambiguity in sanctity-of-life ethics. Traditionally, sanctity-of-life ethics, such as Kantian ethics, emphasize the absolute value of each individual, implying that the physician should at least comfort those who are beyond his help. But utilitarian-triage ethics values life in saving the maximal number of people who can live.

Social Contract Theories

Englishman Thomas Hobbes (1588–1679) emphasized a social contract as the basis of ethics and politics. Social contract theory is essentially secular, independent of belief in God. It assumes self-interest and that moral rules evolved for humans to get along. For Hobbes, humans agreed to rules because otherwise, everyone fared worse. For him, human society runs better under almost any rules, even despotism, than everyone taking up the sword. Hobbes would approve of the 40 years of such rule in modern Singapore.

Social contract theory does not separate ethics from politics. Hypothetical political bargaining creates the rules we call ethics. Also, notice that contract theories implicitly give up on people agreeing about answers to, "What makes an act right?" That is, they give up on agreement on *content* and instead, substitute a *fair process* for people who disagree about content to get along.

Hobbes believed that humans lived worst in a *state of nature,* a premoral agglomeration of self-interested individuals for whom life, he said famously, was "solitary, poor, nasty, brutish, and short." By the use of reason, people realize that each will live better in a society of rules backed by mutual agreement. So they bind themselves under a social contract to create "society" to better themselves and the lives of their children.

Rawlsian contractarianism carries the name of John Rawls, a philosopher of the twentieth century. Rawls believed that moral constraints should be imposed on the social contract. He called his most important constraint "the veil of ignorance"—in the hypothetical social contract, no one should know his or her age, gender, race, health, number of children, income, wealth, or other arbitrary personal information. *Rawlsian contractarianism* assumes that people are self-interested and choose the basic institutions of their society in a social contract; it is Kantian in imposing impartiality or fairness on the choosers by ruling out arbitrary information on choosers.

Rawls argues that the only rational way to choose under his veil of ignorance is as if, when the veil lifts, one might be the least well-off person in society. Because you don't know anything personal under the veil, you don't know what place in society you will occupy. This justifies the choice of his famous *difference principle:* choosers should opt for institutions creating equality unless a difference favors the least well-off group.

So with medicine, *everyone* should be trained in medicine unless training only a few is better for the least well-off. Mandating the difference principle imposes the Golden Rule on the structure of society.

Rawlsian justice entails that every citizen should have equal access to medical care unless unequal access favors the poor. It reduces the inequalities of fate; hence, children and those with genetic disease must get good medical care *as a matter of justice.*

Advocates of free markets favor private medical insurance plans in which the healthy do not subsidize the unhealthy. Rawlsians see "healthy" and "unhealthy" as arbitrary distinctions, due more to genetics than individual merit. Libertarians would allow for-profit companies to practice experience rating, whereby citizens with preexisting illness may be excluded. Rawlsians favor community rating, whereby risk and premium rates are spread over all members of a large community, such as a state or nation.

Four Principles, Principlism

One modern method of analysis is to investigate a medical case in terms of four principles. These principles are (patient) autonomy, beneficence, nonmaleficence, and justice.

Autonomy refers to the right to make decisions about one's own life and body without coercion by others. It honors the value that democracies place on allowing individuals to make their own decisions about whom to marry, whether to have children, how many children to have, what kind of career to pursue, and what kind of life they want to live. Insofar as is possible and to the extent that their decisions do not harm others, individuals should be left alone to make fundamental medical decisions that affect their own bodies and lives.

John Stuart Mill was a political theorist as well as an ethical theorist. In his most famous work of politics, *On Liberty* (1859), he defended this ideal of autonomy against the growing powers of government. He there defends "one simple principle," his so-called *harm principle:* "that the only purpose for which power can rightfully be exercised over any member of a civilized community, against his will, is to prevent harm to others. His own good, either physical or moral, is not a sufficient warrant. . . . Over himself, over his own body and mind, the individual is sovereign."

Such political individualism parallels valuing personal autonomy in ethics. Since the beginning of modern medical ethics in the early 1960s, autonomy has meant the patient's right to make his or her own decisions about his or her body, including dying and reproduction.

Autonomy rejects paternalistic ethics. During the patient's rights movement in the early 1960s in America, feminists scorned paternalistic physicians as sexist octogenarians who imposed their rigid ideas on a more enlightened, free-thinking, younger generation.

In the first two decades of bioethics (1962–1982), bioethicists exalted autonomy above other values, emphasizing the right of competent adults to end their lives, to control their own bodies and reproduction, and to decline to participate in experiments. Since then, bioethicists have realized that other values matter, such as good of the family and the physician's character.

Beneficence, or helping others, grounds compassion. It grounds the moral difference between therapeutic and nontherapuetic experiments. If physicians intend to help diabetics, beneficence justifies experiments on diabetics, but if they have no such intent, the experiment may be unjustified.

Beneficence can be seen both as a principle and as a virtue for physicians. Physicians receive special powers, income, and prestige from society, and in return, are asked to help patients. Medical training requires this trait, as demands on a student increase on a slope between premedical years and residency. Self-sacrifice is part of medicine. Ideally, physicians should want to help others, but if the internal desire is lacking, they should act this way out of duty. The principle of beneficence spells out this duty.

Beneficence may conflict with autonomy (as any of these principles may conflict with each other). Consider the involuntary psychiatric commitment of schizophrenic, homeless people. Is it better to let such people wander the cold streets of a big city, or to incarcerate and medicate them against their will? Should we let them "die with their rights on" or inject them with sedatives and antipsychotic drugs "for their own good"? Maybe we should do nothing at all and not risk making them worse off. After all, who are we to say that it is beneficent to do so? Maybe homeless schizophrenics want to stay as they are.

How beneficence and autonomy are balanced in particular cases is not easy to understand. Indeed, when John Stuart Mill advocated both utilitarianism and personal autonomy, critics wondered whether he contradicted himself.

Nonmaleficence, not harming others, echoes an ancient maxim of professional medical ethics, "First, do not harm." Above all, this maxim implies that physicians not technically competent to do something shouldn't do it. So medical students should not harm patients by practicing on them without consent: patients are there to be helped, not to help students learn.

Patients should not leave encounters with physicians worse off than they were before. This crucial principle of medical ethics prohibits corruption, incompetence, and dangerous, nontherapeutic experiments. It explains why the 80,000 deaths per year in American hospitals horrify critics.

The principle of nonmaleficence also accords with Mill's harm principle: the state and society should not attempt to shape all citizens for the better. In a fundamental sense, the first obligation we have is to leave each other alone, especially those who don't want our help. That means that physicians should not harm patients by unsolicited intrusions.

The last principle, *justice*, has both a social and a political meaning. Socially, it means treating similar kinds of people similarly (this is the so-called formal element of the larger principle). A just physician treats each patient the same, regardless of his insurance coverage.

Politically, the principle refers to distributive justice, and in medicine, to the allocation of scarce medical resources. Because there are many theories of justice, this principle is not self-evident. For example, Rawls's theory of justice demands that medicine serve the worse-off people.

But another view equates justice with simple egalitarianism: medicine is just if it treats each patient equally. Of course, that goal would not be easy to achieve either, and doing so would go a long way toward realizing Rawls's ideal. At the least, it would mean a guarantee of equal access to medical care for every citizen, such that insurance coverage would not be a factor in selection of which patient receives a liver transplant.

In the most minimal sense, justice requires physicians to treat patients impartially, without bias on account of gender, race, sexuality, or wealth. Even in such a minimal sense, justice requires a high standard of behavior among physicians.

These four principles were chosen as a distillation of the ethical theories described above. Their use in medical ethics is controversial. Critics say they are often invoked at the start of the talk, and then forgotten. More substantially, critics say that champions of the four principles do not tell us how to balance them to find the correct answer in a case. Finally, critics of *principlism* claim that champions do not tell us how to resolve conflicts between principles in particular cases.

Feminist Ethics

In the mid-1970s, dissatisfied female patients in Boston wrote the classic *Our Bodies, Ourselves.* Although they had access to the grandest medical centers, the authors couldn't get the information they wanted in down-to-earth, patient-friendly language. So they published a how-to manual covering every women's issue from breast cancer to abortion. Successive editions sold millions of copies and gave rise in publishing to what is now called "alternative medicine" and "self-help" books. In bioethics, the movement gave rise to a new emphasis on the autonomy, especially that of female patients.

During the 1980s feminist philosophers questioned whether traditional ethical theories were the ways to think of ethics or merely *male* ways. Kantianism, Greek ethics, social contract theories, and utilitarianism all looked like male theories: too abstract, too intellectual, and too false to the experience of women. What previous theories ignored were values such as trust, cooperation, nurturing, and bonding.

Carol Gilligan claimed—on scant evidence—that many women analyzed ethical dilemmas differently from men. Subsequent feminist theorists explored topics of caring, trust, and family relationships in moral theories.

This *Ethics of Care* promotes female virtues of caring, nurturing, trust, intimate friendship, and love. Its emphasis on the family contrasts with the atomistic individual confronting medicine.

Other feminists believe that only traditional gender roles make these virtues female and that the theory reinforces stereotypes of women as only mothers. As one female wit quipped, "Their ethics scream, 'Mommy!'"

When emphasizing empowering women to stop the spread of HIV, other feminists address concerns far beyond the family or one's network of caring.

The ethics of care may be a balance against abstract, semilegalistic concepts, such as rights. It also reflects a turning inward in ethics to the family.

The ethics of care does not tell us how to treat people we do not know or people we do not care about. This is important because much of medicine is about treating strangers, at least when patients first meet physicians. Nor does this theory tell us how to resolve conflicts among those we care about, such as when a female physician is torn between caring for a patient or being with her own daughter at childbirth.

Case-Based Reasoning

Since 1990, some bioethicists, including the author of this text, have advocated using seminal cases to teach bioethics and to generalize from paradigms to other cases. Both the Wharton Business School and the traditional teaching in medical schools use cases to teach.

Karen Quinlan in 1975 and Nancy Cruzan in 1990 went into persistent vegetative states. After many months, parents of both women decided that their daughter's biography had ended. Karen's case focused on removal of a respirator, Nancy's on removal of a feeding tube; both resulted in landmark legal decisions.

By understanding issues in these two cases about killing and letting die, ordinary versus extraordinary treatment, forgoing versus withdrawing treatment, standards of brain death, and proxy consent we understand these issues for future cases, such as the Terri Schiavo case in 2005.

Case-based reasoning does not deny that ethical theories play a role in moral life. When these are relevant to a case, they must be discussed. Case-based reasoning does deny that any overarching ethical principle of morality will guide physicians in making day-to-day decisions. Each situation or case will present a unique array of people, interests, conflicting principles, incompatible roles and duties, strong passions and concerns about the larger good, about resources, about institutional policies, and about political consequences. Each set of circumstances will require what the Greeks called *phronesis*, or practical judgment, to find the optimal solution for all parties.

From the viewpoint of case-based ethics, the four principles express four interests or values that appear in some cases in bioethics. But the problem is that many cases contain far more than four factors. For example, feminists rightly emphasize that many analyses in bioethics omit the family and exploitation of women. Certainly no good analysis of AIDS in Africa, or new reproductive technologies, could occur without such viewpoints.

Indeed, perhaps the typical case in bioethics involves *dozens* of conflicting values and *many* parties who have interests in the case, such as the patient himself, his family, his physician, the nonmedical staff, the agency paying for the medical treatment, and society itself. Any theory that tried to reduce all these values and interests to one simple value inevitably would exclude most values and the interests of some participants. Hence, simplistic theories most likely will harm some people by omitting them from consideration.

Political Ideas and Bioethics: Libertarianism

Libertarians favor government for defense and for limited public works, perhaps not even including national parks or a public interstate road system (we could have private toll roads). They disfavor government programs such as Medicare, Medicaid, disability insurance, food stamps, and welfare. Libertarians oppose forced taxation by the government, especially when it redistributes property and income from rich to poor. They champion the property rights of the status quo, but tend to be silent about how those enjoying the status quo acquired their property. Libertarian philosophers such as Harvard's Robert Nozick see forced taxation as equivalent to forced labor, that is, to slavery.

Accordingly, libertarians oppose mandatory FICA taxes on workers' pay and taxes for Medicare and for the Hospital Insurance Trust Fund. Even though federal programs such as Medicare have made American physicians rich, libertarian physicians would rather have no government control over their business. In a libertarian society, physicians would be reimbursed only in cash.

Critics say that in such a system, fewer hospitals would be built, elderly patients would frequently forgo procedures for lack of money, and physicians would earn far less money. In such a system, physicians would be controlled by few federal regulations.

CONCLUSION

It would be nice if one idea could solve all ethical problems. We might have a decision-procedure for discovering right answers. But that is likely a quixotic quest. Any theory that asks, "What makes an act right?" is probably asking the wrong question in assuming that one monistic thing makes all right acts moral. But rather than moral acts sharing one form (e.g., universal) or being an expression of one value (such as utility) it is likely that one could do so only at the most abstract levels of description.

A wrinkle here is that conflicts among traditional ethical theories in medicine often generate intriguing cases. Clashes over distribution of organs for transplant, or studying vertical transmission from mother to child in Africa, express conflicts between Kantian and utilitarian ethical theories. Clashes over the rule of rescue express conflicts between partial and impartial ethical theories.

For example, the rule of rescue (discussed in Chapters 1 and 13) exemplifies the larger clash in medicine between kinds of ethical theories. On one side are partial theories that favor special regard to identified people such as patients in the hospital, members of one's family, or members of one's country. The ethics of care illustrates one such partial theory.

On the other side are impartial theories, such as Kantian ethics or utilitarianism, that regard each person as having the same moral worth regardless of his geographical location or other nonmorally relevant criteria. It is precisely the partiality of the rule of rescue toward an identified person that impartial theories despise, for such partiality seems to disvalue the worth of all the anonymous people who do not receive the medical resource.

This clash looms throughout medicine. Admission to the hospital may illustrate the rule of rescue when a powerful physician decides to admit a patient without medical insurance and to care for him. Obviously, the hospital cannot do so for everyone or it will be sought out by other patients without insurance and go bankrupt. Such an admission may give the patient hundreds of thousands of dollars worth of treatment that she would otherwise not get.

But the important point here is that the *theories themselves* are creating the above problems and cases in medical ethics. Only some super- or metatheory could conceivably solve such clashes, but that is unlikely.

The study of ethical theories enlightens the study of modern medical ethics, but the study of modern medical ethics is not the same as merely applying one ethical theory to a case. The study of these theories does not give us a definitive, absolute answer to each case in medical ethics. Our society has inherited many different ethical theories from the past, the most important of which have been sketched above. Although each theory has its champions who believe that it alone is completely correct, most sophisticated people today believe that the best part of each of these theories needs to guide us in a particular case, such that in analyzing some cases, we will use parts of many different theories together.

FURTHER READING AND RESOURCES

Michael Slote, "Ethics," *Encyclopedia of Bioethics*, 2005.
Alasdair MacIntyre, *A Short History of Ethics*, New York, Macmillan, 1982.
Hugh LaFollette, ed., *The Blackwell Guide to Ethical Theory*, Oxford, Wiley-Blackwell, 2000.
David Copp, ed., *The Oxford Guide to Ethical Theory*, New York, Oxford University Press, 2007.
Peter Singer, ed., *A Companion to Ethics*, Oxford, Blackwell, 1993.
Peter Singer, ed., *A Companion to Bioethics*, 2nd edition, Oxford, Blackwell, 2009.

DISCUSSION QUESTIONS

1. Is it fair to ask, "What makes an act right?" in thinking about ethical theories? What are the limitations of this approach?
2. How do utilitarianism and Kantian ethics typically clash in bioethics? Cite some examples.
3. How do partial and impartial ethics clash in bioethics? Cite some examples.
4. How do ancient Greek ethics agree with Christian ethics that the most important thing in medical ethics is the character of the physician?
5. How does increased knowledge from genetics about predispositions to disease or superior athletic performance reinforce Rawls' idea that everyone does not start out equally?
6. Does case-based reasoning degenerate to moral relativism? Can we objectively give reasons for a position and balance people's interests without being relativists? Or is "being relative to the case" not a vice but a virtue?

Notes

Chapter 1

1. Associated Press, October 16, 1983.
2. Robert Steinbrock and Bernard Lo, "The Case of Elizabeth Bouvia: Starvation, Suicide, or Problem Patient?" *Archives of Internal Medicine* 146 (January 1986), p. 161.
3. Quoted in George Annas, "When Suicide Prevention Becomes Brutality: The Case of Elizabeth Bouvia," *Hastings Center Report* 14, no. 2 (April 1984), p. 20.
4. Associated Press, in *Birmingham Post-Herald*, December 14, 1984, p. A2.
5. Quoted in Arthur Hoppe, *San Francisco Examiner*, December 20, 1983.
6. Steinbrock and Lo, "The Case of Elizabeth Bouvia," p. 161.
7. *Bouvia v. County of Riverside*, California Superior Court, December 16, 1983.
8. Richard Scott, in "Patient's Suicide Wish Troubles Hospital MDs," *American Medical News*, January 20, 1984, p. 5.
9. Hoppe, *San Francisco Examiner.*
10. Annas, "When Suicide Prevention," p. 46.
11. George Annas, "Elizabeth Bouvia: Whose Space Is This Anyway?" *Hastings Center Report* 16, no. 2 (April 1986), p. 20.
12. Steinbock and Lo, "The Case of Elizabeth Bouvia," p. 162.
13. Annas, "Elizabeth Bouvia," pp. 24–25.
14. Derek Humphrey and Ann Wickett, *The Right to Die: Understanding Euthanasia*, Harper and Row, 1986, p. 150.
15. Paul Longmore, "Elizabeth Bouvia, Assisted Suicide, and Social Prejudice," in *Issues in Law and Medicine*, no. 2 (Fall 1987), p. 158.
16. The hospital's rationale in its brief to Judge Deering is quoted in Annas, "Elizabeth Bouvia," p. 24.
17. *Bouvia v. Glenchur*, Los Angeles Superior Court, *California Reporter* 225 (1986), pp. 296–308.
18. *Bouvia v. Superior Court* (Glenchur), *California Reporter* 297, California Appellate 2 District, 1986.
19. In *Bartling v. Superior Court* (1984), California court recognized the constitutional right of a competent patient to refuse life-sustained treatment, as it did in a 1983 criminal case, *Barber v. Superior Court*. A Florida court in 1978 recognized a competent patient's right to remove a life-sustaining device in *Satz v. Perlmutter*, 362 So.2nd 160. Thanks to Bonnie Steinbock and Alicia Ouellette for these references.
20. Jeff Wilson (AP), "Precedent-Setter Lives On after Plea to Die," *Indianapolis Star*, December 19, 1993, p. H7.
21. Elaine Woo, "Obituary: Harlan Hahn; USC Professor Fought for Disability Rights, Sued University to Improve Its Access," *Los Angeles Times*, May 10, 2008.
22. B. D. Colen, "His Life, to Take or Not," *Newsday*, September 25, 1989, pp. 5–19.
23. Susan Schindehette and Gail Wescott, "Deciding Not to Die," *People*, January 18, 1993, p. 86.
24. Susan Schindehette and Gail Wescott, "Deciding Not to Die," p. 86.
25. Russ Fine, *UAB Report*, September 4, 1992, p. 4.
26. Fine, *UAB Report*.
27. Russ Fine, personal communication to author, May 16, 1994.
28. Cowart's case became the topic of famous videotape, "Please Let Me Die," and a later film, *Dax's Case*. See also L. Kliever, *Dax's Case—Essays in Medical Ethics and*

Human Meaning, Dallas, TX, SMU Press, 1989.
29. Dax Cowart, personal communication to author at meeting of American Association of Medical Colleges, Chicago, Ill., October 1989.
30. Quotations are from Phaedo, in E. Hamilton and H. Cairns, eds., *Plato: The Collected Dialogues*, Princeton, NJ, Princeton University Press, 1961.
31. Epictetus, Dissertations, 1.9, p. 16. Quoted by James Rachels, "Euthanasia," in T. Regan, ed., *Matters of Life and Death,* 3rd ed., New York, McGraw-Hill, 1993, p. 35.
32. Seneca, *De Ira,* quoted in Rachels, "Euthanasia."
33. Jean Paul Sartre, *Existentialism Is a Humanism*, New York, Philosophical Library, 1947.
34. Frederick Russell, *The Just War in the Middle Ages,* Cambridge, England, Cambridge University Press, 1975.
35. Quoted in James Gutman, "Death and Dying in Western Culture," *Encyclopedia of Bioethics* 1, New York, Free Press, 1978, p. 240.
36. Baruch Spinoza, *Ethics,* William White and Amelia Stirling, trans., New York, Hafner, 1949.
37. Quoted in Derek Humphrey and Ann Wickett, *The Right to Die: Understanding Euthanasia,* New York, Harper and Row, 1986, pp. 8–9.
38. David Hume, "On Suicide" (1755), in Eugene Miller, ed., *Collected Essays of David Hume,* Indianapolis, IN, Liberty Classics, 1986.
39. Hume, "On Suicide."
40. "To deprive oneself of an integral part or organ (to mutilate oneself), for example, to give away or sell a tooth so that it can be implanted in the jawbone of another person, or to submit oneself to castration in order to gain an easier living as a singer, and so on, belongs to partial self-murder."
41. Immanuel Kant, "On Suicide" (1755–1780), *Lectures on Ethics*, L. Enfield, trans., New York, Harper and Row, 1963, pp. 148–154.
42. Kant, "On Suicide."
43. John Stuart Mill, *On Liberty* (1859), New York, Appleton-Century-Crofts, 1974.
44. Quoted in Humphrey and Wickett, *The Right to Die*, p. 16.
45. Alan Meisel, *The Right to Die*: Cumulative Supplement 1, New York, Wylie, 1991, p. x.
46. For a decade, Michigan had a loophole with no explicit law banning assisted suicide, but after Jack Kevorkian's actions, later corrected this omission.
47. T. Woody, "Was His Act of Mercy Also Murder?" *New York Times*, November 7, 1988.
48. Art Kleiner, "Life after Suicide," *High Wire,* Summer 1982, p. 30.
49. Tad Friend, "Jumpers," *New Yorker,* October 13, 2003.
50. H. Hendin, "Suicide in America," *Miami News*, August 30, 1982, p. B1.
51. Humphrey and Wickett, *The Right to Die,* p. 152.
52. Humphrey and Wickett, *The Right to Die,* p. 155.
53. Humphrey and Wickett, *The Right to Die,* p. 154.
54. Kevin D. O'Rourke, "Value Conflicts Raised by Physician-Assisted Suicide," *Linacre Quarterly* 57, no. 3 (August 1990), pp. 38–49.
55. SUPPORT Principal Investigators, "A Controlled Trial to Improve Care of Seriously Ill Hospitalized Patients. The Study to Understand Prognoses and Preferences for Outcomes and Risks of Treatment (SUPPORT), *Journal of the American Medical Association* 274 (1995), pp. 1591–1598.
56. Andrea Phelps et al., "Religious Coping and Use of Intensive Life-Prolonging Care Near Death in Patients With Advanced Cancer. *JAMA.* 301, no. 11 (2009), pp. 1140–1147.
57. John Shuster, talk at UAB Medical School, August 14, 1995.
58. Paul Longmore, Column in *Electric Edge*, January/February 1997.
59. Paul Longmore, "Elizabeth Bouvia, Assisted Suicide, and Social Prejudice," in *Issues in Law and Medicine* 2, no. 2 (Fall 1987), p. 158.
60. Longmore, "Elizabeth Bouvia," p. 158.
61. Fine, *UAB Report*, p. 12.
62. Fine, *UAB Report*, p. 4.
63. "McAfee Tries to Cut Red Tape," *Birmingham Post-Herald*, June 18, 1990, p. C1.
64. J. Hogeland and L. Sellars, "McAfee Shouldn't Get Special Treatment," (letter) *Birmingham Post-Herald,* July 9, 1990.
65. Douglas Martin, "Disability Culture: Eager to Bite the Hands That Would Feed Them," *New York Times*, June 1, 1997, p. A1.

Chapter 2

1. Robert Morse, *In the Matter of Karen Quinlan: The Complete Legal Briefs, Court Proceedings, and Decisions in Superior Court of New Jersey*, vols. 1 and 2, Frederick, MD, University Publications of America, 1982, p. 236 (hereafter, *Proceedings 1*, *Proceedings 2*). The later court transcript contradicts itself about the exact drugs Karen consumed. Attending physician Robert Morse testified that, "She had some barbiturates, which was normal, 0.6 milligrams; toxic is 2 milligrams, and the toxic dose is about 5 milligrams percent" [sic]. Julius Korein, in *Proceedings 1*, pp. 34–35. Consulting neurologist Julius Korein, whom the Quinlans hired, testified that Karen's drug screen "was positive for quinine, negative for morphine, barbiturates and other substances. A subsequent test for Valium and Librium was positive." (No one else mentioned Librium.) Court prosecutor George Daggett testified that Karen had taken tranquilizers with alcohol shortly before becoming unconscious. George Daggett, *New York Times*, September 20, 1975, New Jersey sec. The Quinlans denied that the drug screen showed barbiturates: "The early urine and blood samples, taken on the day Karen was brought to the hospital, revealed only a 'normal therapeutic' level of aspirin and the tranquilizer Valium in her system." Joseph and Julia Quinlan with Phyllis Battelle, *Karen Ann: The Quinlans Tell Their Story*, 1977, New York, Doubleday Anchor, p. 22.
2. Quinlan and Quinlan, *Karen Ann*, p. 27.
3. Daniel Coburn, in *Proceedings 1*, p. 17.
4. Julius Korein, in *Proceedings 1*, p. 329.
5. Fred Plum, in Quinlan and Quinlan, *Karen Ann*, p. 198.
6. Robert Morse, in Quinlan and Quinlan, *Karen Ann*, pp. 188–189.
7. Quinlan and Quinlan, *Karen Ann*, pp. 272–273 (the nun is not named).
8. Gino Concetti, quoted in Quinlan and Quinlan, *Karen Ann*, p. 284.
9. Quoted in Quinlan and Quinlan, *Karen Ann*.
10. Hentoff, "The Deadly Slippery Slope," *The Village Voice*, September 1, 1987.
11. Hentoff, "The Deadly Slippery Slope."
12. *Cruzan v. Director, Missouri Dept. of Health*, 110 S. Ct. 2841, 1990.
13. George Annas, "Nancy Cruzan and the Right to Die," *New England Journal of Medicine* 323, no. 10 (September 6, 1990), p. 670.
14. "Love and Let Die," *Time*, March 19, 1990, pp. 62ff.
15. Andrew M. Malcolm, "Nancy Cruzan: End to Long Goodbye," *New York Times*, December 29, 1990, p. A3. See also, "A Conversation with Mr. and Mrs. Cruzan," Midwest *Medical Ethics: The Nancy Cruzan Case* 5, nos. 1–2 (Winter/Spring 1989).
16. Charles Baron, "On Taking Substituted Judgment Seriously," *Hastings Center Report* 20, no. 5 (September-October 1992), p. 7.
17. John Robertson, "Cruzan: No Rights Violated," *Hastings Center Report* 20, no. 5 (September-October 1992), p. 7.
18. Ronald Cranford, lecture at UAB Medical School, January 19, 1991.
19. Joanne Lynn and Jacqueline Glover, Cruzan and Caring for Others," *Hastings Center Report* 20, no. 5 (September-October 1992) p. 11.
20. Annas, "Nancy Cruzan and the Right to Die," p. 672.
21. Irwin Molotsky, "Wife Wins Right-to-Die Case; Then a Governor Challenges It," *New York Times*, October 2, 1998, p. A20.
22. Timothy E. Quill, "Terri Schiavo—A Tragedy Compounded," *New England Journal of Medicine* 352 (April 21, 2005), pp. 1630–1633.
23. Jane Brody, "Preserving a Delicate Balance of Potassium," *New York Times*, June 22, 2004, p. 12. Low-carbohydrate high-protein diets do not create the right kind and amount of potassium for the body, nor do sports drinks replenish potassium lost in exercising nearly as well as fresh fruits and vegetables.
24. According to Kenneth Goodman, M.D., of the Department of Bioethics at the University of Miami, personal communication, November 14, 2004.
25. Arian-Camp-Flores, "The Legacy of Terri Schiavo," *Newsweek*, April 4, 2005, p. 26.
26. Austrian physician Semmelweis correctly charged his colleagues with spreading child-birth fever by not washing their hands and going from birth to birth; he was subsequently regarded by his fellow physicians as crazy.
27. Arian-Camp-Flores, "The Legacy," p. 26.
28. Quoted from William Colby, *The Long Goodbye: The Deaths of Nancy Cruzan*, Carlsbad, CA, Hay House Publishing, 2002.
29. Manuel Roig-Franzia, "Florida High Court Overrules Governor in Schiavo Case," *Washington Post*, September 24, 2004, p. A3.

30. Manuel Roig-Franzia, "Court Lets Right-to-Die Ruling Stand," *Washington Post*, January 24, 2005, A12.
31. Roig-Franzia, "Court Lets Right-to-Die Ruling Stand."
32. Walter F. Roche and Same Werhover, "DeLay Family Decided to End Life of His Father After Injury in 1988," *Washington Post*, March 28, 2005, p. A3.
33. Charles Babington and Mike Allen, "Congress Passes Schiavo Measure," *Washington Post*, March 2, 2005, p. A1.
34. Democrat Jim Jordan, quoted by Charles Babington, "Viewing Videotape, Frist Disputes Fla. Doctors' Diagnosis of Schiavo," *Washington Post*, March 20, 2005, p. A3.
35. Tamara Lipper, "Between Life and Death," *Newsweek*, March 28, 2005, p. 30.
36. Manuel Roig-Franzia, "Schiavo's Parents Take 'Final Shot' to Keep Her Alive," *Washington Post*, March 26, 2005, p. A4.
37. Nancy Weaver Teichert, "Experts: Lack of Food, Water, Does Not Cause Pain for Dying," *Sacramento Bee*, March 28, 2005; *Birmingham News*, March 29, 2005, p. A6.
38. "Report of Autopsy: Schiavo, Terri, Case #5050439," March 31, 2005, p. 5. See: http://www.sptimes.com/2005/06/15/schiavoreport.pdf#search=%22Terri%20Schiavo%20autopsy%22
39. Author's note: Colleagues in physical therapy report that "H.O." on such an autopsy probably means heterotopic ossification, formation of bone in muscle and soft tissue. It often occurs in persons with head injury and spinal cord injury and indicates that forceful passive range of motion may be a causative factor especially when there is severe spasticity. Microtrauma related to aggressive passive range of motion is only one of the theories of its etiology. It can lead to joint anklyosis, immobility, and consolidation of a joint.
40. "Report of Autopsy," p. 7.
41. "Report of Autopsy," p. 8.
42. President's Commission for the Study of Ethical Problems in Medicine and Biomedical and Behavioral Research, *Defining Death*, Superintendent of Documents, Washington, D.C., 1981, p. 14.
43. P. Mollaret and M. Goulon, "Le Coma Depasse," *Revue Neurologie* 101, no. 3 (1959).
44. Ad Hoc Committee of the Harvard Medical School to Examine the Definition of Brain Death, "A Definition of Irreversible Coma," *Journal of the American Medical Association* 205, no. 337 (1968).
45. The characteristics listed by the philosopher Mary Anne Warren in Chapter 5 (with regard to whether an aborted fetus is a person) might be used in a similar way to define the higher person standard: If all these characteristics are lacking we do not have a person.
46. Robert Morrison, "Death: Process or Event?" *Science* 173 (1971), pp. 694–698.
47. Lance Stell, "Let's Abolish 'Brain-Death,'" *Community Ethics* (University of Pittsburgh Center for Medical Ethics) 4, no. 1 (Winter 1997).
48. David Hammer, "Different Cases Cast Light on US Right-to-Die Cases," Associated Press, *Birmingham Post-Herald*, November 10, 2003, C5; Associated Press, "Arkansas Man Wakes After 19 Years in Coma," July 9, 2003; Benedict Carey, "Man Recovering from Brain Injury after 19 Lost Years," *New York Times*, July 4, 2006, reprinted in *Birmingham News*, July 4, 2006, A1.
49. AP, "Policeman Who Briefly Emerged from Coma-like State in '96 Dies," *Birmingham News*, April 16, 1997, p. 7A.
50. Benedict Carey, "Inside the Injured Brain."
51. Multi-Society Task Force on PVS, "Medical Aspects of the Persistent Vegetative State," parts 1 and 2, *New England Journal of Medicine* 330, no. 22 (May 26, 1994; June 2, 1994), pp. 1572–1579.
52. I. Dubroja et al., "Outcome of Post-traumatic Unawareness Persisting for More Than a Month," *Journal of Neurological Neurosurgery Psychiatry* 58, no. 4 (1995), pp. 465–466. R. Chen et al., "Prediction of Outcome in Patients with Anoxic Coma: a Clinical and Electrophysiologic Study," *Critical Care Medicine* 24, no. 4 (April 1996), pp. 672–678. Associated Press, "Policeman Who Briefly Emerged from Coma-like State in '96 Dies," *Birmingham News*, April 16, 1997, p. 7A.
53. I. Dubroja et al., "Outcome of Post-traumatic Unawareness Persisting for More Than a Month." *Journal of Neurological Neurosurgery Psychiatry* 58, no. 4 (1995), pp. 465–66.
54. R. Chen et al., "Prediction of Outcome in Patients with Anoxic Coma: A Clinical and Electrophysiologic Study," *Critical Care Medicine* 24, no. 4 (April 1996), pp. 672–78.

55. Benedict Carey, "Inside the Injured Brain, Many Kinds of Awareness," *New York Times*, April 5, 2005.
56. Carl Zimmer, "What If There's Something Going On in There?" *New York Times Magazine*, September 29, 2003.
57. Zimmer, "What If There's . . ."
58. Owen, Adrian, "Using Functional MRI Imaging to Detect Covert Awareness in the Vegetative State," *Archives of Neurology* 64, no. 8 (August 2007), p. 1098.
59. Morgan Peck, "Brain-wave Test Challenges Vegetative-State Diagnosis," August 6, 2008, *IEEE Inside Technology Spectrum*, p. 1. http://www.spectrum.ieee.org/biomedical/diagnostics/brainwave-test-challenges-vegetativestate-diagnosis
60. In 2009, Belgian researcher Steven Laureys awoke Rom Houben, who for 23 years had been conscious and falsely diagnosed as in a vegetative state, but unable to move. "Once someone is labeled as being without consciousness, it is very hard to get rid of that," Laureys said.
61. Her CT scan is on the website of University of Miami Department of Bioethics:http://www.miami.edu/ethics2/schiavo/CT%20scan.png
62. Rita Rubin, "Doctors Work to Understand Vegetative States," *USA Today*, March 21, 2005, 3A.
63. Cathy Lynn Grossman, "Pope Declares Feeding Tubes a 'Moral Obligation,'" *USA Today*, April 2, 2004, A1.
64. John Paris, quoted by Lisa Greene, "At Pope's Word, New Schiavo Cases?" *St. Petersburg/Tampa Bay Times*, May 1, 2004. http://www.sptimes.com/2004/05/01/Tampabay/At_pope_s_word__new_S.shtml
65. Mike Allen, "Conservative Groups."
66. Manuel Roig-Franzia, "Catholic Stance on Tube-Feeding Is Evolving," *Washington Post*, March 27, 2005, A7.
67. Frank Savage, quoted in the *Birmingham Post-Herald*, March 28, 2005, D1.
68. Harriet McBryde Johnson, "Overlooked in the Shadows," *Washington Post*, March 25, 2005.
69. Lisa Belkin, "As Family Protest, Hospital Seeks End to Woman's Life Support," *New York Times*, January 10, 1991, pp. A1-2.
70. Steven Miles, "Interpersonal Issues in the Wanglie Case," *Kennedy Institute of Ethics Journal* 2, no. 1 (March 1992), pp. 61–72.
71. For a review of these cases, see *Law, Medicine, and Health Care* 20 (1993), pp. 310–315.
72. R. Knox, "Americans' New Way of Dying: Don't Fight It," *Boston Globe*, June 5, 1994.
73. Knox, "New Way of Dying," app. B, p. 288.
74. Daniel Callahan, "On Feeding the Dying," *Hastings Center Report* 13, no. 5 (October 1983), p. 22; Gilbert Meillander, "On Removing Food and Water: Against the Stream," *Hastings Center Report* 14, no. 6 (December 1984), pp. 11–13.
75. W. May, R. Barry, O. Greise, et al., "Feeding and Hydrating the Permanently Unconscious and Other Vulnerable Persons," *Issues in Law and Medicine* 3, no. 3 (Winter 1987), pp. 203–217; C. Sprung, "Changing Attitudes and Practices in Forgoing Life-Sustaining Treatments," *Journal of the American Medical Association* 263, no. 16 (April 25, 1990), pp. 2211–2221.
76. American Medical Association, *Opinions of the Judicial Council*, Chicago, Ill. 1973.
77. Linda Greenhouse, "Right to Reject Life," *New York Times*, June 27, 1990.
78. SUPPORT Principal Investigators, "A Controlled Trial to Improve Care of Seriously Ill Hospitalized Patients. The Study to Understand Prognoses and Preferences for Outcomes and Risks of Treatment (SUPPORT). *Journal of the American Medical Association* 274 (1995) pp. 1591–1598.
79. R. F. Uhlmann, R. A. Pearlman, and K. C. Cain, "Physicians and Spouses' Predictions of Elderly Patients' Treatment Preferences," *Journal of Gerontology* 43 (1988), pp. 115–121.
80. Rick Weiss, "Patients' Surrogates Often Wrong about Preferred Treatment," *Washington Post*, March 14, 2006, p. A3.

Chapter 3

1. Johannes J. M. van Delden et al., "The Remmelink Study: Two Years later," *Hastings Center Report* 23, no. 6 (November-December 1993), p. 24.
2. http://www.euthanasia.cc/dutch.html#remm
3. Tara Burghart, Associated Press, "1 in 18 Opt Out of Assisted Suicide," August 18, 2005, *Birmingham News*, p. A11.
4. Veronica English et al., "Ethics Briefings," *Journal of Medical Ethics* 32 (2006), pp. 371–372.
5. Isabel Wilkerson, "Physician Fulfills a Goal: Aiding a Person in Suicide," *New York Times*, June 7, 1990.

6. Timothy Quill, "Death and Dignity: A Case of Individualized Decision Making," *New England Journal of Medicine* 327 (1992), pp. 1380–1384.
7. Susan Okie, "Dr. Pou and the Hurricane: Implications for Patient Care during Disasters," *New England Journal of Medicine* 358, no. 1 (January 3, 2008), pp. 1–5.
8. Okie, "Dr. Pou and the Hurricane," p. 1.
9. Susan Tolle, "Care of the Dying: Clinical and Financial Lessons from the Oregon Experience," *Annals of Internal Medicine* 128, no. 7 (April 1, 1998).
10. Tolle, "Care of the Dying."
11. Ezekiel Emanuel and Margaret Battin, "What Are the Potential Cost-Savings of Legalizing Physician-Assisted Suicide?" *New England Journal of Medicine* 339 (1998), pp. 167–172.
12. Susan Tolle et al., The Oregon Death with Dignity Act: A Guidebook for Health Professionals (PDF document), p. 7: http://www.ohsu.edu/ethics/toc.pdf#search=%22Susan%20Tolle%20Guidebook%20Oregon%22
13. Number of DWDA Prescription Recipients and Deaths, by Year, Oregon, 1998–2007. Oregon Death with Dignity Act, http://www.oregon.gov/DHS/ph/pas/docs/year10.pdf
14. *Seventh Annual Report on Oregon's Death with Dignity Act*, Office of Disease Prevention and Epidemiology, Department of Human Services, State of Oregon, March 10, 2005, 800 N.E. Oregon Street, Portland, OR 97232.
15. Tolle et al., *A Guidebook* p. 23–25.
16. Dave Parks, "Study: Ill Oregonians Refuse Food to Die, Rejecting Suicide Law," *Birmingham News*, July 24, 2003, p. A12.
17. Ludwig Edelstein, *Ancient Medicine: Collected Essays of Ludwig Edelstein*, O. Temkin and L. Temkin, eds. Baltimore, MD, Johns Hopkins University Press, 1967.
18. G. E. R. Lloyd, *Hippocratic Writings*, trans. Chadwick and W. N. Mann, New York, Penguin, 1950, p. 13.
19. Leo Alexander, "Medical Science under Dictatorship," *New England Journal of Medicine* 42 (July 14, 1949).
20. Robert Jay Lifton, *The Nazi Doctors*, New York, Basic Books, 1986.
21. J. C. Wilke, *Assisted Suicide and Euthanasia: Past and Present, Hayes Publications*, 1998, p. 9. I am indebted to Stephen W. Poff, M.D., for this reference and for points made in this paragraph.
22. Timothy Egan, *New York Times*, May 5, 1994, p. A1.
23. "Excerpts from Court's Decision," *New York Times*, June 27, 1997, p. A18.
24. Gina Kolata, "'Passive Euthanasia' in Hospitals Is the Norm, Doctors Say," *New York Times*, June 28, 1997, p. A1.
25. Christine Cassell, quoted in Michael Specter, "Suicide Device Fuels Debate," *Washington Post*, June 8, 1990.
26. James Rachels, "Active and Passive Euthanasia," *New England Journal of Medicine* 29 (January 9, 1975), pp. 78–80.
27. Baruch Brody, "Ethical Questions Raised by the Persistent Vegetative Patient," *Hastings Center Report* 18, no. 1 (1988), p. 35.
28. Jean Davies, "Raping and Making Love Are Different Concepts: So Are Killing and Voluntary Euthanasia," *Journal of Medical Ethics* 14 (1988), pp. 148–149.
29. Quoted in Barnard White Stack, "Doctors Divided Over the Very Ill, *Pittsburgh Post Gazette*, June 11, 1990.
30. Timothy Quill and Margaret Pabst Battin, "Excellent Palliative Care as the Standard, Physician-Assisted Dying as a Last Resort," in Timothy Quill and Margaret Pabst Battin, eds. *Physician-Assisted Dying: The Case for Palliative Care and Patient Choice*, Baltimore, MD, Johns Hopkins Press, 2004 pp. 323–330.
31. Quoted in Alan Parachini, "A Dutch Doctor Carries Out a Death Wish," *Los Angeles Times*, July 5, 1987, sec. 6, p. 9.
32. Joan Teno and Joanne Lynn, "Voluntary Active Euthanasia: The Individual Case and Public Policy," *Journal of the American Geriatrics Society* 39 (1991), pp. 827–830.
33. Quill and Pabst Battin, "Excellent Palliative Care," p. 325.
34. Quoted in Barnard White Stack, "Doctors Divided Over the Very Ill," *Pittsburgh Post Gazette*, June 11, 1990.
35. Margaret Battin, "The Least Worst Death," *Hastings Center Report* 13, no. 2 (April 1983), pp. 13–16.
36. Douglas Walton, *Slippery Slope Arguments*, New York, Oxford University Press, 1992.
37. Alexander, "Medical Science Under Dictatorship," p. 47.
38. Alexander, "Medical Science Under Dictatorship," p. 44.
39. Charlie LeDuff, "Prosecutors Say Ex-Doctor Killed Because It Thrilled Him," *New York Times*, September 7, 2000, p. A29.

40. Yale Kamisar, quoted in Earl Ubell, "Should Death Be a Patient's Choice?" *Parade Magazine*, February 9, 1992, p. 27.
41. T. Curiel, "Murder or Mercy? Hurricane Katrina and the Need for Disaster Training," *New England Journal of Medicine* 355, no. 20 (November 2006), p. 2067.
42. Michael Specter, "Suicide Device Fuels Debate," *Washington Post*, June 8, 1990.
43. Quoted in Peter Steinfels, "Dutch Study Is Euthanasia Vote Issue," *New York Times*, September 20, 1991.
44. Nat Hentoff, "The Deadly Slippery Slope," *Village Voice*, September 1, 1987.
45. Timothy Egan, "Assisted Suicide Comes. . . ."
46. Nat Hentoff, "The Coat Hanger of Assisted Suicide," *Washington Post*, December 12, 1997.
47. Christiaan Barnard, *One Life*, New York, Macmillan, 1965.
48. Alto Charo, quoted by Okie, "Dr. Pou and the Hurricane," p. 4.
49. L. Ganzini et al., "Prevalence of Depression and Anxiety in Patients Requesting Physicians Aid in Dying: Cross Sectional Survey," *British Medical Journal* 337 (2008), pp. 973–975.

Chapter 4

1. Maggie Scarf, "The Fetus as Guinea Pig," *New York Times Magazine* (October 19, 1975), pp. 194–200.
2. Scarf, "The Fetus as Guinea Pig."
3. A. Philipson et al., "Transplacental Passage of Erythomycin and Clindamycin," *New England Journal of Medicine* 288, no. 23 (June 7, 1973), pp. 1219–1221.
4. Paul Ramsey, *The Ethics of Fetal Research*, New Haven, CT, Yale University Press, 1975.
5. William Nolen, *The Baby in the Bottle*, New York, Coward, McCann, and Geoghegan, 1978, p. 203.
6. Nolen, *The Baby in the Bottle*.
7. "The Edelin Trial," transcript of a WBGH re-creation of Edelin's trial for a television documentary by Bill Moyers. Project of Legal-Medical Studies, Inc., Box 8219, John F. Kennedy Station, Government Station, Boston, MA 12134.
8. *Commonwealth v. Kenneth Edelin*, Mass. Supreme Court 359, N.E. 2nd, 1976.
9. Kenneth Edelin, quoted in *Ob. Gyn. News*, January 1, 1977, p. 1.
10. Quoted from Paul Ramsey, *Ethics at the Edges of Life*, New Haven, CT, Yale University Press, 1978, p. 94.
11. Nolen, *The Baby in the Bottle*, p. 174.
12. Nolen, *The Baby in the Bottle*, p. 175.
13. Paul Badham, "Christian Beliefs and the Ethics of In Vitro Fertilization," *Bioethics News* 6, no. 2 (January 1987), p. 10.
14. Michael Luo, "On Abortion, It's the Bible of Ambiguity," *New York Times*, November 13, 2005, Ideas and Trends Section, pp. 1, 3.
15. Paul Johnson, *A History of Christianity*, New York, Atheneum, 1983, Ch. 3.
16. John Connery, "Abortion: Roman Catholic Perspectives," *Encyclopedia of Bioethics* 1, New York, Macmillan, 1978.
17. Robert W. Mulligan, S.J., Jesuit Community at St. Louis University, personal letter to author.
18. Over the last 30 years, the Church has moved closer to immediate animation, especially with its emphasis on the value of the human embryo.
19. *Roe v. Wade*, Supreme Court Reporter 93, 410 U.S. 151, pp. 709–762.
20. Barbara Ehrenreich and Deirdre English, *For Her Own Good: 150 Years of Experts' Advice to Women*, New York, Doubleday, 1987, pp. 319–320.
21. Melanie Zurek and Silvia Henriquez, "Abortion Access Project and National Latina Institute for Reproductive Health," letter, *New York Times*, January 12, 2009.
22. Allan F. Guttmacher Institute, *Abortion and Women's Health*, New York and Washington, D.C., 1990, p. 27.
23. *A Private Affair*, a 1992 movie about this case, starred actress Sissy Spacek as Sherry Finkbine.
24. Peter Steinfels, "Papal Birth-Control Letter Retains Its Grip," *New York Times*, July 29, 1993, pp. A1, 13.
25. Norma McCorvey, *I Am Roe—My Life: Roe v. Wade and Freedom of Choice*, New York, Harper Collins, 1993.
26. Fact Sheet: Abortion Surveillance, June 7, 2002, Centers for Disease Control, Atlanta, Ga. For updates, see: www.cdc.gov/mmwr/preview/mmwrhtml/ss5407a1.htm
27. Mary Anne Warren, "On the Moral and Legal Status of the Fetus," *Monist* 57 (1973), pp. 43–61.
28. Don Marquis and Warren Quinn, "Why Abortion Is Immoral," *Journal of Philosophy* 86 (1989), pp. 183–202.

29. John T. Noonan, Jr. "An Almost Absolute Value in History," in John T. Noonan, Jr. ed., *The Morality of Abortion: Legal and Historical Perspectives*, Cambridge, MA, Harvard University Press, 1970, pp. 51–59.
30. Judith Jarvis Thomson, "A Defense of Abortion," *Philosophy & Public Affairs* 1, no. 1 (Fall 1971), pp. 47–66.
31. Francis Kamm, *Creation and Abortion*, New York, Oxford University Press, 1992.
32. John Connery, "Abortion: Roman Catholic Perspectives," pp. 9–13.
33. Ellen Willis, "*Harper's* Forum on Abortion," *Harper's* (July 1986), p. 38.
34. "Explosions Over Abortion," *Time*, January 14, 1985, p. 17.
35. Jeff Lyon, "Doctor's Dilemma: When Abortion Gives Birth to Life, Physicians Become Troubled Saviors," *Chicago Tribune*, August 15, 1982, Sec. 12, pp. 1, 3. (A 2.5 pound baby may be viable; jockey Willie Shoemaker, born prematurely, weighed this much and was kept warm in a shoebox in an oven.)
36. Linda Villanova, "Newest Skill for Future OB/GYN's Abortion Training," *New York Times*, June 11, 2002.
37. Susan Lee et al., "Fetal Pain: A Systematic Review of the Literature," *Journal of the American Medical Association* 294 (2005), pp. 947–954.
38. Consultants to the Advisory Committee to the Director, National Institutes of Health, *Report of the Human Fetal Tissue Transplantation Research Panel*, 1, National Institutes of Health, Bethesda, MD, 1988.
39. For costs and various kinds of pills, Google "Planned Parenthood" and "Emergency Contraception."
40. "Mother versus Child," Kenneth Jost, *American Bar Association Journal* (April 1989), p. 86.
41. E. Abel and Robert Sokol, "Fetal Alcohol Syndrome Is Now the Leading Cause of Mental Retardation" (letter), *Lancet* 8517, pp. 898–899.
42. Associated Press, "Mother Gets 6 Years for Drugs in Breast Milk," *New York Times* October 28, 1992, p. A11.
43. Harold Morowitz, "*Roe v. Wade* Passes a Lab Test," *New York Times*, November 25, 1992, p. A13.
44. *Planned Parenthood v. Casey*, excerpts quoted from *New York Times*, June 30, 1992, p. A8.
45. "Restrictions on Young Women's Access to Reproductive Services," Center for Reproductive Rights, June 2006, Item F010. www.crlp.org/tools
46. Hadley Arkes, "Courts Strike Down Laws Against Partial-Birth Abortion," *Wall Street Journal*, December 17, 1998, p. A31.

Chapter 5

1. Patrick Steptoe and Robert Edwards, *A Matter of Life*, London, Morrow, 1980.
2. *Time*, August 7, 1978, p. 68.
3. Richard Blandau, quoted in *Time*, November 13, 1978, p. 89.
4. Walter Kornberg, "Playing God in Laboratory: Question of Man's Wisdom," *Los Angles Times*, 16 March 1969, p. G3.
5. Audrey Smith, quoted in Steptoe and Edwards, *A Matter of Life*, p. 48.
6. Stephanie Saul, "In Vitro Clinics Face Questions Over Multiple Births," *New York Times*, February 12, 2009.
7. Sheryl Gay Stolberg, "For the Infertile, A High-Tech Treadmill of Despair," *New York Times*, December 14, 1997.
8. Centers for Disease Control, *Assisted Reproductive Technology Success Rates in the United States: 1996 National Summary and Fertility Clinic Reports*. (CDC website)
9. Seale Harris, *A Women's Surgeon: The Life Story of J. Marion Sims*, New York, Macmillan, 1950, p. 245; Barron Lerner, "Scholars Argue over Legacy of Surgeon Who Was Lionized, Then Vilified," *New York Times*, 28 October 2003, p. D7.
10. Elaine Tyler, *Barren in the Promised Land: Childless Americans and the Pursuit of Happiness*, Cambridge, MA, Harvard University Press, 1995, pp. 65–69.
11. Sheryl Gay Stolberg, "Quandary on Donor Eggs: What to Tell the Children," *New York Times*, January 18, 1998.
12. Gina Kolata, "New Pregnancy Hope: A Single Sperm Injected," *New York Times*, August 11, 1993, p. B7.
13. Peggy Orenstein, "Your Gamete, Myself," *New York Times*, 15 July 2007.
14. Richard Paulson, Mark Sauer, and Rogerio A. Lobo, "Reversing the Natural . . . of Pregnancy," *New England Journal of Medicine* 322 (1990), pp. 644–659.
15. Gina Kolata, "Successful Births Reported with Frozen Human Eggs," *New York Times*, October 17, 1997, p. A1.
16. David Colker, "It's a Boy—Embryo Is Viable after 1990 Freezing," *Los Angeles Times*, February 17, 1998.

17. Kirsty Horsey, "Twins Born 16 Years Apart," *Daily Mail* (England), May 30, 2006, p. A1.
18. Richard Jerome, "In the Band," *People*, July 1, 2002, pp. 48–50.
19. Sylvia Westphal, "New Way to Extend Fertility," *Wall Street Journal*, 20 April 2007, p. A1.
20. Denise Grady, "Parents Torn Over Extra Frozen Embryos from Fertility Procedures," *New York Times*, December 4, 2008, p. A22.
21. Laura Mansnerud, "The Baby Bazaar: How Bundles of Joy Not for Sale Are Sold," *New York Times*, October 26, 1998.
22. Mansnerud, "The Baby Bazaar."
23. The American Surrogacy Center, "Legal Overview of Surrogacy Laws by State," 2002. www.surrogacy.com
24. The Ethics Committee of the American Society for Reproductive Medicine, American Society for Reproductive Medicine, "Financial Compensation of Oocyte Donors," 2006.
25. Gina Kolata, "Soaring Price of Donor Eggs Sets Off Debate," *New York Times*, February 25, 1998, p. A1; Adrienne Knox, "Brokers and Fertility Clinics in Bidding War for Women Willing to Sell Eggs from Ovaries," *Birmingham News*, March 15, 1998, p. A3.
26. Richard Jerome, "Mortal Choices," *People*, October 7, 1996, pp. 96–102.
27. "McCaughey Septuplets Turn Four," *Dateline NBC*, November 20, 2001, reproduced at: www.msnbc.com/news/660542.asp
28. Robert Samuels, "Nine Years After Birth of Sextuplets, Now-Single Mom Struggles," *Washington Post*, 1 October 2006.
29. "Grandmother," *People*, June 28, 2006.
30. Reproductive Health and Early Life Changes," http://www.unfpa.org/modules/intercenter/cycle/earlylife.htm
31. Henry Chu, "China: Too Many Men, Too Few Women," *Birmingham News*, February 23, 2001.
32. "Text of Vatican's Statement on Human Reproduction," *New York Times*, March 11, 1987, pp. 10ff.
33. Laurie Goodstein and Elisabeth Povoledo, "Vatican Issues Instructions for Bioethics," *New York Times*, 12 December 2008.
34. Paul Ramsey, *Fabricated Man*, New Haven, CT, Yale University Press, 1970.
35. Steptoe and Edwards, *A Matter of Life*, p. 113.
36. Paul Ramsey, *The Ethics of Fetal Experimentation*, New Haven, CT, Yale University Press, 1975.
37. Joseph Fletcher, *Ethics of Genetic Control: Enduring Reproductive Roulette*, New York, Doubleday Anchor, reprinted by Prometheus, Buffalo, NY, 1984, p. 36.
38. Joseph Fletcher, "Ethical Aspects of Genetic Controls," *New England Journal of Medicine* 285, no. 14 (1971), pp. 776–781.
39. *Time*, November 13, 1978, p. 89.
40. John Marlow, quoted in *U.S. News and World Report*, August 7, 1978, p. 24.
41. John Marshall, quoted in *Time*, July 31, 1978, p. 59.
42. Leon Kass, "The New Biology: What Price Relieving Man's Estate?" *Journal of the American Medical Association* 174 (November 19, 1971), pp. 779–788.
43. James Watson, "Moving towards the Clonal Man," *Atlantic*, May 1971, p. 53.
44. Max Perutz, quoted in Steptoe and Edwards, *A Matter of Life*, p. 117.
45. Daniel Callahan, *New York Times*, July 27, 1978, p. A16.
46. M. Hansen et al., "The Risk of Major Birth Defects after Intracytoplasmic Sperm Injection and In Vitro Fertilization," *New England Journal of Medicine* 346 (March 7, 2002), pp. 725–730.
47. M. Hansen et al., "The Risk."
48. Examination of leftover embryos created by IVF reveals a good deal of genetic abnormalities, such as mosaicism and morphological problems (Yamada Shita, "ART and Birth Defects," *Congenital Abnormalities* 45 (2005), pp. 39–43. IVF may contribute to aberrant imprinting and DNA methylation, or epigenetic changes in the embryo's DNA. Scientists need to study whether different methods of stimulating superovulation or culturing embryos, as well as different times of transferring embryos to the uterus, affect epigenetic alternations (M. Hansen, "ART and Risk of Birth Defects—A Systematic Review," *Human Reproduction* 20 (2005), pp. 328–338.
49. Amy Docker Marcus, "A Registry for Test-Tube Babies," *Wall Street Journal*, September 16, 2003, pp. D1, D9.
50. Jeremy Rifkin and Ted Howard, *Who Shall Play God?* New York, Dell, 1977, pp. 115.
51. Hans Tiefel, "In Vitro Fertilization: A Conservative View," *Journal of the American Medical Association* 247, no. 23 (June 18, 1982), pp. 3235–3242.
52. Jeff Minerd, ESHRE: Birth Defect Risk Preferable to Childlessness in IVF Survey," *MedPage Today*, June 23, 2005.

53. Sheryl Gay Stolberg, "Quandary on Donor Eggs: What to Tell the Children," *New York Times*, January 18, 1998.
54. Cynthia Cohen, "Parents Anonymous," Cynthia Cohen, (ed.) *Egg Donation*, Baltimore, MD, Johns Hopkins University Press, 1997.
55. Susan Schindelhette, "My Life as a Sperm Donor," *People*, June 5, 2006, pp. 135–137.
56. Helen Ragone, *Conception from the Heart*, Bloomington, IN, Indiana University Press, 1994.
57. Rick Weiss, "Bioethics Panel Calls for Ban on Radical Reproductive Procedures," *Washington Post*, January 16, 2004.
58. Gina Kolata, "With Help of Science, Infertile Couples Can Even Pick Traits," *New York Times*, November 23, 1997, p. A1.
59. Frederic Golden, "Good Eggs, Bad Eggs," *Time*, January 11, 1999, p. 58.
60. Mary Rutz, "Selling Eggs: Cost and Consent in the Bull Market," *Bulletin of the University of Illinois at Chicago Department of Medical Education* 5, no. 2 (January, 1999), p. 3.
61. *Newsday*, February 8, 2009, p. A46.

Chapter 6

1. Maggie Scarf, "The Fetus as Guinea Pig," *New York Times Magazine*, October 19, 1975, pp. 194–200; Paul Ramsey's *The Ethics of Fetal Research*, New Haven, CT, Yale University Press, 1975.
2. Associated Press, "Ex-Husband Has Embryos Destroyed," June 16, 1993.
3. "The Science and Application of Cloning," National Bioethics Advisory Commission, *Cloning Human Beings: Report and Recommendations of the National Bioethics Advisory Commission*, Rockville, MD, June 1997, p. 20.
4. I. Wilmut et al., "Viable Offspring Derived from Fetal and Adult Mammalian Cells," *Nature* 385 (February 27, 1997), pp. 810–813.
5. Arnold Kriegstein, director, University of California Institute of Regenerative Medicine, quoted in "What a Bush Veto Would Mean for Stem Cells," Nancy Gibbs and Alice Park, *Time*, July 24, 2006, p. 36.
6. Douglas Melton, quoted in "What a Bush Veto Would Mean for Stem Cells," Gibbs and Park, *Time*, July 24, 2006, p. 36.
7. Justin Gillis and Rick Weiss, "NIH: Few Stem Cell Colonies Likely Available for Research," *Washington Post*, March 3, 2004, p. A3.
8. Chee Yoke Heong, "Malaysia New Dream: Biovalley," *Asia Times*, 2003.
9. "China, A Cloning Paradise," *Asia Times*, February 24, 2005.
10. "State Cloning Laws," The National Conference of State Legislators, April 18, 2006. http://ncls.org/programs/health/Genetics/rt-shcl.htm
11. "State Human Cloning Laws," April 18, 2006, The National Conference of State Legislatures. http://www.ncls.org/rorams/health/Genetics/rt-shel.htm.
12. Rick Weiss, "Mature Human Embryos Cloned," *Washington Post*, 12 February 2004, p. A28.
13. Gina Kolata, "Koreans Report Ease in Cloning for Stem Cells," *New York Times*, May 20, 2005, p. A1.
14. David Stout, "In First Veto, Bush Blocks Stem Cell Bill," *New York Times*, July 19, 2006, p. A1.
15. Paul Basken, "NIH Pleases Scientists with New Rules for Stem Cell Research," *Chronicle of Higher Education*, July 7, 2009 (web edition).
16. Rob Stein, "Researches May Have Found the 4 Equivalent of Embryonic Stem Cells," *Washington Post*, July 24, 2009, p. A5.
17. Rob Stein, "Lab Produces Monkeys with Two Mothers," *Washington Post*, August 27, 2009.
18. Richard McCormick, "Who or What Is a Preembryo?" *Kennedy Journal of Ethics* 1, no. 1 (March 1991), p. 5.
19. Richard McCormick, "Who or What Is a Preembryo?" It is also true that some Catholic theologians hold out for personhood as beginning some short time after conception. For our purposes here, and since their view has been de-emphasized of late, that view will not be discussed.
20. Richard McCormick, "Who or What Is a Preembryo?" p. 12.
21. Bonnie Steinbock, "Moral Status, Moral Value and Human Embryos: Implications for Stem Cell Research," ed. Bonnie Steinbock, New York, *Oxford Handbook of Bioethics* (2007).
22. Brian Leiberman, "Use of In-Vitro Fertilisation Embryos Cryopreserved for 5 Years or More," *Lancet* 15, no. 4 (October 4, 2000).
23. http://www.snowflakes.org/

24. "Committee Decides 'Therapeutic Cloning' Can Go Ahead," *BioNews* 147, 3 May 2002, p. 2.
25. David Ozar, "The Case for Not Unthawing Frozen Embryos," *Hastings Center Report* 15, no. 4 (August 1985), pp. 7–12.
26. Gene Outka, "The Ethics of Human Stem Cell Research," *Kennedy Institute Journal of Ethics* 12 (2002), pp. 175–213.
27. Lee Silver, *Re-Making Eden: Cloning and Beyond in a Brave New World*, New York, Avon, 1997.
28. Leon Kass, "Cloned Embryos," *First Things*, June 2002.

Chapter 7

1. Laurie Tarkan, "Too Many Interventions, and Too Many Preemies," *New York Times*, August 6, 2002.
2. National Center for Health Statistics, November 15, 2005, March of Dimes Press Release, same day.
3. N. Marlow, "Neurologic and Developmental Disability at Six Years of Age After Extremely Preterm Birth," *New England Journal of Medicine* 352, no. 1 (January 6, 2005).
4. John Boswell, *The Kindness of Strangers: The Abandonment of Children in Western Europe from Late Antiquity to the Renaissance*, New York, Pantheon, 1989; Robert Weir, *Selected Nontreatment of Handicapped Newborns*, New York, Oxford University Press, 1984.
5. William Lecky, *A History of European Morals from Augustus to Charlemagne*, II, New York, Braziler, 1955, pp. 25–56 (originally published 1869).
6. Marlow, "Neurologic and Developmental Disability at Six Years of Age After Extremely Preterm Birth."
7. A famous movie in medical ethics follows a case that is a collage of these three cases: *Who Should Survive?* Produced by the Joseph P. Kennedy Foundation, Film Service, 999 Asylum Avenue, Hartford, CT 10605.
8. James Gustafson, "Mongolism, Parental Desires, and the Right to Life," *Perspectives on Biology and Medicine* 16 (Summer 1973), p. 529.
9. R. Duff and A. Campbell, "Moral and Ethical Dilemmas in the Special-Care Nursery," *New England Journal of Medicine* 289, no. 17 (October 25, 1973), pp. 890–894.
10. John Lorber, "Results of Treatment of Myelomeningocele: An Analysis of 524 Unselected Cases, with Special Reference to Possible Selection for Treatment," *Developmental Medicine and Child Neurology* 13, no. 2 (1971), pp. 279–303.
11. Mary Tedeschi, "Infanticide and Its Apologists," *Commentary*, November 1984, p. 34.
12. Shari Staaver, "Siamese Twins' Case Devastates M.D.s," *American Medical News*, October 9, 1981, pp. 15–16.
13. Bonnie Steinbock, "Whatever Happened to the Danville Siamese Twins? *Hastings Center Report* 17, no. 4 (August-September, 1987), pp. 3–4. See also John Robertson, "Dilemma in Danville," *Hastings Center Report* 11, no. 5 (October 1981), p. 7.
14. U.S. Commission on Civil Rights, *Medical Discrimination Against Children with Disabilities*, Washington, D.C., September 1989, p. 391.
15. U.S. Commission on Civil Rights, *Medical Discrimination*, pp. 36, 323.
16. C. Everett Koop, "The Seriously Ill or Dying Child: Supporting the Patient and the Family," in D. Horan and D. Mall, eds., *Death, Dying and Euthanasia*, Frederick, MD, University Publications of America, 1977, pp. 537–539.
17. Adrian Peracchio, "Government in the Nursery: New Era for Baby Doe Cases," *Newsday*, November 13, 1983. Reprint, *The Baby Jane Doe Story: Winner of the 1984 Pulitzer Prize for Local Reporting, Newsday*, 1983.
18. Kathleen Kerr, "An Issue of Law and Ethics," *Newsday*, October 26, 1983; B. D. Colen, "A Life of Love—and Endless Pain," *Newsday*, October 26, 1983. (Available from *Newsday* in the reprint "The Baby Jane Doe Story: Winner of the 1984 Pulitzer Prize for Local Reporting"); "Baby Jane Doe," *Wall Street Journal*, November 21, 1983.
19. Kathleen Kerr, "Legal, Medical Legacy of Case," *Newsday*, December 7, 1987.
20. Kerr, "Legal, Medical Legacy of Case."
21. Bonnie Steinbock, "Baby Jane Doe in the Courts," *Hastings Center Report* 14, no. 1 (February 1984), p. 15; *Hastings Center Report* 14, no. 4 (August 1984).
22. Kerr, "Legal, Medical Legacy of Case"; see also Kerr, "Reporting the Case of Baby Jane Doe."
23. "Baby Jane Doe Has Surgery to Remove Water from Brain," *New York Times*, April 7, 1984, p. 28.

24. "Baby Jane Doe Has Surgery," *New York Times*.
25. Kerr, "Legal, Medical Legacy of Case."
26. Steven Baer, "The Half-Told Story of Baby Jane Doe," *Columbia Journalism Review*, November-December 1984, pp. 35–38; Mary Tedeschi, "Infanticide and Its Apologists," *Commentary*, November 1984, p. 34.
27. *Hastings Center Report* 24, no. 3 (May-June 1984), p. 2.
28. Rhoda Amon, "A Long-Running Morality Play," www.lihistory.com/9/hs9oral.htm
29. Gustafson, "Mongolism, Parental Desires."
30. C. Everett Koop, "The Slide to Auschwitz," *Whatever Happened to the Human Race?* Old Tappan, NJ, Revell, 1979.
31. *Who Should Survive?*
32. Fred Bruning, "The Politics of Life," *MacLean's*, December 12, 1983, p. 17.
33. James Rachels, "Active and Passive Euthanasia," *New England Journal of Medicine*. Vol. 292, January 9, 1975, pp. 78–80.
34. Koop, "The Slide to Auschwitz."
35. R. McCormick, "To Save or Let Die: The Dilemma of Modern Medicine," *Journal of the American Medical Association* 229, no. 8, July 1974, pp. 172–176.
36. Peter Singer, *Practical Ethics*, New York, Cambridge University Press, 1979, p. 137; Tristam Engelhardt, "Ethical Issues in Aiding the Death of Young Children," in Marvin Kohl, ed., *Beneficent Euthanasia*, Buffalo, NY, Prometheus, 1975; Michael Tooley, "Abortion and Infanticide," *Philosophy and Public Affairs* 2, no. 1 (Fall 1972), pp. 37–65.
37. Kerr, "Legal, Medical Legacy of Case."
38. Robert Weir, *Selected Nontreatment of Handicapped Newborns*, New York, Oxford University Press, 1984.
39. R. B. Zachary, "Life with Spina Bifida," *British Medical Journal* 2 (1977), p. 1461.
40. David Gibson, "Dimensions of Intelligence," in *Down Syndrome: The Psychology of Mongolism*, New York, Cambridge University Press, 1978, pp. 35–77; Janet Carr, "The Development of Intelligence," in David Lane and Brian Stafford, eds., *Current Approaches to Down Syndrome*, New York, Praeger, 1985, pp. 167–186.
41. Carr, "The Development of Intelligence."
42. Tom Regan, *The Case for Animal Rights*, Berkeley, CA, University of California Press, 1985.
43. Mathew Rarey, "Wrongful-Birth Lawsuits Put Doctors in Ethical Dilemma," *Washington Times*, August 5, 1999, p. A20.
44. "High Court Rules 'Wrongful Birth' Suits Invalid," *Atlanta Journal-Constitution*, July 7, 1999, p. E1.
45. Suzanne Daley, "France Bans Damages for 'Wrongful Births,'" New *York Times*, Jan. 2002, p. A8.
46. Loretta Kopelman, "Do the 'Baby Doe' Rules Ignore Suffering?" *Second Opinion* 18, no. 4 (April 1983), pp. 101–113.
47. John Robertson, "Extreme Prematurity and Parental Rights After Baby Doe," *Hastings Center Report* (July/August 2004), p. 33.
48. Brenda Coleman, "Moral Floodgates Opened by Father Pulling Plug on Son," Associated Press, May 1, 1989; 49. Gregg Levoy, "Birth Controllers," *Omni*, August 1987, p. 31.
49. *In the Matter of Baby K*, United States District Court, E. D. Virginia, July 7, 1993, no. Civ. A. 93-104-A; see also "The Case of Baby K," *Trends in Health Care, Law, and Ethics* 9, no. 1 (Winter 1994), pp. 1–48.
50. Gina Kolata, "Parents of Tiny Infants Find Care Choices Are Not Theirs," *New York Times*, September 30, 1991, p. A1.
51. Laurie Tarkan, "Too Many Interventions, and Too Many Preemies," *New York Times*, April 6, 2002.
52. John Robertson, "Extreme Prematurity and Parental Rights After Baby Doe," *Hastings Center Report* (July/August 2004), p. 34.
53. Bill Bartholomene, personal communication, who also read an earlier version of this chapter and who was a resident at the time and narrated the movie *Who Should Survive?* Also John Freeman, "On Learning Humility: A Thirty-Year Journey," *Hastings Center Report* (May-June, 2004), pp. 13–16.
54. A. Gallo, "Spina Bifida: The State of the Art of Medical Management," *Hastings Center Report* 14, no. 1 (February 1984), pp. 10–13.
55. Gallo, "Spina Bifida."
56. Spina Bifida Association, *Brief Amicus Curiae of the Spina Bifida Association of America, Weber v. Stony Brook Hospital*, New York State Supreme Court, Appellate Division, 2nd Department, *New York Law Journal*, October 28, 1983; quoted in Steinbock, "Baby Jane Doe in the Courts," p. 19.
57. Bob Meadows, Lorna Grisby, "Precious Child, Impossible Choice, *People*, May 15, 2006, p. 123.
58. Anita Silvers, "Rights Are Still Rights: The Case for Disability Rights," *Hastings Center Report* (November/December 2004), pp. 39–40.

Chapter 8

1. http://en.wikipedia.org/wiki/Unnecessary_Fuss
2. Quoted from the tape by W. Robbins, "Animal Rights: A Growing Movement in the U.S.," *New York Times*, June 15, 1984, p. A16.
3. *Evaluation of Experimental Procedures Conducted at the University of Pennsylvania Experimental Head-Injury Laboratory 1981–1984 in Light of the Public Health Science Animal Welfare Policy*, Office for Protection of Research Risks, National Institutes of Health, 1985, p. 37.
4. Quoted in "Animals in the Middle," in the television series *Innovation*, sponsored by Johnson and Johnson on A and E Network, September 5, 1987.
5. W. Robbins, "Animal Rights: A Growing Movement in the U.S.," *New York Times*, June 15, 1984, p. A16.
6. Robert Marshak, quoted in *New York Times*, July 29, 1984, p. A12.
7. Donald Abt, quoted in *New York Times*, August 12, 1984, p. B1.
8. *New York Times*, December 10, 1984, p. A10.
9. *New York Times*, December 10, 1984.
10. "Of Pain and Progress," *Newsweek*, December 26, 1988, p. 53.
11. Lila Guterman, "New Attacks on Animal Researchers Provoke Anger and Worry," *Chronicle of Higher Education*, August 15, 2008, p. A6.
12. Quoted in J. Duschek, "Protestors Prompt Halt in Animal Research," *Science News*, July 27, 1985, p. 53.
13. Edward Taub, "The Silver Spring Monkey Incident: The Untold Story," *Coalition for Animals and Animal Research Newsletter* 4, no. 1 (Winter-Spring 1991), pp. 1–8.
14. Tony Dajer, "Monkeying with the Brain," *Discover*, January 1992, pp. 70–71. See also Warren E. Leary, "Sharp Brain Healing Found in Disputed Monkey Tests, *New York Times*, June 28, 1991, p. A9.
15. Joachim Liepert, Heike Bauder, Wolfgang H. R. Miltner, Edward Taub, and Cornelius Weiller, "Treatment-Induced Cortical Reorganization After Stroke in Humans," *Stroke: The Journal of the American Heart Association* 31 (June 2000), pp. 1210–1216.
16. Edward Taub, *Topics in Stroke Rehabilitation*, 3, pp. 38–61.
17. Sandra Blakeslee, "Pushing Injured Brains and Spinal Cords to New Paths," *New York Times*, August 28, 2001, p. D6.
18. "Stroke Rehab Therapy Shows Benefits in 2-Year Follow-up," *UAB Reporter*, April 12, 2006.
19. "Taub Wins American Psychological Association Scientific Award," *UAB Synopsis*, February 16, 2004.
20. Edward Taub, Gitendra Uswatte, Danna Kay King, David Morris, Jean E. Crago, and Anjan Chatterjee, "A Placebo-Controlled Trial of Constraint-Induced Movement Therapy for Upper Extremity After Stroke," *Stroke: The Journal of the American Heart Association* 37 (April 2006), pp. 1045–1049.
21. John Durant, quoted in John Hargrove, "Bush Signs Heflin Bill to Protect Researchers," *Birmingham Post-Herald*, August 28, 1992.
22. Biomedical Research Education Trust, http://www.bret.org.uk/num.htm
23. Bernard Rollins, *Animal Rights and Human Morality*, Buffalo, NY, Prometheus, 1981, pp. 97–99.
24. D. Carvajal, "A New Science, at First Blush," *New York Times*, November 20, 2007, pp. C1, 4.
25. http://www.bret.org.uk/num.htm
26. Press Release, National Academies of Science, 29 May 2009, http://www8.nationalacademies.org/onpinews/newsitem.aspx?RecordID=12641
27. Office of Technology Assessment, *Animal Usage in the United States*, Superintendent of Documents, Washington, D.C., 1986, p. 12; *Newsweek*, December 26, 1988, p. 51; Andrew Rowan, *Of Mice, Models, and Men: A Critical Evaluation of Animal Research*, Albany, State University of New York Press, 1984, pp. 67–70.
28. Nicholas Fontaine, *Memoires pour servir Ö l'histoire de Port-Royal*, vol. 2, originally published in Cologne in 1738; quoted in L. Rosenfield, From *Best-Machine to Man-Machine: The Theme of Animal Soul in French Letters from Descartes to La Mettrie*, New York, Oxford University Press, 1940, pp. 52–53; also quoted in Peter Singer, *Animal Liberation*, New York Review of Books, 1975.
29. C. S. Lewis, *How Human Suffering Raises Almost Intolerable Intellectual Problems*, New York, Macmillan, 1940, pp. 131–133.
30. David Hume, *A Treatise of Human Nature*, 1789, New York, Oxford University Press.
31. Singer, *Animal Liberation*.
32. Shelly Kagan, quoted from Mark Oppenheimer, "Who Lives, Who Dies?" The Christian Century, July 3–10, 2002. pp. 24–29.
33. Quoted in S. Isen, "Laying the Foundation for Animal Rights: Interview with Tom

Regan," *Animals Agenda*, July-August, 1984, pp. 4–5.
34. Tom Regan, *The Case for Animal Rights*, Berkeley, University of California Press, 1983.
35. Quoted in "Animals in the Middle," in the television series *Innovation*, sponsored by Johnson and Johnson on the A & E Network, September 5, 1987.
36. Quoted in "Animals in the Middle."
37. Carl Cohen, "The Case for Animal Rights," *New England Journal of Medicine* 315, no. 14 (October 4, 1986), pp. 865–870.
38. Wise Young, quoted by Niall Shank, Ray Greek, Nathan Nobis, and Jean Swingle-Greek, "Animals and Medicine: Do Animal Experiments Predict Human Responses?" *The Skeptic* 13, no. 3 (2007), p. 1.
39. Niall Shank et al., "Animals and Medicine: Do Animal Experiments Predict Human Responses?" *The Skeptic* 13, no. 3 (2007), p. 1.

Chapter 9

1. S. Gomer, H. Powell, and G. Rolino, "Japan's Biological Weapons"; H. Powell, "A Hidden Chapter in History," *Bulletin of Atomic Scientists*, October 1981, pp. 43, 44.
2. Eugene Kogon, *The Theory and Practice of Hell*, New York, Farrar, Straus, and Cudahy, 1950; Berkeley reprint, 1980, p. 166.
3. Kogon, *The Theory and Practice of Hell.*
4. Vera Alexander, *The Search for Mengele*, HBO movie, October 1985; interviewed by Central Television (London) and quoted in Posner and Hare, op. cit., p. 37.
5. William Curran, "The Forensic Investigation of the Death of Joseph Mengele," *New England Journal of Medicine* 315, no. 17 (October 23, 1985), pp. 1071–1073.
6. David Rothman, "Ethics and Human Experimentation," *New England Journal of Medicine* 317, no. 19 (November 5, 1987), p. 1198.
7. Robert Bazell, "Growth Industry," *New Republic*, March 15, 1993, p. 14.
8. Constance Pechura, "From the Institute of Medicine," *Journal of the American Medical Association* 269, no. 4 (January 27, 1993), p. 453.
9. David Rothman, "Ethics and Human Experimentation," p. 1198.
10. H. Beecher, "Ethics and Clinical Research," *New England Journal of Medicine* 274 (1966), pp. 1354–1360.
11. H. Pappworth, *Human Guinea Pigs*, Boston, MA, Beacon, 1968.
12. Molly Selvin, "Changing Medical and Societal Attitudes toward Sexually Transmitted Diseases: A Historical Overview," in King K. Holmes et al., eds., *Sexually Transmitted Diseases*, New York, McGraw-Hill, 1984, pp. 3–19.
13. Alan Brandt, "Racism and Research: The Case of the Tuskegee Syphilis Study," *Hastings Center Report* 8, no. 6 (December 1978), pp. 21–29.
14. Paul de Kruif, *The Microbe Hunters*, New York, Harcourt Brace, 1926, p. 323.
15. J. E. Bruusgaard, "öber das Schicksal der nicht spezifisch behandelten Luetiker" ("Fate of Syphilitics Who Are Not Given Specific Treatment"), *Archives of Dermatology of Syphilis* 157, April 1929, pp. 309–332.
16. H. H. Hazen, "Syphilis in the American Negro," *Journal of the American Medical Association* 63 (August 8, 1914), p. 463.
17. James Jones, *Bad Blood*, New York, Free Press, 1981. p. 74.
18. Jones, *Bad Blood.*
19. Jones, *Bad Blood.*
20. Brandt, "Racism and Research."
21. Quoted in E. Ramont, "Syphilis in the AIDS Era," *New England Journal of Medicine* 316, no. 25 (June 18, 1987), pp. 600–601.
22. R. A. Vonderlehr, T. Clark, and J. R. Heller, "Untreated Syphilis in the Male Negro," *Journal of the American Medical Association* 107, no. 11 (September 12, 1936), pp. 856–860.
23. Jean Heller, "Syphilis Victims in U.S. Study Went Untreated for 40 Years," *New York Times*, July 26, 1972, pp. 1, 8.
24. Or worse: in 1988, a malpractice suit brought against a hospital in Vermont was settled out of court for $2.7 million on behalf of a 28-year-old woman who had gone into a coma after being incompetently tapped by a resident. "Malpractice Suit Settled for $2.7 Million," *Burlington Free Press* (Alabama), December 21, 1988.
25. Archives of National Library of Medicine; quoted in Jones, *Bad Blood*, p. 127.
26. W. J. Brown et al., *Syphilis and Other Venereal Diseases*, Cambridge, MA, Harvard University Press, 1970, p. 34.
27. Heller, "Syphilis Victims in U.S. Study."
28. Heller, "Syphilis Victims in U.S. Study."
29. Allison Mitchell, "Survivors of Tuskegee Study Get Apology from Clinton," *New York Times*, May 17, 1997, p. A1.

30. Carol Yoon, "Families Emerge as Silent Victims of Tuskegee Syphilis Experiments," *New York Times*, May 9, 1998, p. A1.
31. Marcia Angell, "The Ethics of Clinical Research in the Third World," *New England Journal of Medicine* 337, no. 12 (September 18, 1997), pp. 847–849.
32. R. H. Kampmeier, "The Tuskegee Study of Untreated Syphilis" (editorial), *Southern Medical Journal* 65, no. 10 (October 1972), pp. 1247–1251.
33. Thomas Benedek, "The 'Tuskegee Study' of Untreated Syphilis: Analysis of Moral Aspects versus Methodological Aspects," *Journal of Chronic Diseases* 31 (1978), pp. 35–50. I have drawn considerably on this excellent article.
34. Kampmeier, "The Tuskegee Study of Untreated Syphilis."
35. "The Deadly Deception" (with George Strait), Nova, January 28, 1992.
36. Thomas Benedek, "The 'Tuskegee Study' of Untreated Syphilis," p. 44.
37. Personal correspondence, April 25, 1985. Benjamin Friedman is Professor Emeritus of Medicine, UAB.
38. Benedek, "The 'Tuskegee Study' of Untreated Syphilis."
39. G. W. Hayes et al., "The Golden Anniversary of the Silver Bullet," *Journal of the American Medical Association* 270, no. 13 (October 6, 1993), p. 1610.
40. R. H. Kampmeier, "Final Report of the 'Tuskegee Study' of Syphilis," *Southern Medical Journal* 67, no. 11 (1974), pp. 1349–1353. Kampmeier advances a fourth argument that is somewhat more technical. Penicillin achieves seroreversal in latent syphilis, but Kampmeier insists that such seroreversal has never been proved to be associated with decreased morbidity or mortality. A related point is possible uncertainty over diagnosis and thus over therapeutic effects. (S. Edberg and S. Berger, *Antibiotics and Infection*, New York, Churchill Livingstone, 1983, pp. 141–142; K. Holmes et al., *Sexually Transmitted Diseases*, New York, McGraw-Hill, 1984, p. 1352; John Hotson, "Modern Neurosyphilis: A Partially Treated Chronic Meningitis," *Western Journal of Medicine* 135 [September 1981], pp. 191–200; Sarah Polt, Professor of Pathology, UAB, personal correspondence.)
41. Benedek, "The 'Tuskegee Study' of Untreated Syphilis."
42. Benedek, "The 'Tuskegee Study' of Untreated Syphilis."
43. Sheryl Gay Stolberg, "U.S. Ends Overseas HIV Studies Involving Placebos," *New York Times*, February 19, 1998.
44. Marcia Angell, "Tuskegee Revisited," *Wall Street Journal*, October 28, 1997.
45. Ellen Goodman, "Is Tuskegee Study OK Abroad?" *Boston Globe*.
46. Ruth Macklin, "Ethics and International Collaborative Research, Part I," *American Society for Bioethics and Humanities Exchange* 1, no. 2, p. 1.
47. Ellen Goodman, "Is Tuskegee OK Abroad?"
48. D. Bagenda and P. Musoke-Mudido, "We're Trying to Help Our Sickest People, Not Exploit Them," *Washington Post*, September 28, 1997, p. C3.
49. Macklin, "Ethics and International Collaborative Research."
50. Marcia Angell, "Tuskegee Revisited," *Wall Street Journal*, October 28, 1997.
51. Goodman, "Is Tuskegee OK Abroad?"
52. Stolberg, "U.S. Ends Overseas HIV Studies."
53. George Annas, "Global Clinical Trials and Informed Consent," *New England Journal of Medicine* 360, no. 20 (May 2009).
54. See my *Elements of Bioethics*, Chapter 8.
55. Dan Stober, Knight-Ridder Newspapers, "Dr. Hamilton Was Enthusiastic Experimenter in Radiation," *Birmingham News*, February 20, 1994, p. 10A; "America's Nuclear Secrets," *Newsweek*, December 27, 1993, p. 15.
56. Keith Schneider, "Scientists Are Sharing the Anguish over Nuclear Experiments on People," *New York Times*, March 2, 1994, p. A9.
57. Robert Burns, "Radiation Experiments Were Far-Reaching," Associated Press, *Birmingham Post-Herald*, August 18, 1995, p. E6.
58. Dennis Domerzalski, Scripps-Howard News Service, "Radiation 'Guinea Pigs' Tell Stories," *Birmingham Post-Herald*, February 3, 1994, p. A8.
59. Philip J. Hilts, "U.S. Is Urged to Repay Some in Radiation Tests," *New York Times*, July 17, 1995, p. A9. See also *Final Report*, Advisory Committee on Human Radiation Experiments, Washington, D.C.: U.S. Government Printing Office.
60. Arthur Caplan, "Rethinking the Cost of War," *Due Consideration*, New York, John Wiley & Sons, 1998, pp. 123–124.
61. Manuel Roig-Franzia, "Probe Opens on Study Tied to Johns Hopkins," *Washington Post*, August 23, 2001, p. B1.

62. Tamar Levin, "U.S. Investigating Johns Hopkins Study of Lead Paint Hazard," *New York Times*, August 24, 2001.
63. Richard Jerome, "Death by Research," *People*, February 21, 2000, p. 123.
64. Deborah Nelson and Rick Weiss, "Hasty Decisions in the Race to a Cure? Gene Therapy Proceeded Despite Safety, Ethics Concerns," *Washington Post*, November 21, 1999, p. A1.
65. Arthur Caplan is quoted extensively in Complaint for Civil Action filed by John Gelsinger for estate of Jesse Gelsinger against Trustees of University of Pennsylvania et al., www.sskrplaw.com/links/healthcare2.html
66. Nelson and Weiss, "Hasty Decisions."
67. Rick Weiss, "Research Volunteers Unwittingly at Risk," *Washington Post*, August 1, 1998, p. A1. See also this article from the on-line journal *Target Health*: *Target Health*, June 14, 1998. http://www.targethealth.com/
68. Institute of Medicine, *Responsible Research: A Systems Approach to Protecting Research Participants*, National Academy Press, Washington, D.C., 2002.
69. For psychiatrists who abused schizophrenic patients in psychiatric research, see Robert Whitaker, "Lure of Riches Fuels Testing," *Boston Globe*, November 17, 1998, p. A1; for another story about abuse of subjects and fraud in medical research, see Douglas M. Birch and Gary Cohn, "How a Cancer Drug Trial Ended in Betrayal," *Baltimore Sun*, June 24, 2001.
70. Steve Stecklow and Laura Johannes, "Drug Makers Relied on Clinical Researchers Who Now Await Trial," *Wall Street Journal*, August 15, 1997, p. A1.
71. *The Olivieri Report: The Complete Text of the Report of the Independent Inquiry Commissioned*, Canadian Association of University Teachers, Halifax, Canada, Lorimer, 2001. Miriam Shuchman, *The Drug Trial: Nancy Olivieri and the Science Scandal that Rocked the Hospital for Sick Children*, New York, Random House, 2005.
72. The Olivieri Report, op. cit.

Chapter 10

1. Thomas Starzl, *The Puzzle People: Memoirs of a Transplant Surgeon*, Pittsburgh, Pittsburgh University Press, 1992, p. 151.
2. Obituary of Norman Shumway, *The Independent* (London, England), February 16, 2006.
3. Christiaan Barnard and Curtiss Bill Pepper, *One Life*, New York, Macmillan, 1969, p. 372.
4. Barnard and Pepper, *One Life*, p. 406.
5. "The Ultimate Operation," *Time*, December 15, 1967, p. 65; "Heart Transplant Keeps Man Alive in South Africa," *New York Times* December 4, 1967, p. A1.
6. Barnard and Pepper, *One Life*, p. 444.
7. Quoted in Connie Chung, "Knife to the Heart," television documentary on heart transplant surgery, January 27, 1997.
8. Donald McRae, *Every Second Counts: The Race to Transplant the First Human Heart*, New York, Putnam, 2006, p. 272.
9. Francis Moore, M.D. quoted in interview with Chung, "Knife to the Heart."
10. Andre Courmand, *New York Times*, December 6, 1967.
11. Norman Staub, quoted in Peter Hawthorne, *The Transplanted Heart*, Johannesburg, South Africa, Keartland Publishing, 1968, p. 188.
12. Denise Grady, "Summary of Discussion of Ethical Perspectives," in Margery Shaw, ed., *After Barney Clark*, Austin, TX, University of Texas Press, p. 52.
13. *Time*, December 9, 1982, p. 43.
14. *Time*, March 14, 1983, p. 74.
15. Thomas Preston, "Who Benefits from the Artificial Heart?" *Hastings Center Report* 15, no. 1 (February 1985), p. 5; *New York Times*, December 5, 1988, p. A2.
16. *Washington Post*, May 1, 1983, p. A2.
17. William A. Check, "Lessons from Barney Clark's Artificial Heart," *Health*, April 1984, pp. 22, 26.
18. Gideon Gill, "Burcham Dies After Blood Accumulates in Chest," *Louisville Courier-Journal*, April 26, 1983.
19. Gill, "Burcham Dies."
20. Michael Vitez, "Marriage of Two Minds: 'World's Smartest Couple' Nears First Anniversary," Knight-Ridder Newspapers, July 3, 1988.
21. Steve Ditlea, "Robert Jarvik Returns," *Red Herring*, October 11, 2002.
22. "Profile: Dr. William C. DeVries, Surgeon," Linda Kozaryn, *Defend America*, American Armed Forces Press Service, August 2002.
23. Donald McRae, *Every Second Counts: The Race to Transplant the First Human Heart*, New York, Putnam, 2006.

24. William Pierce, "Permanent Heart Substitution: Better Solutions Ahead," editorial, *Journal of the American Medical Association* 259, no. 6 (February 12), 1988, p. 891.
25. Werner Forssmann, quoted in Barnard and Pepper, *One Life*, p. 360.
26. Starzl, *The Puzzle People*, p. 148.
27. Donald McRae, *Every Second Counts: The Race to Transplant the First Human Heart*, New York, Putnam, 2006, p. 192.
28. *New York Times*, editorial, December 16, 1982, p. A26.
29. "The Dracula of Medical Technology," Editorial, *New York Times*, May 16, 1988.
30. "Transplants in the U.S. by Recipient ABO," *The Organ Procurement and Transplantation Network*, June 30, 2006, http://optn.transplant.hrsa.gov/latestData/rptData.asp
31. Stacy Burling, "Widow Sues Artificial-Heart Maker," *Philadelphia Inquirer*, October 17, 2002; Sheryl Gay Stolberg, "On Medicine's Last Frontier: The Last Journey of James Quinn," *New York Times*, October 8, 2002.
32. Lauran Neegaard, "FDA Advisers Reject Abiomed's Artificial Heart," Associated Press, *Birmingham News*, June 24, 2005, p. A14.
33. "FDA Approves Artificial Heart Implant," *USA Today*, October 14, 2004, p. A1.
34. Norman Shumway, quoted in *Transplant News*, July 13, 2001, from an interview in the *San Francisco Chronicle*.
35. NIH website, www.nhlbi.nih.gov/health/public/heart/other/hrt_lung.htm#Cost
36. D. P. Lubeck and J. P. Bunker, Office of Technology Assessment, *Case Study 9, The Artificial Heart: Costs, Risks, and Benefits*, Washington, D.C., U.S. Government Printing Office, 1982.
37. *Progressive*, February 1983, pp. 12–13.
38. Rene Fox and Judith Swazey, *The Courage to Fail: A Social View of Organ Transplants and Dialysis*, 2nd ed., rev., Chicago, University of Chicago Press, 1974, 1978.
39. P. M. Park, "The Transplant Odyssey," *Second Opinion*, November 12, 1989, pp. 27–32; quoted in Rene Fox and Judith Swazey, *Spare Parts: Organ Replacement in American Society*, New York, Oxford University Press, 1992, p. 202.
40. A. J. Moskowitz, "The Cost of Long-Term LVAD Implantation," *Annals of Thoracic Surgery* 71, Supplement 3 (March 2001), pp. S195–198, S203–204.
41. Sandeep Jauhar, "The Artificial Heart," *New England Journal of Medicine* (February 5, 2004), pp. 542–544.
42. Denise Grady, "Researchers Find Poor Use of Pumps for Ailing Hearts," *New York Times*, November 6, 2008, p. A19.
43. Rob Stein, "Heart Pump Creates Life-Death Ethical Dilemma," *Washington Post*, 24 April 2008.
44. David Benatar and Don A. Hudson, "A Tale of Two Novel Transplants Not Done: The Ethics of Limb Allografts," *British Medical Journal* 324 (April 20, 2002), pp. 971–975.
45. According to Dr. Nadey Hakim, of London, interviewed by Lawrence K. Altman, "A Pioneering Transplant, and Now an Ethical Storm," *New York Times*, December 6, 2005.
46. Marco Lanzetta et al., "International Registry on Hand and Composite Tissue Transplantation," *Transplantation* 79, no. 9 (May 15, 2005).
47. Susan Okie, "Brave New Face," *New England Journal of Medicine*, 354, no. 9 (March 2, 2006).
48. Ariane Bernard and Craig S. Smith, "French Face-Transplant Patient Tells of Her Ordeal," *New York Times*, February 7, 2006.
49. Lawrence K. Altman, "A Pioneering Transplant, and Now an Ethical Storm," *New York Times*, December 6, 2005.
50. Craig S. Smith, "As a Face Transplant Heals, Flurries of Questions Arise," *New York Times*, December 14, 2005, p. A1.
51. Lawrence K. Altman, "Patient Opted for Transplant as Method to Mend Face," *New York Times*, December 12, 2005, p. A6.
52. Lawrence K. Altman, "A Pioneering Transplant, and Now an Ethical Storm," *New York Times*, December 6, 2005, p. D1.
53. Personal communication to author, September 7, 2006.
54. Jean-Michel Dubernard, "Outcomes 18 Months after the First Human Partial Face Transplantation," *New England Journal of Medicine* 13 (December 2007), pp. 2451–2460.
55. Reuters, "China Performs Its First Human Face Transplant," April 14, 2006.
56. "Boston Hospital Completes World's Seventh Face Transplant." *Red Orbit* 11 (April 2009), Web.1.
57. "Norman Shumway, Heart Transplantation Pioneer, Dies at Age 83," Press Release, February 10, 2006, Stanford Medical Center.

Chapter 11

1. Dale H. Cowan, ed., *Human Organ Transplantation: Social, Medical-Legal, Regulatory, and Reimbursement Issues*, Ann Arbor, MI, Health Administration Press, 1987, p. 60.
2. James Childress, "Who Shall Live When Not All Can Live?" *Soundings* 53, no. 4 (Winter 1970).
3. Belding Scribner, unpublished manuscript, quoted in Renée Fox and Judith Swazey, *The Courage to Fail: A Social View of Organ Transplants and Dialysis*, 2nd ed. rev., Chicago, University of Chicago Press, 1974, 1978, p. 227.
4. Renée Fox and Judith Swazey, *The Courage to Fail*, p. 235.
5. One of the first organized interdisciplinary conferences to discuss such issues took place in 1967, funded by a company, CIBA.
6. H. M. Schmeck, Jr., "Panel Holds Life-or-Death Vote in Allotting of Artificial Kidney," *New York Times*, May 6, 1962, pp. 1, 83.
7. Shana Alexander, "They Decide Who Lives, Who Dies: Medical Miracle Puts a Burden on a Small Committee," *Life* 53, no. 102 (November 9, 1962).
8. Renée Fox and Judith Swazey, *The Courage to Fail*, p. 209.
9. Judith Swazey at "The Birth of Bioethics" conference, Seattle, WA, University of Washington Medical School, September 24, 1992.
10. David Sanders and Jesse Dukeminier, "Medical Advance and Legal Lag: Hemodialysis and Kidney Transplantation," *UCLA Law Review* 15 (1968), pp. 357–412.
11. http://www.cms.hhs.gov/ESRDGeneralInformation/Downloads/2004ProgramHighlights.pdf
12. Fox and Swazey, *The Courage to Fail*, p. 232.
13. David Sanders and Jesse Dukeminier, "Medical Advance and Legal Lag."
14. George Annas, "The Prostitute, the Playboy, and the Poet: Rationing Schemes for Organ Transplantation," *American Journal of Public Health* 75, no. 2 (1985), pp. 187–189.
15. Fox and Swazey, *The Courage to Fail*, chapter 9.
16. Fox and Swazey, *The Courage to Fail*, p. 234.
17. Herbert Fingarette, *Heavy Drinking*, Berkeley, University of California Press, 1988.
18. Alvin Moss and Mark Seigler, "Should Alcoholics Compete Equally for Liver Transplantation?" *Journal of the American Medical Association* 265, no. 10 (March 13), 1992, p. 1295.
19. C. Cohen and M. Benjamin, "Alcoholics and Liver Transplantation," *Journal of the American Medical Association* 265, no. 10 (March 13, 1992), pp. 1295–1301.
20. Nicholas Rescher, "The Allocation of Exotic Medical Lifesaving Therapy," *Ethics* 79 (April 1969).
21. Tracy E. Miller, "Multiple Listing for Organ Transplantation: Autonomy Unbounded," *Kennedy Institute of Ethics Journal* 2, no. 1 (March 1992), pp. 43–57.
22. Munson, Ronald, *Raising the Dead*, New York, Oxford University Press, 2002, pp. 26–45.
23. Munson, *Raising the Dead*, p. 29.
24. Munson, *Raising the Dead*, p. 30.
25. Munson, *Raising the Dead*, p. 36.
26. Munson, *Raising the Dead*, p. 45.
27. Tracy E. Miller, "Multiple Listing for Organ Transplantation."
28. M. Michaels et al., "Ethical Considerations in Listing Fetuses as Candidates for Neonatal Heart Transplantation," *Journal of the American Medical Association* 269, no. 3 (January 20, 1993), pp. 401–402.
29. Rene Fox and Judith Swzey, *Spare Parts: Organ Replacement in American Society*, New York, Oxford University Press, 1992.
30. Albert R. Jonsen, "Bentham in a Box," *Law, Medicine and Health Care* 14 (1986), pp. 172–174.
31. Newsroom Fact Sheets, United Network for Organ Sharing, November 21, 2005, http://www.unos.org/inthenews/factsheets.asp, July 10, 2006.
32. Michael Stoll, "A New Waiting Game for Hearts," *Philadelphia Inquirer*, February 7, 2000.
33. Jeffrey Kahn and Susan Parry, "Organ and Tissue Procurement," *Encyclopedia of Bioethics*, 3rd ed., New York, Macmillan, 2004, p. 1936; see also "A Science Odyssey: People and Discoveries: First Successful Kidney Transplant Performed," http://www.pbs.org/wgbh/aso/databank.entries/dm54ki.html
34. I distinguish here between donors and organs. More organs still come from cadavers (brain dead patients). Cadavers yield 1.7 kidneys on average, but live donors of course can give only one kidney. Each

year, about 8,500 kidneys come from cadavers and about 5,500 from live donors. See www.unos.org

35. A. Bass, "New Liver Transplants; Pressure on Parents," *Boston Globe*, December 17, 1989, 1, 75; quoted in Fox and Swazey, *Spare Parts*.
36. Norman Fost, "Conception for Donation," *Journal of the American Medical Association* 291, no. 17 (May 6, 2004), p. 2126.
37. Charles B. Huddleston et al., "Lung Transplantation in Children," *Annals of Surgery* 236, no. 3 (September 2002), pp. 270–276.
38. S. Quattrucci et al., "Lung Transplantation for Cystic Fibrosis: 6-Year Follow-Up," *Journal of Cystic Fibrosis* 4, no. 2 (May 2005), pp. 107–114.
39. V. Fourbister, "Living Donors Dramatize Risk vs. Need," *American Medical News*, September 20, 1999, p. 1.
40. The death was confirmed by Dr. Jean Edmond in V. Fourbister, "Living Donors Dramatize Risk vs. Need," *American Medical News*, September 20, 1999, p. 1.
41. Debra Shelton's update is "Donor Has Physical Pain, But Peace About Decision," and "Man's Second Chance Hasn't Turned Out Like He Expected," *St. Louis Post-Disptach*, December 21, 2003.
42. Mary Ellison et al., "Living Kidney Donors in Need of Kidney Transplants," *Transplantation* (November 15, 2002), pp. 1349–1351. These 56 patients were out of 140,000 patients. Also, UNOS elevates to top of the list for receiving a kidney anyone who previously donated one and who now needs one.
43. Carole Tarrant, "For Family, Selfless Act Goes Awry," *New York Times*, March 12, 2002.
44. H. N. Ibrahim et al., "Longterm Consequences of Kidney Donation," *New England Journal of Medicine* 360 (2009), pp. 459–469.
45. Richard D. Lamm, "Health Care as Economic Cancer," *Dialysis and Transplantation* 16 (1987), p. 433.
46. Fox and Swazey, *Spare Parts*, p. 10.
47. Fox and Swazey, *Spare Parts*, p. 45.
48. Interview, *Good Morning America*, July 9, 1993.
49. Walter Robinson, *Medical Ethics* (Lahey Clinic Medical Ethics Newsletter) 11, no. 2 (Spring 2004), p. 8.
50. Walter Robinson, *Medical Ethics*, p. 6.
51. Peter Landers, "Longer Dialysis Offers New Hope But Poses a Dilemma," *Wall Street Journal*, October 2, 2003, p. A1.

Chapter 12

1. Rene Fox and Judith Swazey, *The Courage to Fail: A Social View of Organ Transplants and Dialysis*, 2nd ed., rev., Chicago, University of Chicago Press, 1974, 1978; Harmon Smith, "Heart Transplantation," *Encyclopedia of Bioethics*, New York, Free Press, 1978.
2. Richard Howard and J. Najarian, "Organ Transplantion—Medical Perspective," *Encyclopedia of Bioethics* 3, New York, Free Press, 1978, pp. 1160–1165.
3. *Animals Voice* 2, no. 3 (December 1984).
4. Charles Krauthammer, "The Using of Baby Fae," *Time*, December 3, 1984, p. 14.
5. Quoting Kenneth P. Stoller, M.D., "Baby Fae: The Unlearned Lesson," *Perspectives on Medical Research* 2 (1990). www.curedisease.com/Perspectives/vol.2_1990/BabyFae.html
6. "Baby Fae Stuns the World," *Time*, November 12, 1984, p. 72.
7. "Baby Fae Stuns the World," p. 70.
8. Tom Regan, "The Other Victim," *Hastings Center Report* 15, no. 1 (February 1985), pp. 9–10.
9. Thomasine Kushner and Raymond Belotti, "Baby Fae: A Beastly Business," *Journal of Medical Ethics* 11 (1985), pp. 178–183.
10. Denise Breo, "Interview with Baby Fae's Surgeon," *American Medical News*, November 16, 1984, p. 18.
11. "Interview with Dr. Jack Provonsha," *U.S. News and World Report*, November 12, 1984, p. 59.
12. Dan Chu and Eleanor Hoover, "Helped by a Baboon Heart, An Imperiled Infant, Baby Fae, Beat the Medical Odds," *People* November 18, 1984.
13. Breo, "Interview with Baby Fae's Surgeon," p. 18.
14. Chu and Hoover, "Helped by a Baboon Heart," p. 74.
15. Chu and Hoover, "Helped by a Baboon Heart," p. 74.
16. Thomas Starzl, *The Puzzle People: Memoirs of a Transplant Surgeon*, Pittsburgh, University of Pittsburgh Press, 1992, p. 123.
17. Breo, "Interview with Baby Fae's Surgeon," p. 18.
18. Paul Ramsey, "The Enforcement of Morals: Nontherapeutic Research on Children," *Hastings Center Report* 6 (August 1976), pp. 21–30.
19. Richard McCormick, "Proxy Consent in the Experimentation Situation," *Perspectives*

in Biology and Medicine 18, no. 1 (Autumn 1974), pp. 2–20.

20. Alexander Capron, "When Well-Meaning Science Goes Too Far," *Hastings Center Report* 15, no. 1 (February 1985), pp. 8–9.
21. George Annas, "The Anything Goes School of Human Experimentation," *Hastings Center Report* 15, no. 1, February 1985, pp. 15–17.
22. "Celebrity surgery" was a term coined in a *New Republic* editorial, December 17, 1984.
23. Keith Reemtsma, *Hastings Center Report* (February 1985), p. 10.
24. Alex Capron, *Hastings Center Report* (February 1985), p. 8.
25. Charles Krauthammer, "The Using of Baby Fae," *Time*, December 3, 1984, pp. 87–88.
26. Breo, "Interview," p. 18.
27. Breo, "Interview," p. 13.
28. Starzl, *The Puzzle People*, p. 123.
29. "Baby Fae Stuns the World," p. 70.
30. Jacques Loman, *Journal of Heart Transplantation* 4, no. 1 (November 1984), pp. 10–11.
31. Annas, "The Anything Goes School."
32. *Nature* 88, no. 312 (November 8, 1984), p. 59–90.
33. Krauthammer, "The Using of Baby Fae."
34. "Judicial Council Offers New Guidelines," *American Medical News* 27, December 14, 1984, p. 46.
35. Associated Press, "Hospital Sets Policy on Organ Donor Use," February 23, 1988.
36. Joan Heilman, "Tiny Gabriel's Gift of Life," *Redbook*, December 1988, p. 162. (Article given to me by Lynn Bondurant.)
37. J. Peabody et al., "Experience with Anencephalic Infants as Prospective Organ Donors," *New England Journal of Medicine* 321, no. 6 (August 10, 1989), pp. 344–350.
38. Debra Berger, "The Infant with Anencephaly: Moral and Legal Dilemmas," *Issues in Law and Medicine* 5 (1989), p. 68.
39. Medical Task Force on Anencephaly, "The Infant with Anencephaly," *New England Journal of Medicine* 332, no. 10 (March 8, 1990), p. 669.
40. Robert D. Trough and John D. Fletcher, "Can Organs Be Transplanted before Brain Death? *New England Journal of Medicine* 321, no. 6 (1989), p. 388.
41. A. Kantrowitz et al., "Transplantation of the Heart in an Infant and an Adult," *American Journal of Cardiology* 22, no. 782 (1968).
42. Associated Press, "Ethicists Debate Death and Baby's Lacking Brain," March 31, 1992; in *Birmingham News*, p. A1.
43. Brian Udell, quoted in *USA Today*, March 30, 1992, p. 3A.
44. *In Re T.A.C.P., Southern (Law) Reporter*, 2nd Series, Supreme Court of Florida, November 12, 1992, pp. 588–595.
45. D. Shewmon, "Anencephaly: Selected Medical Aspects," *Hastings Center Report* 18, no. 5 (1988), pp. 11–19.
46. Laurie Abraham, "The Use of Anencephalic Infants as Organ Sources," *American Medical News* 261, no. 12 (March 24–31, 1989), pp. 1773–1781.
47. Debra H. Berger, *Issues in Law and Medicine* 67 (1989), pp. 84–85; quoted by Estella Moriarty in *In Re T.A.C.P.*, p. 595.
48. D. Medearis and L. Holmes, "On the Use of Anencephalic Infants as Organ Donors," *New England Journal of Medicine* 321, no. 6 (August 10, 1989), p. 392.
49. Beth Brandon, "Anencephalic Infants as Organ Donors: A Question of Life and Death," *Case Western Law Review* 40 (1989–1990), p. 781; quoted by Estella Moriarty in *In Re T.A.C.P.*
50. *In Re T.A.C.P.*, p. 590.
51. A. Capron, "Anencephalic Donors: Separate the Dead from the Dying," *Hastings Center Report* 17, no. 1 (February 1987), pp. 5–8; John Arras, "Anencephalic Newborns as Organ Donors: A Critique," *Journal of the American Medical Association* 259, no. 15 (April 15, 1986), pp. 2284–2285.
52. Shewmon, "Anencephaly: Selected Medical Aspects."
53. Alice Dregger, *One of Us: Conjoined Twins and the Future of Normal*, Cambridge, MA, Harvard University Press, 2004.
54. Alice Dregger, "Jarring Bodies: Thoughts on the Display of Unusual Anatomies," *Perspectives in Biology and Medicine* 43, no. 2 (Winter 2000), pp. 161–172.
55. Ben Carson, *Gifted Hands: The Ben Carson Story*, Grand Rapids, MI, Zondervan Press, 1990.
56. Press Release, "Conjoined Twin Fact Sheet," Johns Hopkins Children's Center, www.hopkinschildrens.org/pages/news/twins_factsheet.html
57. Alice Dregger, *One of Us: Conjoined Twins and the Future of Normal*, Cambridge, MA, Harvard University Press, 2004, p. 66, quoting Rowena Spencer, *Conjoined Twins: Developmental Malformations and Clinical*

Implications, Baltimore, MD, Johns Hopkins University Press, 2003, pp. 310–311.
58. Dregger, *One of Us*, p. 67.
59. Press Release "Hopkins Team Separates Conjoined Twins," Johns Hopkins International, September 16, 2004.
60. From a discussion of evolution between Richard Dawkis, Francis Collins, Danel Dennett, and Ben Carson recorded at: http://www.archive.org/details/RichardDawkinsDanielDennettVs.FrancisCollinsBenjaminCarson
61. Dregger, *One of Us*, p. 63.
62. David Wasserman, "Killing Mary to Save Jodie: Conjoined Twins and Individual Rights," *Philosophy and Public Affairs Quarterly* 21, no. 1 (Winter 2001), pp. 9–14.
63. Dregger, *One of Us*, p. 93.
64. Dregger, *One of Us*, p. 65.

Chapter 13

1. *New York Times*, November 6, 1987, p. B1.
2. Ibid.
3. *New York Times*, November 13, 1987, p. B21.
4. Ibid.
5. *New York Times*, November 13, 1987, p. A1.
6. Ibid.
7. "Brown versus Koch," *60 Minutes*, 1988.
8. "Court Backs Treatment of Woman Held under Koch Plan," *New York Times*, December 19, 1987, p. A1.
9. "Brown versus Koch," *60 Minutes*, interview with Ed Bradley, 1988.
10. "Brown versus Koch."
11. *New York Times*, January 20, 1988, p. A16.
12. Julian Jaynes, *The Origin of Consciousness and the Breakdown of the Bicameral Mind*, Boston, Houghton Mifflin, 1976.
13. Thomas Szasz, "Involuntary Mental Hospitalization: A Crime against Humanity," in *Ideology and Insanity*, New York, Doubleday, 1970.
14. D. Rosenhan, "On Being Sane in Insane Places," *Science* 179 (1973), pp. 250–258.
15. *O'Conner v. Donaldson*, 422 U.S. 563. 95 S. Ct. 2486, June 26, 1975.
16. John Petrilia, "Mental Health Therapies," Biolaw, Frederick, MD, University Publications of America, 1986, pp. 177–215.
17. Quoted in Charles Krauthammer, "How to Save the Homeless Mentally Ill, *New Republic*, February 8, 1988, p. 24.
18. Saul Feldman, "Out of the Hospitals, into the Streets: The Overselling of Benevolence," *Hastings Center Report* 13, no. 3 (June 1983), pp. 5–7.
19. C. Dugger, "Judge Orders Homeless Man Hospitalized," *New York Times*, December 23, 1992, p. B1.
20. Treatment Advocacy Center, "State Standards for Assisted Treatment: State by State Chart," December 12, 2004. www.psychlaws.org
21. E. Rosenthal, "Who Will Turn Violent? Hospitals Have to Guess," *New York Times*, April 7, 1993, p. A1.
22. *"Tarasoff v. Regents of University of California,"* 17 Cal. 3d 425, 551 P.2d 334, 131 *California Reporter* 14 (Cal. 1976).
23. Virginia Abernethy, "Compassion, Control, and Decisions about Competence," *American Journal of Psychiatry* 141, no. 1 (1984), pp. 53–58.
24. Abernethy, "Compassion, Control, and Decisions."
25. *New York Times*, November 13, 1987, p. A1.
26. Robert Levy and Robert Gould, "Psychiatrists as Puppets of Koch's Round-Up," *New York Times*, November 27, 1987.
27. Paul Chodoff, "The Case for Involuntary Hospitalization of the Mentally Ill," *American Journal of Psychiatry* 133, no. 5 (May 1976).
28. Ellen Goodman, "Before They Die with Their Rights On," WP, November 21, 1987.
29. J. Livermore, C. Malmquist, and P. Meehl, "On the Justification of Civil Commitment, *University of Pennsylvania Law Review* 117 (November 1968), pp. 75–96.
30. Alice Baum and Donald Burnes, *A Nation in Denial: The Truth about Homelessness*, Boulder, CO, Westview, 1993.
31. Clifford J. Ivy, "The State Is Failing the Mentally Ill in Adult Homes, Pataki Administration Study Says," *New York Times*, September 15, 2002, p. 21.
32. J. Livermore, C. Malmquist, and P. Meehl, "On the Justification of Civil Commitment, *University of Pennsylvania Law Review* 117 (November 1968), pp. 75–96.
33. Livermore, Malmquist, and Meehl, "On the Justification of Civil Commitment."

Chapter 14

1. Natalie Angier, "Team Reports Genetic Cause of Huntington's, *New York Times*, March 24, 1993, p. A1.

2. Rita Rubin, "Ray of Hope for Huntington's, *USA Today*, p. A1–2.
3. Benjamin A. Pierce, *Genetics: A Conceptual Approach*, 2nd ed., New York, W. H. Freeman, 2006, p. 123.
4. "DNA Links to Breast Cancer Found," *The Tennessean*, May 28, 2007, p. A4.
5. Daniel Kevles, *In the Name of Eugenics: Genetics and the Uses of Human Heredity*, New York, Knopf, 1985, pp. 3–19.
6. Kevles, *In the Name of Eugenics*, pp. 93–94.
7. Robert Lacey, *Ford: The Man and the Machine*, New York, Little, Brown, 1987.
8. Kevles, *In the Name of Eugenics*, p. 97.
9. Kevles, *In the Name of Eugenics*, p. 97.
10. Herman Muller, *Out of the Night: A Biologist's View of the Future*, New York, Vanguard, 1935; Kevles, *In the Name of Eugenics*, p. 164.
11. Ronald W. Clark, *The Life and Work of J. B. S. Haldane*, New York, Coward-McCann, 1968, p. 70; quoted in Kevles, p. 127.
12. B. S. Haldane, "Toward a Perfected Posterity," *The World Today* 45 (December 1924); quoted in Kevles, p. 127.
13. "Maria Lopez" is a composite, based on a 4-part series in the *New York Times* on the emerging epidemic in diabetes, January 9–12, 2006.
14. N. R. Kleinfield, "Diabetes and Its Awful Toll Quietly Emerge as a Crisis," *New York Times*, January 9, 2006, p. A1.
15. World Health Organization, Department of Noncommunicable Disease Surveillance. *Definition, Diagnosis and Classification of Diabetes Mellitus and Its Complications.* Geneva: WHO, 1999.
16. Marc Santora, "East Meets West, Adding Pounds and Peril," *New York Times*, January 12, 2006, p. A1.
17. Kleinfield, "Diabetes and Its Awful Toll."
18. Kleinfield, "Living at the Epicenter of Diabetes, Defiance and Despair," *New York Times*, January 10, 2006, p. A1.
19. Kleinfield, "Diabetes and Its Awful Toll."
20. "Diabetes gene detected," *Sydney Morning Herald*, January 19, 2006.
21. Peter Kraft et al., "Genetic Risk Prediction—Are We There Yet?" *New England Journal of Medicine* 360, no. 17 (April 2009), p. 1701.
22. R. Caselli et al., "Longitudinal Modeling of Age-Related Memory Decline and the APOE 4 Effect," *New England Journal of Medicine* (July 16, 2009), p. 256.
23. Denise Grady, "Study Shows Few Women Rue Preventive Breast Operation," *New York Times*, April 17, 1999, p. A14.
24. Paul Recer, "Studies May Have Exaggerated Breast Cancer Risk," *Birmingham News*, (August 21, 2002), p. 5A.
25. Denise Grady, "The Ticking of a Time Bomb in the Genes," *Discover*, June 1987, p. 34.
26. G. Meissen et al., "Predictive Testing for Huntington's Disease with Use of a Linked DNA Marker," *New England Journal of Medicine* 318, no. 9 (March 3, 1988), pp. 538ff.
27. Meissen, "Predictive Testing."
28. Danish Council of Ethics, *Ethics and Mapping of the Human Genome*, 1993.
29. Catherine Hayes, "Genetic Testing for Huntington's Disease"; Natalie Angier, "Vexing Pursuit of Breast Cancer Gene," *New York Times*, July 12, 1994.
30. C. Muir, *Cancer Incidence in Five Continents* vol. 5, Lyon, International Agency for Research on Cancer, 1987, Table 12-2.
31. Kleinfield, "Diabetes and Its Awful Toll."
32. L. R.Vartanian et al., "Effects of Soft Drink Consumption on Nutrition and Health: A Systematic Review and Meta-Analysis," *American Journal of Public Health* 97, no. 4 (2007).
33. "Cancer Genetics," Benjamin A. Pierce, *Genetics: A Conceptual Approach*, 2nd ed., New York, W. H. Freeman, 2006, pp. 627–637.
34. D. Craufurd and R. Harris, "Ethics of Predictive Testing for Huntington's Disease: The Need for More Information," *British Medical Journal* 293 (July 26, 1986), pp. 249–251.
35. M. Waldoz, "Probing the Cell: The Diagnostic Power of Genetics Is Posing Hard Medical Choices," *Wall Street Journal*, April 1986, p. A1.
36. Grady, "The Ticking of a Time Bomb."
37. Arthur Beaudet of Baylor College of Medicine, quoted in M. Waldoz, "Probing the Cell."
38. President's Commission for the Study of Ethical Problems in Medicine and Biomedical and Behavioral Research, *Screening and Counseling for Genetic Conditions: The Ethical, Social, and Legal Implications for Genetic Screening, Counseling, and Educational Problems*, Washington, D.C., U.S. Government Printing Office, 1983.
39. C. Norton, "Absolutely Not Confidential," *Hippocrates*, March-April 1989, pp. 53–59; see also *Medical Records: Getting Yours*, Washington, D.C., Public Citizen, 1986.

40. Genetic Information Nondiscrimination Act (GINA) of 2008: Information for Researchers and Health Care Professionals; http://www.genome.gov/24519851.
41. Ian Urbina, "In the Treatment of Diabetes, Success Often Does Not Pay," *New York Times*, January 11, 2006, p. A1.
42. Urbina, "In the Treatment of Diabetes."
43. Nicholas Wade, "Gene Identified as Risk Factor for Heart Ills," *New York Times*, May 4, 2007, p. A1.
44. Sharon Begley, "Reading the Book of Jim," *Newsweek*, June 4, 2007, p. 50.
45. Natalie Angier, "Gene for Mental Illness Proves Elusive," *New York Times*, January 13, 1993, p. B3.
46. Miron Baron, quoted in Angier, "Gene for Mental Illness Proves Elusive."
47. Sharon Begley, "Reading the Book of Jim," *Newsweek*, June 4, 2007, p. 50.
48. "New Research Shows Second-hand Smoke Raises Diabetes Risk, *British Medical Journal* April 17, 2006.
49. Begley, "Reading the Book of Jim," p. 48.

Chapter 15

1. World Health Organization *Data and Statistics*, http://www.who.int/hiv/data/en/.
2. Barbara Tuchman, *A Distant Mirror*, New York, Knopf, 1978, p. 119.
3. B. Hahn, G. Shaw, and F. Gao, *Nature* 397 (February 4, 1999), pp. 436–441. The authors also offered proof that the three major phylogenetic groups of HIV-1 (M, N, and O) arose from three independent transmissions to man of simian immunodeficiency virus, SIVcpz, which they hypothesized had existed in chimps for hundreds of thousands of years.
4. Centers for Disease Control, "Overview of HIV/AIDS" and "Human Immunodeficiency Virus Type 2," www.cdc.gov/hiv/hivinfo
5. Randy Shilts, *And the Band Played On*, New York, St. Martin's, 1987.
6. Greg Dixon "Stop Homosexuals before They Infect Us All," *USA Today*, January 16, 1983.
7. "Television evangelists Jerry Falwell and Pat Robertson, two of the most prominent voices of the religious right, said liberal civil liberties groups, feminists, homosexuals, and abortion rights supporters bear partial responsibility for Tuesday's terrorist attacks because their actions have turned God's anger against America. God Gave U.S. 'What We Deserve,' Falwell Says," John F. Harris, *Washington Post*, September 14, 2001, p. C3.
8. Charles Stanley, quoted in Scripps-Howard News Service, *Birmingham Post-Herald*, January 21, 1986.
9. Interviewed on *Cross Fire*, CNN, November 16, 1987.
10. Shilts, *And the Band Played On*, p. 311.
11. Jonathan Lieberson, "The Reality of AIDS," *New York Review of Books*, January 16, 1986.
12. Margaret Heckler, quoted in Shilts, *And the Band Played On*, p. 345.
13. Joseph Bove, quoted in Shilts, *And the Band Played On*, p. 345.
14. Bove, quoted in Shilts, *And the Band Played On*, p. 345.
15. Jane Gross, "AIDS Patients Face Downside of Living Longer," *New York Times*, January 6, 2008.
16. John Boswell, *Christianity, Social Tolerance, and Homosexuality; Gay People in Western Europe from the Beginning of the Christian Era to the Fourteenth Century*, Chicago, University of Chicago Press, 1980.
17. 539 U.S. 558 (2003) http://www.law.cornell.edu/supct/html/02-102.ZS.html
18. Larry Kramer, "Who Says AIDS Is Hard to Get?" *Newsweek*, 1992.
19. Nick Wadhams, "World Falls Short on AIDS Goals, U.N. Warns," *Birmingham News*, June 2, 2006, p. 4A.
20. Robert Steinbrook, "The AIDS Epidemic: A Progress Report from Mexico City," *New England Journal of Medicine* 359, no. 9 (August 28, 2008), pp. 886–887.
21. Figures on AIDS in Africa and worldwide are notoriously vague and political. See Alan Whiteside, "AIDS in Africa: Facts, Figures and the Extent of the Problem," pp. 1–15. Anton A. Van Niekerk and Loretta M. Kopelman, *Ethics and AIDS in Africa*, Walnut Creek, CA, Left Coast Press, 2006. According to the World Health Organization, 33 million people live with HIV as of July 4, 2009. http://www.who.int/hiv/en/
22. "A Global Menace," *Newsweek*, May 15, 2006, p. 52.
23. Alexander Irwin, Joyce Millen, and Dorothy Fallows, *Global AIDS: Myths and Facts*, Cambridge, MA, South End Press, 2003, p. 52.

24. Irwin, Millen, and Fallows, *Global AIDS*, p. 55.
25. Kent Sepkowitz, "One Disease, Two Epidemics—AIDS at 25," *New England Journal of Medicine* 354, no. 23 (June 8, 2006), pp. 2413–2414.
26. The case is taken from Irwin, Millen, and Fallows, *Global AIDS*, pp. 21–22.
27. Quoted in Irwin, Millen, and Fallows, *Global AIDS*.
28. Michael Merson, "The HIV-AIDS Pandemic at 25—The Global Response," *New England Journal of Medicine* 354, no. 23 (June 8, 2006), p. 2414.
29. J. Decosas et al., "Migration and AIDS," *Lancet* 346, no. 8978 (1995), pp. 826–828. Quoted in Irwin et al., *Global AIDS*.
30. Jeffrey Fisher, quoted in L. A. McKeown, "Preventing AIDS in the Next Generation," *WebMD Medical News*, December 1, 1999.
31. Irwin, Millen, and Fallows, *Global AIDS*.
32. Philippe Bourgois, "In Search of Horatio Alger: Culture and Ideology in the Crack Economy," in *Crack in America: Demon Drugs and Social Justice*, eds., B. Rienarman and H. Levine, Berkeley, CA, University of California Press, 1997.
33. Sepkowitz, "One Disease, Two Epidemics," p. 2413.
34. William Easterly, *White Man's Burden: Why the West's Efforts to Aid the Rest Have Done So Much Ill and So Little Good*, New York, Penguin, 2006.
35. Kevin Fenton, quoted at the World Aids Conference in Mexico City in August 2008. See R. Steinbrook, "The AIDS Epidemic—A Progress Report . . . ," p. 887.

Chapter 16

1. Lisa Belkin, "Twice a Victim: of Both Cancer and Care System," *New York Times*, March 26, 1993, p. B12.
2. Personal communication from Lisa Belkin to author, June 17, 2006.
3. This case stemmed from a 1993 (above) story by Lisa Belkin. In 2006, an email to her revealed that one of her children said that Rosalyn had died "several years before."
4. Quoted by Paul Krugman, "Death By Insurance," *New York Times*, May 1, 2006, A25.
5. Steve LeBlanc, "Mass. Health Care Plan Riles Some Liberals," Associated Press, April 7, 2006.
6. Robert Steinbrook, "Health Care Reform in Massachusetts—A Work in Progress," *New England Journal of Medicine* 543, no. 20 (May 18, 2006), p. 2095.
7. This has been repeatedly claimed by members of Physicians for a National Health Program; see, e.g., John V. Walsh, *Providence Journal* (Scripps-Howard), column, July 14, 1993. See also Paul Krugman, "Death By Insurance."
8. The name is misleading. It is an acronym for the Consolidated Budget Reconciliation Act of 1985, under which this provision became law.
9. The act allows both workers and their immediate family members who had been covered by a health care plan to maintain their coverage if a "qualifying event" causes them to lose coverage. Among the qualifying events listed in the statute are loss of benefits coverage due to (1) the death of the covered employee, (2) a reduction in hours (which can be the result of resignation, discharge, layoff, strike or lockout, medical leave, or simply a slowdown in business operations) that causes the worker to lose eligibility for coverage, (3) divorce, which normally terminates the ex-spouse's eligibility for benefits, or (4) a dependent child reaching the age at which he or she is no longer covered. COBRA imposes different notice requirements on participants and beneficiaries, depending on the particular qualifying event that triggers COBRA rights. COBRA also allows for longer periods of extended coverage in some cases, such as disability or divorce, than others, such as termination of employment or a reduction in hours. COBRA does not apply, on the other hand, if employees lose their benefits coverage because the employer has terminated the plan altogether." Consolidated Omnibus Budget Reconciliation Act of 1985, Wikipedia. http://en.wikipedia.org/wiki/Consolidated_Omnibus_Budget_Reconciliation_Act_of_1985
10. Jack K. Shelton and Julia Mann Janosi, "Unhealthy Health Care Costs," *Journal of Medicine and Philosophy* 17, no. 1 (February 1992), p. 8.
11. Cost of retirement coverage for car employees.
12. "Medicare Enrollment Reports," December 14, 2005, http://www.cms.hhs.gov/MedicareEnrpts/, July 11, 2006.

13. Kaiser Family Foundation, "Medicare Spending and Financing," April 2005, http://www.kff.org/medicare/upload/7305.pdf, July 10, 2006.
14. "Health Care Costs," *USA Today*, May 12, 1993, p. A2.
15. Robert Pear, "Bailout Provides More Mental Health Coverage," *New York Times*, October 6, 2008, p. A1.
16. CHAMPUS website.
17. Paul Krugman, "Health Care Confidential," *New York Times*, January 26, 2006, p. A23.
18. Robert Steinbrook, "Health Care Reform in Massachusetts—A Work in Progress," *New England Journal of Medicine* 543, no. 20 (May 18, 2006), p. 2095.
19. Allan Guttmacher Institute, quoted in AP, December 15, 1987.
20. Clifford Krauss, "In Blow to Canada's Health System, Quebec Law is Voided," *New York Times*, June 10, 2005, A3.
21. Krauss, "In Blow to Canada's Health System."
22. Krauss, "In Blow to Canada's Health System."
23. Courtney S. Campbell, "Gridlock on the Oregon Trail," *Hastings Center Report* 23, no. 4 (July-August 1993), p. 6.
24. Matthew J. Carson, "Results of Oregon Health Plan Study Released," The Commonwealth Fund, July 29, 2005. http://www.cmwf.org/newsroom/newsroom_show.htm?doc_id=288798, July 10, 2006.
25. Steve LeBlanc, "Mass. Health Care Plan Riles Some Liberals," Associated Press, April 7, 2006.
26. Patricia Barry, "Coverage," *AARP Bulletin* (July-August, 2006), pp. 8–10.
27. Stuart Altman and Michael Doonan, "Can Massachusetts Lead the Way in Health Care Reform?" *New England Journal of Medicine* 354, no. 20 (May 18, 2006), p. 2094.
28. Altman and Doonan, "Can Massachusetts Lead the Way?"
29. Olga Pierce, "Analysis: Can Mass. Plan Stay Solvent?" United Press International Story, July 6, 2006.
30. Kevin Sack, "In Massachusetts, Universal Coverage Strains Care," *New York Times*, April 5, 2008, p. A1.
31. Sack, "Massachusetts Faces Costs."
32. Consumers Union, "Medicare for All Americans," *Consumer Reports*, September 1992, p. 592.
33. Consumers Union, "Medicare for All Americans," *Consumer Reports*, September 1992, p. 592.
34. Milt Freudenheim, "The Check Is Not in the Mail," *New York Times*, May 2, 2006, p. C1.
35. Garrett Hardin, "The Tragedy of the Commons," *Science* 162 (1968), pp. 1243–1248.
36. Consumers Union, "The Crisis in Health Insurance," *Consumer Reports*, August 1990, p. 543.
37. Ibid, p. 40.
38. Consumers Union, "Wasted Health Care Dollars," *Consumer Reports*, July 1992, p. 436.
39. Lila Guterman, "As the Rich Get Richer, Do People Get Sicker?" *Chronicle of Higher Education*, November 28, 2003, p. A22.
40. Amy Goldstein, "Forecast Dire for Medicare Fiscal Health," *Washington Post*, May 2, 2006, reprinted in *Birmingham News*, p. 3A.
41. Robert Pear, "In Medicare Debate, Massaging the Facts," *New York Times*, May 23, 2006, A19.
42. Richard Epstein, remarks made at UAB, Conference on the Ethics of Managed Care, April 12, 1997. See also his *Mortal Peril*, Reading, MA, Addison-Wesley, 1997, especially Chapters 7 and 8.
43. David Blumenthal et al., "The Future of Health care," *New England Journal of Medicine* 314, no. 11 (March 13, 1986), p. 723.
44. David Orentlicher, "Rationing and the Americans with Disabilities Act," *Journal of the American Medical Association* 271, no. 4 (January 26, 1994), pp. 308–314.
45. Orentlicher, "Rationing."
46. Long Lamm quotation.
47. Paul Starr, *The Social Transformation of American Medicine*, New York, Basic Books, 1982.
48. Julia Preston, "Texas Hospitals' Separate Paths Reflect the Debate on Immigration," *New York Times*, July 18, 2006, A18.
49. Preston, "Texas Hospitals' Separate Paths."
50. Shikha Dalmia, "Who's Milking Who?" *Reason*, August/September 2006, p. 44.
51. Ewardo Porter, "Here Illegally, Working Hard and Paying Taxes," *New York Times*, June 19, 2006, A1–14.

Chapter 17

1. I am indebted to UAB surgeon David Joseph for comments on this chapter and for Kenneth Kipnis's suggesting the idea

for it to me over ten years ago and for sharing his PowerPoint slides for his lecture on this case and intersex children.

2. Associated Press, "Runner Reported to Have Internal Male Sex Organs," September 12, 2009, *Birmingham News*, Section D, p. 2.
3. Consortium on the Management of Disorders of Sex Development, *Clinical Guidelines of the Management of Disorders of Sex Development in Childhood*, 2006, Intersex Society of North America.
4. L. Sax, "How Common Is Intersex?" A Response to Ann Fausto-Sterling, *Journal of Sex Research* 39, no. 3 (2002), pp. 174–178.
5. John Colapinto, *As Nature Made Him: The Boy Who Was Raised as a Girl*, New York, Harper Collins, 2000, p. 22.
6. Rick Weiss, "Mature Human Embryos Cloned," *Washington Post*, February 12, 2004, p. A28.
7. Mel Grumbach, pediatric endocrinologist at the University of California, San Francisco, quoted in Colapinto, *As Nature Made Him*, p. 75.
8. Colapinto, *As Nature Made Him*, p. 180.
9. Cheryl Chase, 1998, interviewed by Robin Whites (November 28, 1997). Intersexuals (interview with Chase). *All Things Considered*, NPR. See also Elizabeth Weil (September 2006). What If It's (Sort of) a Boy and (Sort of) a Girl?" *New York Times Magazine*.
10. Alice Dregger, *One of Us: Conjoined Twins and the Future of the Normal*, Cambridge, MA, Harvard University Press, 2005.
11. American Academy of Pediatrics (2000).
12. In particular, Colapinto mentions two male twins with botched circumcisions born in Atlanta in 1985 and cases cited by Toronto child psychiatrist Kenneth Zucker, pp. 249, 274.
13. Ken Kipnis and Milton Diamond, "Pediatric Ethics and the Surgical Assignment of Sex," *Journal of Clinical Ethics* 9, no. 3 (1988).
14. Linda Geddes, "Puberty Blockers Recommended for Transsexual Teens," *New Scientist*, December 10, 2008.
15. Peter Lee et al., "Consensus Statement on Management of Intersex Disorders," *Pediatrics* 188, no. 2 (August 2006), e488–e500.

Chapter 18

1. See my "Recent Work on Virtues," *American Philosophical Quarterly*.
2. Lewis White Beck, *Six Secular Philosophers*, South Bend, IN, St. Augustine's Press, 1997.
3. James Rachels may have invented this example. See Stuart Rachels's introduction to *The Legacy of Socrates*, ed. Stuart Rachels, New York, Columbia University Press, 2006.

Name Index

Subject Index